The Nurse Preceptor Toolkit

PREPARING NURSES AND ADVANCED PRACTICE NURSES FOR CLINICAL PRACTICE

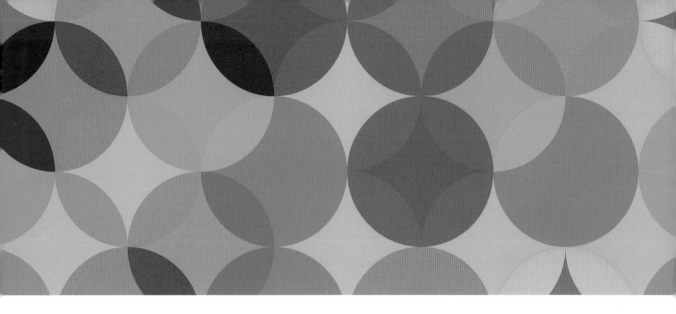

The Nurse Preceptor Toolkit

PREPARING NURSES AND ADVANCED PRACTICE NURSES FOR CLINICAL PRACTICE

1st Edition

BETH HEUER, DNP, CRNP, CPNP-PC, PMHS, FAANP
Pediatric Nurse Practitioner and Associate
  Professor of Clinical Instruction
Temple University College of Public Health/
  School of Nursing
Philadelphia, Pennsylvania

CYNTHIA A. DANFORD, PhD, CRNP, PPCNP-BC, CPNP-PC, FAAN
Nurse Scientist II
Office of Nursing Research and Innovation
Cleveland Clinic
Cleveland, Ohio
Consultative Staff
Lerner Research Institute
Cleveland Clinic

ELSEVIER

ELSEVIER
3251 Riverport Lane
St. Louis, Missouri 63043

THE NURSE PRECEPTOR TOOLKIT: PREPARING NURSES AND   ISBN: 978-0-443-10736-8
ADVANCED PRACTICE NURSES FOR CLINICAL PRACTICE

Executive Content Strategist: Lee Henderson
Senior Content Development Manager: Laura Schmidt
Senior Content Development Specialist: Kristen Helm
Publishing Services Manager: Deepthi Unni
Senior Project Manager: Kamatchi Madhavan
Design Direction: Brian Salisbury

Working together
to grow libraries in
developing countries

www.elsevier.com • www.bookaid.org

Printed in India

Last digit is the print number: 9 8 7 6 5 4 3 2 1

*To my amazing husband, Douglas, for his unwavering love and
support. To my son, Stephen, who graciously shared his mother
with entirely too many writing projects over the years.
To my mom, who always believed that I could accomplish
anything. And to the best writing partner ever,
Dr. Cindy Danford. "We can do hard things."*
–Beth Heuer

*In memory of my parents, Ed and Julie Danford, who by
example taught me the significance of service to others; they
gave me the foundation and courage to devote my life to the
health and well-being of children and families. To my brother,
Dave, for his constant and unwavering support, guidance, and
patience. To my remarkable co-editor, Dr. Beth Heuer, for her
renowned expertise, insight, and wonderful sense of humor.*
–Cindy Danford

*To all preceptors committed to sharing their expertise while
educating present and future generations of nurses and
advanced practice nurses. We admire and appreciate your
contributions to advancing the profession of nursing.*
–Beth and Cindy

Larissa Africa, MBA, BSN, RN, FAAN
President and CEO
Versant Healthcare Competency Solutions
Las Vegas, Nevada

Abiola Akamo Aghakasiri, DNP, FNP-C
NOELA Community Health Center,
New Orleans East, LA

Nancy M. Albert, PhD, CCNS, CHFN, CCRN, NE-BC, FAHA, FCCM, FHFSA, FAAN
Associate Chief Nursing Officer
Nursing Institute, Office of Research and Innovation
Cleveland Clinic
Chesterland, Ohio;
Clinical Nurse Specialist
Heart, Vascular & Thoracic Institute
Cleveland Clinic
Cleveland, Ohio;
Consultant Staff
Lerner Research Institute
Cleveland Clinic
Cleveland, Ohio

Patricia Nicole Anders, BSN, RN
School Nurse
Health Services
Lake Washington School District
Redmond, Washington

Gabriella Anderson, BSN, RN, SANE-A
Assistant Nurse Manager
Forensic Nursing Program
Cleveland Clinic
Cleveland, Ohio

Sue Anderson, PhD, RN, FNP-BC
Director, Nursing Science and Graduate Nursing Programs
Nursing
Saint Mary's College
Notre Dame, Indiana

Heather L. Bartlett, MSN, RN, CPNP-PC
Pediatric Nurse Practitioner
Department of General Pediatrics and Adolescent Medicine
University Pediatricians, Children's Hospital of Michigan
Detroit, Michigan;
Clinical Faculty
Pediatric Primary Care PNP Program
Wayne State University College of Nursing
Detroit, Michigan

Jennifer Beigie, MSN, RN, SANE-A
Assistant Nurse Manager
Forensic Nursing
Cleveland Clinic Hillcrest Hospital
Mayfield Heights, Ohio

Amy Bieda, PhD, APRN, PCPNP-BC, NNP-BC
Associate Professor
College of Public Health, Department of Nursing
Temple University
Philadelphia, PA

Jennifer M. Brown, DNP, MSN, RN, APN
Assistant Professor
College of Public Health, Department of Nursing
Temple University
Philadelphia, Pennsylvania

Petra Brysiewicz PhD, MN, FAAN, fANSA, ASSAf
Professor
School of Nursing & Public Health
University of KwaZulu-Natal, South Africa
Editor: International Emergency Nursing

Stacy Buchanan, DNP, RN, CPNP-PC
Senior Clinical Instructor
Nell Hodgson Woodruff School of Nursing
Emory University
Atlanta, Georgia

Kelly Calvey, BSN, RN
Forensic Nurse
Cleveland Clinic - Fairview Hospital
Cleveland, Ohio

Cynthia Ann Chew, DNP, CPNP-PC, IBCLC
Assistant Professor and Director of Nurse Practitioner
    Programs
Health Promotion and Development
University of Pittsburgh School of Nursing
Pittsburgh, Pennsylvania;
Pediatric Nurse Practitioner and Lactation Consultant
Pediatric Associates of Westmoreland
Greensburg, Pennsylvania

Daniel Crawford, DNP, ARNP, CPNP-PC, CNF, FAANP
Associate Professor (Clinical) & Director, Pediatric
    Primary Care Nurse Practitioner Program
College of Nursing
The University of Iowa
Iowa City, Iowa;
Pediatric Nurse Practitioner
Child Neurology
The University of Iowa Stead Family Children's Hospital
Iowa City, Iowa

Shayna Dahan, BSN, RN, MSN, CPNP, PMHS
Nurse Practitioner
School Health
Montefiore Hospital
Bronx, New York

**Cynthia A. Danford, PhD, CRNP, PPCNP-BC,
    CPNP-PC, FAAN**
Nurse Scientist II
Office of Nursing Research and Innovation
Cleveland Clinic
Cleveland, Ohio
Consultative Staff
Lerner Research Institute
Cleveland Clinic

Susan B. Dickey, PhD, RN
Associate Professor
College of Public Health, Department of Nursing
Temple University
Philadelphia, PA

Shayla Dressler, BSN, RN, NCSN
School Nurse
Health Services
Lake Washington School District
Redmond, Washington

Heather Dunn, PhD, ACNP-BC, ARNP
Assistant Professor (Clinical)
College of Nursing
The University of Iowa
Iowa City, Iowa

Daniela Edson, DNP, MSN, RN, AGACNP-BC, CCRN
Director of the Adult-Gerontology Acute
    Care Program
Nursing
Saint Mary's College
Notre Dame, Indiana;
Nurse Practitioner
ICU
Beacon Medical Group
Elkhart, Indiana;
Nurse Practitioner
Trauma/Surgical Services
Beacon Medical Group
South Bend, Indiana

Caerissa Fawkes, BSN, RN
School Nurse
Health Services
Lake Washington School District
Redmond, Washington

Nanne M. Finis, MS
Chief Nurse Executive
UKG
Inverness, Illinois

Dr. Judith M. Fouladbakhsh, PhD, RN, PHCNS-BC, AHN-BC, CHTP, SGAHN
Public Health Clinical Nurse Specialist, ANCC Board Certified
Advanced Practice Holistic Nurse, AHNCC Board Certified
Certified Healing Touch Practitioner, Advanced Reiki Master
Creating Health through Healing Practices LLC, Executive Director
Complementary Integrative Therapies Research, Education, Clinical Practice
NIH Funded Researcher
Friends of the National Institute of Nursing Research (FNINR) Ambassador
Global Academy of Holistic Nursing (SGAHN) Scholar

Christina Gabele, DNP, FNP, ENP
Coordinator, Family NP Program and Clinical Assistant Professor
Byers School of Nursing
Walsh University
North Canton, Ohio

Angela Gager, DNP, FNP-BC
Clinical Assistant Professor
Byers School of Nursing
Walsh University
North Canton, Ohio

Amalia Elizabeth Gedney-Lose, DNP, ARNP, FNP-C
Clinical Assistant Professor
College of Nursing
University of Iowa
Iowa City, Iowa

Barbara Giambra, PhD, RN, CPNP-BC
Assistant Professor
Research in Patient Services, Department of Patient Services, Nursing
Cincinnati Children's Hospital Medical Center
Cincinnati, Ohio;
Volunteer Assistant Professor
James M. Anderson Center for Health Systems Excellence, Department of Pediatrics
Cincinnati Children's Hospital Medical Center
Cincinnati, Ohio;
Assistant Professor, Research Affiliate
College of Nursing
University of Cincinnati
Cincinnati, Ohio

Kristin Hittle Gigli, PhD, RN, CPNP-AC
Assistant Professor
Graduate Nursing, College of Nursing and Health Innovation
University of Texas at Arlington
Arlington, Texas

Tish Gill, DNP, MSN, RN, CNE
Associate Professor
College of Public Health, Department of Nursing
Temple University
Philadelphia, PA

Jess Gordon, BSN, RN, NCSN
School Nurse
Health Services
Lake Washington School District
Kirkland, Washington

Stacia Marie Hays, DNP, APRN, CPNP-PC, CNE, CCTC, FAANP
Clinical Associate Professor
Nursing
Baylor University, Louise Herrington School of Nursing
Dallas, Texas;
Associate Dean of the Graduate Program;
Baylor University, Louise Herrington School of Nursing
Dallas, Texas

Anna Herbert, MSN, BA, RN, CPHON, NPD-BC
Education Consultant
The Center for Professional Excellence
Cincinnati Children's Hospital Medical Center
Cincinnati, Ohio

Beth Heuer, DNP, CRNP, CPNP-PC, PMHS, FAANP
Pediatric Nurse Practitioner and Associate Professor of Clinical Instruction
Temple University College of Public Health/School of Nursing
Philadelphia, Pennsylvania

Lauren Gabrielle Johnson, PhD, RN
Assistant Professor
College of Public Health, Department of Nursing
Temple University
Philadelphia, PA

Brayden Kameg, DNP, PMHNP-BC
Assistant Professor of Nursing
Health and Community Systems
University of Pittsburgh
Pittsburgh, Pennsylvania

Kirstyn Kameg, DNP, PMHNP-BC
Professor
Nursing
Robert Morris University
Moon Township, Pennsylvania

Andrea M. Kline-Tilford, PhD, CPNP-AC/PC, FCCM, FAAN
Nurse Practitioner Director
APRN Nursing
University of Michigan Health
Ann Arbor, Michigan

Marjorie Hart Lehigh, MSN, MHed, MHA
Professor
Nursing
Temple University
Philadelphia, Pennsylvania;
Nursing Administrative Coordinator
Nursing
Penn Presbyterian Medical Center
Philadelphia, Pennsylvania

Michelle Levay, MSN, RN
Nurse Research Manager
Office of Nursing Research & Innovation
Cleveland Clinic
Cleveland Ohio

Maria Lofgren, DNP, ARNP, NNP-BC, CPNP, FAANP
Clinical Associate Professor
Director of Faculty Practice
University of Iowa College of Nursing
Iowa City, Iowa;
Director of Advanced Practice Providers
Administration
University of Iowa Health Care
Iowa City, Iowa

Donna J. Marvicsin, PhD, PNP-BC, CDE
Clinical Associate Professor Emerita
Department of Health Behavior and Biological Sciences
School of Nursing
University of Michigan
Ann Arbor, MI

Bernadette Mazurek Melnyk, PhD, APRN-CNP, EBP-C, FAANP, FNAP, FAAN
Vice President for Health Promotion
Chief Wellness Officer
The Ohio State University
Helene Fuld Health Trust Professor of Evidence-based Practice
Founder, the Helene Fuld Health Trust National Institute for EBP
Former Dean, College of Nursing
Professor of Pediatrics and Psychiatry, College of Medicine
Editor, Worldviews on Evidence-based Nursing
President, the National Consortium for Building Healthy Academic Communities
Columbus, Ohio

Anne Marie Michon, MSN, RN, CPNP-PC
Pediatric Nurse Practitioner-PC
Pediatric Epilepsy/Neurology Division
Beaumont Children's
Royal Oak, Michigan;
Clinical Faculty for PNP-PC Program
College of Nursing
Wayne State University
Detroit, Michigan

Elizabeth Mollard, PhD, CNM, WHNP, IBCLC
Assistant Professor
College of Nursing, Lincoln Division
University of Nebraska Medical Center
Lincoln, Nebraska

Natasha North, PhD
Research Director
Children's Nursing Development Unit
University of Cape Town
City of Cape Town, Western Cape, South Africa

Lorraine M. Novosel, PhD, RN, APRN-CNP, AGPCNP-BC, NEA-BC
Nurse Scientist I
Nursing Research and Innovation
Cleveland Clinic
Cleveland, Ohio;
Consultant Staff
Lerner Research Institute
Cleveland Clinic
Cleveland, Ohio

Charlotte Nwogwugwu, DrPH, MSN, MPH, PMHNP-BC, CPH-BC
Assistant Professor, Global Health
Department of Partnerships, Professional Education, and Practice (PPEP)
University of Maryland Baltimore
Baltimore, Maryland

Annette Peacock-Johnson, DNP, RN
Associate Professor of Nursing - Emerita
Department of Nursing Science
Saint Mary's College
Notre Dame, IN

Audra Rankin, DNP, APRN, CPNP
Clinical Assistant Professor
School of Nursing
University of North Carolina at Chapel Hill
Chapel Hill, North Carolina

Laura Rauth, MSN, CNS, RN
Clinical Faculty
Department of Nursing
Temple University
Philadelphia, Pennsylvania

Michele Reali-Sorrell, DNP, RN, BA, SANE-A, SANE-P
Forensic Nurse Manager
Emergency Service
Cleveland Clinic
Cleveland, Ohio

Imelda Reyes, DNP, MPH, APRN, FAANP
Associate Dean of Advanced Education/Professor in Residence
Graduate Nursing
University of Nevada, Las Vegas
Las Vegas, Nevada

Celeste M. Schultz, PhD, RN-BC, CPNP-PC
Clinical Assistant Professor
Human Development Nursing Science
University of Illinois Chicago College of Nursing
Chicago, Illinois

Danielle Sebbens, DNP, CPNP-AC/PC
Associate Director DNP Program
Associate Professor
Coordinator, Acute Care Pediatric Nurse Practitioner Program
Edson College of Nursing and Health Innovation
Arizona State University
Phoenix, Arizona;
Pediatric Critical Care Nurse Practitioner
Pediatric Intensive Care Unit
Phoenix Children's Hospital
Phoenix, Arizona

Vatula Marie Seward, ADN
Registered Nurse
Post Anesthesia Care Unit
Cleveland Clinic
Cleveland, Ohio

Carol Ann Shaw, DNP, RN
Education Consultant
Center for Professional Excellence
Cincinnati Children's Hospital
Cincinnati, Ohio;
RN Residency Program Coordinator
Center for Professional Excellence
Cincinnati Children's Hospital
Cincinnati, Ohio

B. Elias Snyder, PhD, FNP-C, ACHPN
Director & Assistant Professor
Office of Global Health
University of Maryland School of Nursing
Baltimore, Maryland;
Nurse Practitioner
Palliative Care

Jennifer Sonney, PhD, APRN, PPCNP-BC, FAANP, FAAN
Joanne Montgomery Endowed Professor
Child, Family, and Population Health Nursing
University of Washington School of Nursing
Seattle, Washington

Jessica L. Spruit, DNP, RN, CPNP-AC, CPHON, BMTCN, FAANP
Certified Pediatric Nurse Practitioner, Acute Care
Pediatric Palliative Care
C.S. Mott Children's Hospital
Ann Arbor, Michigan;
Certified Pediatric Nurse Practitioner, Acute Care
Pediatric Blood and Marrow Transplant
C.S. Mott Children's Hospital
Ann Arbor, Michigan

Shelley Spurr, BSN, MBA, PhD
Associate Professor
College of Nursing
University of Saskatchewan
Saskatoon, Saskatchewan, Canada

Kristen Starr, RN, BSN
Fox Chase Cancer Center
Temple University Health System
Philadelphia, PA

Mary Frances Terhaar, PhD, RN, ANEF, FAAN
Professor
Nursing
Villanova University
Philadelphia, Pennsylvania

Heather M. Tripp, MEd, BSN, RN, SANE-A, SANE-P
Assistant Nurse Manager
Forensic Nursing
Cleveland Clinic
Cleveland, Ohio

Susan Nickel Van Cleve, DNP, CPNP-PC, PMHS, FAANP, FAAN
Pediatric Mental Health Specialist
Behavioral Health
Children's Community Pediatrics
Pittsburgh, Pennsylvania;
Adjunct Faculty
Health Promotion and Development
University of Pittsburgh School of Nursing
Pittsburgh, Pennsylvania

Kristen Marie Vargo, DNP, MSN, BNS
Director of Nursing
Neurological Institute & Orthopaedic and
   Rheumatology Institute
Cleveland Clinic
Cleveland, Ohio

Sara Williams, BScN, MN, RN
Indigenous Curriculum and Pedagogy Advisor
Faculty of Nursing
University of Windsor
Windsor, Ontario, Canada

Rosie Zeno, DNP, APRN-CNP, CPNP-PC
Associate Clinical Professor
College of Nursing
The Ohio State University
Columbus, Ohio

FOREWORD

Beth Heuer and Cynthia Danford hit it out of the park with their resource entitled *The Nurse Preceptor Toolkit: Preparing Nurses and Advanced Practice Nurses for Clinical Practice*. This toolkit is a must-have for anyone who desires to be an outstanding preceptor, or even for those who have been fulfilling the role for quite some time. There has never been a more urgent need for high-caliber preceptors, yet the demands of the current healthcare system often make precepting a daunting role to consider, given current challenges with staffing and system issues that lead to burnout throughout so many hospitals, primary care practices, long-term care settings, and community health agencies. The preparation of outstanding nurses and advanced practice nurses, which are desperately needed today, depends on high-quality academic programming with outstanding faculty, as well as skilled preceptors who serve as excellent role models for students.

Precepting students affords so many great professional and personal rewards when done well. Heuer and Danford's toolkit contains all of the essential elements for a great precepting and student experience, including a wide variety of best practices. This comprehensive step-by-step guide offers key elements of providing an exceptional preceptor–student journey. The appendices are chock-full of helpful resources, such as preceptor expectation checklists, one-minute preceptor examples, and a mentoring contract. Real-life exemplars also are highlighted in the book that provide helpful insights on how to deal with what I call "character-building" situations. I have no doubt that this toolkit will be a game changer for preceptors, faculty, and students. Congratulations on an awesome resource that I intend to make available for my preceptors and faculty!

Bernadette Mazurek Melnyk, PhD, APRN-CNP, EBP-C, FAANP, FNAP, FAAN
Vice President for Health Promotion
Chief Wellness Officer
The Ohio State University
Helene Fuld Health Trust Professor of Evidence-based Practice
Founder, the Helene Fuld Health Trust National Institute for EBP
Former Dean, College of Nursing
Professor of Pediatrics and Psychiatry, College of Medicine
Editor, Worldviews on Evidence-based Nursing
President, the National Consortium for Building Healthy Academic Communities
Columbus, Ohio

The publication of this first edition of *The Nurse Preceptor Toolkit* began several years ago with a simple conversation between the editors, who identified that formal information was lacking on "how to precept graduate nursing students." Precepting learners in the clinical setting is not commonly discussed in educational programs. Yet nurses are expected to "pay it forward" and help guide students (and others new to a clinical field) to gain valuable clinical experience while maintaining their own patient care assignments. Given the conundrum of being expected to teach others yet not having the foundational tools, we developed a preceptor workshop with a team of experienced nurse practitioners representing a variety of specialties from across the country. While developing the workshop, we gathered many resources and created an accompanying workbook. The workshop and workbook were well received, and the overwhelmingly positive input led to the genesis of this book. Our initially small endeavor grew into this comprehensive resource on precepting not only graduate students, but also undergraduate students, new nurses, and nurses transitioning to a new clinical site or specialty area.

The Nurse Preceptor Toolkit is organized into five sections that we believe present the content in a practical, user-friendly manner. The first section, *Setting the Stage*, provides background information on precepting given the changing landscape of healthcare. We address the growing demand for preceptors and present elements foundational for effective precepting. The second section, *Defining the Preceptor*, reviews basic concepts of precepting, explores the benefits of precepting, and describes coaching and mentoring. The third section, *Framing the Precepting Experience*, provides content on the learning process, social and communication styles, and the learning curve that influences both the learner and the preceptor. The fourth section, *Clinical Judgment Skills and Precepting Models*, provides concrete tools that preceptors can use to enhance learning and promote role development. The fifth section, *Preceptor Toolkit*, provides information on the "nuts and bolts" of precepting. Topics include expectations for academic programs, well-rounded experiences for undergraduate and graduate students, onboarding and orientation for new and experienced nurses, management of challenging students, professional development, and self-care.

We are pleased to include several unique features in this book. We address precepting in leadership roles, global health and school settings, forensics and trauma, and indigenous populations. Precepting for faculty roles and when developing non-research projects, as well as considerations for addressing health policy, are also included.

Most chapters include at least one pop-out box (sometimes two or three) with highlighted information. Many chapters have exemplars written by a variety of experienced preceptors to illustrate real-life application of concepts or issues. The book also includes appendices of ready-to-use practical tools and suggestions for preceptors to use in the clinical site. The authors of the chapters, exemplars, and boxes represent diverse perspectives from universities and healthcare institutions across the country.

We believe the book will be of use to a variety of audiences, including those new to precepting and those who have precepted for many years. Faculty and schools of nursing will be able to use this book to provide direction for the nurses on whom they rely to precept students. Faculty are encouraged to provide preceptors with this book as a roadmap for their ventures into clinical education. This book is a foundational resource for health leadership courses addressing the preceptor role. Given the breadth of knowledge this book provides, preceptors outside the discipline of nursing can also benefit from the content and resources within this book. The content is relevant for teaching all healthcare providers caring for patients and families across the life course.

Finally, we are indebted to the chapter and exemplar authors, who are our fellow colleagues from across the country, for their contributions to this book. We also greatly appreciate the guidance, diligence, and support provided by our Elsevier team who have been kind and directive as we navigated the trials and tribulations of developing, writing, and editing our first book. Of course, we are grateful to our fellow preceptors who were the inspiration for the creation of this book and who continue to "pay it forward," resulting in the development of a well-prepared nursing workforce.

Beth Heuer
Cynthia A. Danford

ACKNOWLEDGMENTS

The following authors contributed to the original Precepting Workshop and Preceptor Toolkit presented at the National Association of Pediatric Nurse Practitioners National Conference Workshops in 2018 and 2019. We appreciate the help you provided to build the vision that became this book.

Jay M. Hunter, DNP, RN, CPNP-AC, CCRN, CPEN, CPN
UCSF Benioff Children's Hospitals and
School of Nursing
Oakland, California

Imelda Reyes, DNP, MPH, CPNP-PC, FNP-BC, FAANP
UNLV School of Nursing
Las Vegas, Nevada

Jessica L. Spruit, DNP, RN, CPNP-AC, FAANP
C.S. Mott Children's Hospital
Ann Arbor, Michigan

Jodi Bloxham, DNP, APRN, PNP-AC, PNP-PC
University of Iowa College of Nursing
Iowa City, Iowa

Daniel Crawford, DNP, RN, CPNP-PC, CNE, FAANP
University of Iowa College of Nursing
Iowa City, Iowa

Shayna Dahan, MSN, CPNP, PMHS
Montefiore School Health Program
Bronx, New York

Amanda Lee, MSN, PPCNP-BC
ACCESS Community Health Network
Chicago, Illinois

Maria Lofgren, DNP, ARNP, NNP-BC, CPNP, FAANP
University of Iowa College of Nursing
Iowa City, Iowa

Audra Rankin, DNP, APRN, CPNP
University of North Carolina at Chapel
Hill School of Nursing
Chapel Hill, North Carolina

CONTENTS

1

Introduction to Precepting

Beth Heuer and Cynthia A. Danford

CHAPTER OBJECTIVES

- Identify the growing need for well-prepared preceptors in nursing education and facility onboarding
- Describe factors within the healthcare landscape that impact access to preceptors in clinical nursing education
- Differentiate elements of effective precepting in the clinical setting

INTRODUCTION

Precepting in nursing is an art involving an interaction between a knowledgeable, experienced nurse and an individual learning a new role. During the preparation of this book, we identified that a variety of terms have been used to reflect preceptors, nurses, and students. For consistency and to lend clarity throughout the book, the following terminology will be used. *Preceptors* are experienced registered nurses (RNs) or advanced practice RNs (APRNs) who provide clinical nursing experience and role model clinical skills for learners within a healthcare setting. *Learners* may include undergraduate or graduate students, new program graduates, or new employees. We use the term "orientee" and "learner" to refer to both students and RNs who are working directly with a preceptor. Adult learning principles and communication skills apply to all orientees. The terms "undergraduate" or "graduate" student, "nursing student,"

"APRN student," or "nurse practitioner (NP) student" will be used in specific instances when describing preceptor interactions with students and nursing school faculty to address required educational objectives and other student issues. The term "RN orientee" will be used to refer to licensed RNs or APRNs who are learning a new role.

BACKGROUND

Preceptors are essential to the growth of the nursing profession. The value preceptors bring to the clinical learning environment is immense, as without preceptors, the translation and application of knowledge to healthcare settings could not effectively occur. Nursing preceptors play a critical role in helping to create a safe learning environment where orientees are taught how to be proficient in their skills, in their new role, and sometimes in a new healthcare setting (Fulton et al., 2017).

Undergraduate and advanced practice nursing students must complete hundreds of direct clinical practice hours with expert nurse clinicians to bridge the gap between their formal education and real-life practice. Subsequently, students need competent and confident preceptors to provide real-time educational experiences and to facilitate the transition from student to RN or APRN. Additionally, healthcare settings are always onboarding new nursing professionals, whether graduate nurses, experienced RNs, or APRNs. As a result, all healthcare settings seek qualified, enthusiastic preceptors to orient novice or seasoned nurses to new roles or new work environments. To accommodate variations in learning needs and work environments, versions of the preceptor–student one-to-one learning model are modified for use within nursing residency programs, in addition to didactic (classroom learning) and simulation-based education (Walsh, 2018).

Since the "art" of how to precept is not typically addressed in formal educational programs, preceptors may lack the necessary knowledge and skills about clinical teaching to provide students with optimal learning experiences (Horton et al., 2012). Studies have shown that preceptor training can help increase confidence and knowledge of the role and expectations (Bazzell & Dains, 2017; Fincham et al., 2019; Martinez-Linares et al., 2019; Warren et al., 2022). Education and training that covers teaching and learning strategies, reflective and clinical reasoning, communication, and the preceptor role are vital components of preceptor preparation (Bengtsson & Carlson, 2015; Windey et al., 2015). This book will address each of these issues to help build an effective skill set and comfort level in the clinical preceptor role.

PRECEPTING IN CHANGING HEALTHCARE AND EDUCATIONAL LANDSCAPES

The nursing profession is in a state of continuous change. The U.S. Bureau of Labor Statistics (2020) reports that there will be approximately 194,500 openings for RNs each year, on average, through the year 2030. Many openings are expected to result from the need to replace workers who leave the nursing workforce for many reasons, including but not limited to those retiring or transferring to different occupations. The need to fill the vacancies in nursing is now more important and more needed than ever, which adds to

the demand for and challenge of finding qualified preceptors. In 2020 alone, there were over 82,000 graduates from entry-level baccalaureate nursing (BSN) programs and 69,000 graduates from RN-to-BSN programs who entered the workforce and filled some of these vacancies. Moreover, schools of nursing are experiencing surges in enrollment. Following the onset of the COVID-19 pandemic, there was a 3.3% increase in entry-level BSN program enrollment (American Association of Colleges of Nurses [AACN], 2021a). In graduate nursing education, more than 36,000 new NPs completed academic programs in 2019–2020 (American Association of Nurse Practitioners [AANP], 2022). In addition to the need for preceptors at the undergraduate level, graduate APRN educational programs require expert clinical preceptors for a variety of roles such as NP, clinical nurse specialist (CNS), certified nurse midwife (CNM), and certified registered nurse anesthetist (CRNA) programs. Given the specialization of CNM and CRNA programs, this book will not detail clinical precepting skills for these roles, although the education principles are applicable for all who want to learn more about how to precept, mentor, and coach students and new colleagues.

Contributing to the anticipated growth in healthcare services is the increasing emphasis on preventive care across the life course, from addressing prenatal care and early childhood vaccinations to reducing the burden of chronic disease in older patients. More educational experiences and more nurse providers are needed in primary practice sites that emphasize chronic disease prevention and management (Martinez Rogers et al., 2021). Unfortunately, the numbers of clinicians willing and able to serve as preceptors is far less than the number of schools of nursing and students requesting clinical placements (American College of Nurse Midwives, 2020; Gigli & Gonzalez, 2022; Miller & Kennedy, 2016). As the nursing workforce ages, the growth of the profession often falls to newer preceptors who must be willing and able to train and onboard students and orientees. Consequently, adequate preparation of preceptors is critically important.

Numerous factors need to coalesce to create an effective precepted clinical education experience for students. "Access to Clinical Nursing Education," a model originally developed by Penchansky and Thomas (1981) and modified by Dr. Kristin Gigli, provides a schematic image of factors considered during the clinical

ACCESS TO CLINICAL NURSING EDUCATION

Kristin Hittle Gigli

Conceptual framework: Access to clinical nursing education framed by healthcare system factors.

This model is adapted from the Penchansky and Thomas "Access to Clinical Nursing Education" model (1981) (Figure 1.1), which frames key factors influencing access to clinical preceptors. The definition and elements of the domains of access to clinical nursing education include:

Affordability related to the direct and indirect costs of clinical nursing education experiences. Costs to the student include: tuition, lodging and transportation, and private clinical placements. Costs to the school of nursing include: paperwork processing, contract fees, and support for academic affiliation coordinators. Costs to the preceptor include: decreased productivity and contract fees.

Acceptability related to characteristics of students and preceptors. Exposure to a variety of preceptors and clinical sites provides diverse learning experiences. Certification concordance between student and preceptor should be ensured.

Attitudes of those engaged in clinical nursing education experiences. This includes attitudes of students toward specific clinical settings, attitudes of preceptors toward the responsibility of precepting, and attitudes of clinical sites toward creating a learning environment for students.

Availability of precepted clinical nursing education experiences. Key considerations include: acceptable preceptor-to-student ratios and the number of preceptors accepting students. Such factors may be influenced by institutional and regulatory policies.

Accessibility related to geographic locations. This takes into consideration the physical location of a clinical site and opportunities to participate in telehealth and simulation learning.

Accommodation in terms of how clinical nursing education experiences are organized and delivered. This includes opportunities to complete clinical hours to complement full-time or part-time student work schedules and meet learners' needs (e.g., setting specific needs [inpatient/outpatient, rural/urban] and specialty experiences).

Healthcare environment provides context and influences the clinical nursing education experience. The surrounding environmental factors are dynamic and changeable. Included are increases in student academic enrollment and learning needs, a focus on interdisciplinary clinical education, consideration of workforce stressors (e.g., mental health burden and influence of pandemics), attention to healthcare delivery changes, consumer preferences, and evolving reimbursement policies.

Reference

Penchansky, R., & Thomas, J. W. (1981). The concept of access: Definition and relationship to consumer satisfaction. *Medical Care, 19*(2), 127–140. https://doi.org/10.1097/00005650-198102000-00001

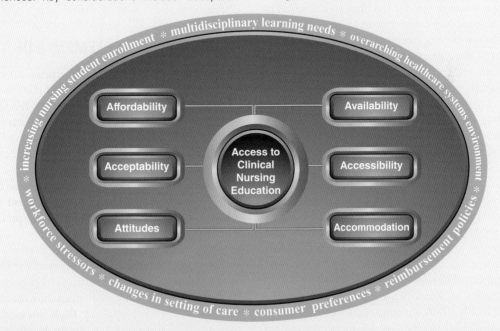

Figure 1.1. Access to clinical nursing education model. (Adapted from Penchansky, R., & Thomas, J. W. (1981). The concept of access: Definition and relationship to consumer satisfaction. *Medical Care, 19*(2), 127–140.)

placement process. Interaction issues may contribute to constraints, confusion, or stress for both students and preceptors, especially as the precepted clinical experience commences. Knowledge of the interaction between workplace environmental factors and student–preceptor issues leads to greater understanding of how clinical education is accessed, thus emphasizing the importance of the preceptor role.

THE GROWING DEMAND FOR ADVANCED PRACTICE REGISTERED NURSE (APRN) PRECEPTORS

Clinical education for APRNs has traditionally used a one-to-one preceptor–student model (Fulton et al., 2017), which allows the student to apply theoretical principles to actual practice in the clinical setting under the guidance of a seasoned provider. As the number of APRN students grows exponentially, high-quality clinical educational experiences from acute, primary, and other healthcare education programs also becomes a greater need. Preceptor demand is at an all-time high to meet the need, resulting in competition for clinical sites from both local and distance-learning APRN students, medical students, medical residents, medical fellows, and physician assistant students. Competition for clinical experiences in various teaching arenas needs to be recognized and addressed to meet current and future demands for the nursing workforce.

There is a need to create sustainable processes to recruit, train, retain, and recognize preceptors for APRN students. Part of the process in securing effective preceptors involves overcoming superimposed barriers to precepting. Gigli and Gonzalez (2022) identified that 60% of surveyed APRNs did *not* precept. Reasons that APRNs gave for not precepting varied and included not being asked (37.6%), not receiving approval by employers (32.8%), lacking the desire (12.9%), and experiencing decreased work productivity (12.4%). The development of academic partnerships between hospitals or clinics and schools/colleges of nursing to acknowledge and discuss barriers to precepting can create mutually beneficial outcomes for all involved: students, schools, preceptors, and employers.

The logistics of identifying and assigning preceptors to work with APRN students occurs in a variety of ways. While clinical faculty may use their professional network to contact preceptors directly, many universities have designated academic affiliations or clinical placement coordinators who contact preceptors on behalf of the academic program. The intent of using a clinical placement coordinator is to streamline the clinical placement process by efficiently identifying a suitable match between student and preceptor at a clinical site, while respecting the time and role demands of faculty and preceptors. In other programs, students are responsible for finding their own preceptors and may post requests for clinical experiences through APRN group list serves, on social media, or at local, state, and national professional events. According to Doherty et al. (2019), 40% of APRN students put forth all or most of the effort to find their own preceptors. Gigli and Gonzalez (2022) reported that 46% of APRN student survey respondents were required to find their own clinical placements while only 19.5% of respondents reported that these placements were arranged by their school or university. Many health systems and clinics require an online application process to manage student placement requests both locally and at a distance. Some medical centers act as gatekeepers and use a medical or advanced practice provider liaison to manage student requests for preceptors. In recent years, a business model has arisen where fee-for-service agencies contract with preceptors on behalf of students (see Chapter 3 Box: *Paid Preceptors*).

UNDERSTANDING ELEMENTS OF EFFECTIVE PRECEPTING

Effective precepting includes many elements such as effective communication, addressing different learning styles of adult learners, flexibility, provision of feedback and support, and the ability to evaluate student knowledge and competencies (Burns et al., 2006). At the same time, preceptors are often expected to refine their own time management skills and maintain productivity within the clinical setting (Bloomingdale & Darmody, 2019).

A significant challenge for novice preceptors can be knowing what is expected as they interact with students or orientees. The AACN (2021b) highlights that nursing students should be engaged in active learning, which means that they are *applying* their knowledge rather than passively absorbing it. Clear information regarding what students and orientees have learned and what they need to learn helps the preceptor guide student experiences as the student builds competency in the RN or APRN role (AACN, 2021b). Identifying competencies that are realistic and manageable to achieve during the learner's clinical rotation is a key to a successful precepting experience.

Given its complexity, precepting, like nursing, is an art. Consider the visual image of a patchwork quilt. The artistry is such that there are many separate parts that, individually, are beautiful and can stand alone; yet, when they come together, become a unified whole. The art of precepting can be broken down into the themes of communication, preparation and approach, engagement and safety, interaction challenges, and evaluation. Individually, these are important concepts to understand and consider. When these concepts are collectively applied and balanced, the result is a strong, effective, and comprehensive precepting experience. The overall outcomes are happier, successful preceptors; improved job satisfaction; retention of new employees (Loughran & Koharchik, 2019); and a means to strengthen the nursing workforce.

REFERENCES

American Association of Colleges of Nursing (2021a). *Nursing schools see enrollment increases in entry-level programs, signaling strong interest in nursing careers*. https://www.aacnnursing.org/News-Information/Press-Releases/View/ArticleId/25183/Nursing-Schools-See-Enrollment-Increases-in-Entry-Level-Programs

American Association of Colleges of Nursing (2021b). *The essentials: Core competencies for professional nursing education*. American Association of Colleges of Nursing. https://www.aacnnursing.org/Portals/42/AcademicNursing/pdf/Essentials-2021.pdf

American Association of Nurse Practitioners. (2022). *NP facts*. https://www.aanp.org/about/all-about-nps/np-fact-sheet

American College of Nurse Midwives (2020). *Preceptors for midwifery clinical education: A call to action in this unprecedented time*. https://www.midwife.org/preceptors-for-midwifery-clinical-education-a-call-to-action-in-this-unprecedented-time

Bazzell, A. F., & Dains, J. E. (2017). Supporting nurse practitioner preceptor development. *The Journal for Nurse Practitioners*, 13(8), e375–e382. https://doi.org/10.1016/j.nurpra.2017.04.013

Bengtsson, M., & Carlson, E. (2015). Knowledge and skills needed to improve as preceptor: Development of a continuous professional development course — a qualitative study part I. *BMC Nursing*, 14(1). https://doi.org/10.1186/s12912-015-0103-9

Bloomingdale, R., & Darmody, J. V. (2019). Clinical Nurse Specialist preceptor protocol. *Clinical Nurse Specialist*, 33(5), 228–236. https://doi.org/10.1097/nur.0000000000000470

Burns, C., Beauchesne, M., Ryan-Krause, P., & Sawin, K. (2006). Mastering the preceptor role: Challenges of clinical teaching. *Journal of Pediatric Health Care*, 20(3), 172–183. https://doi.org/10.1016/j.pedhc.2005.10.012

Fincham, S. J., Smith, T., & Purath, J. (2019). Implementation of an educational program to improve precepting skills. *Journal of the American Association of Nurse Practitioners*, 1. https://doi.org/10.1097/jxx.0000000000000326.

Fulton, C. R., Clark, C., & Dickinson, S. (2017). Clinical hours in nurse practitioner programs equals clinical competence. *Nurse Educator*, 42(4), 195–198. https://doi.org/10.1097/nne.0000000000000346

Gigli, K. H., & Gonzalez, J. D. (2022). Meeting the need for nurse practitioner clinicals: A survey of practitioners. *Journal of the American Association of Nurse Practitioners*, 34(8), 991–1001. https://doi.org/10.1097/jxx.0000000000000749

Horton, C. D., DePaoli, S., Hertach, M., & Bower, M. (2012). Enhancing the effectiveness of nurse preceptors. *Journal for Nurses in Professional Development*, 28(4), E1–E7.

Loughran, M. C., & Koharchik, L. (2019). Ensuring a successful preceptorship: Tips for nursing preceptors. *American Journal of Nursing (AJN)*, 119(5), 61–65. https://doi.org/10.1097/01.naj.0000557917.73516.00

Martinez-Linares, J. M., Parra-Saez, C., Tello-Liebana, C., & Lopez-Entrambasaguas, O. M. (2019). Should we be trained to train? Nursing students' and newly qualified nurses' perception on good lecturers and good clinical preceptors. *International Journal of Environmental Research and Public Health*, 16(24), 4885. https://doi.org/10.3390/ijerph16244885

Martinez Rogers, N. E., Zamora, H., & Ornelas, D. (2021). Teaching baccalaureate nursing students to practice in primary care settings. *Journal of Nursing Education*, 60(3), 129–135. https://doi.org/10.3928/01484834-20210222-02

Miller, J., & Kennedy, O. (2016). Barriers and incentives to precepting nurse practitioner students in a pediatric facility. *Journal of Pediatric Health Care*, 30(4), 302–303. https://doi.org/10.1016/j.pedhc.2016.04.004

U.S. Bureau of Labor Statistics. (2020). *Registered Nurses: Occupational Outlook Handbook: U.S. Bureau of Labor Statistics*. https://www.bls.gov/ooh/healthcare/registered-nurses.htm

Walsh, A. (2018). Nurse residency programs and the benefits for new graduate nurses. *Pediatric Nursing, 44*(6), 275–279.

Warren, J. I., Harper, M. G., MacDonald, R., Ulrich, B., & Whiteside, D. (2022). The impact of preceptor education, experience, and preparation on the role. *Journal for Nurses in Professional Development*, published ahead of print. https://doi.org/10.1097/nnd.0000000000000822

Windey, M., Lawrence, C., Guthrie, K., Weeks, D., Sullo, E., & Chapa, D. W. (2015). A systematic review on interventions supporting preceptor development. *Journal for Nurses in Professional Development, 31*(6), 312–323. https://doi.org/10.1097/nnd.0000000000000195

2

Starting With the Basics

Beth Heuer

CHAPTER OBJECTIVES

- Recognize how preceptors are identified and describe their role in undergraduate, graduate, and institutional onboarding education
- Describe attributes of effective preceptors
- Recognize how to avoid horizontal violence and microaggression as applied to precepting

- Apply concepts of diversity, inclusion, and equity in precepting practice
- Identify standardized clinical education accreditation requirements and state board regulations

When beginning the precepting experience, it is helpful to understand the basics of the process. Multiple layers are intertwined, from the general precepting landscape to embracing preceptor qualifications and readiness to appreciating clinical education regulations. The preceptor has little control over changes to the landscape and education regulations, but awareness contributes to an informed experience. Understanding qualifications can highlight the nurse's readiness to engage in precepting as a professional responsibility or to identify ways to strengthen their abilities in preparation for future precepting experiences.

UNDERSTANDING THE PRECEPTING LANDSCAPE

Navigating the precepting landscape is complex and involves understanding the essence of the preceptor–learner relationship, general nursing education responsibilities, and role transition. Precepting involves the development of a professional relationship built on mutual trust, communication, and respect (Kantar, 2021). Preceptors agree to share their expertise with students and new nurses through dialogue, observation, and role modeling (Ke et al., 2017). Clinical education responsibilities include demonstrating and assessing skills, providing instruction and feedback, observing, delegating, and initiating challenging conversations to gently correct errors. Preceptors are integral in helping the learner transition to a new role along various career continuums. Role transitions may include moving from student to generalist-trained registered nurse (RN), becoming a specialty-trained RN, shifting to a new clinical setting, or seeking further education in an advanced practice RN (APRN) role.

Preceptor Selection and Development

The preparation and educational development of preceptors is critical to growing and maintaining a qualified RN and APRN workforce. Some preceptors volunteer their expertise or may be identified by a nurse leader or faculty member who strongly encourages them to assume the role. However, serving as a preceptor is often a job requirement and a mandatory expectation for nurses seeking advancement within their workplace. Clinical preceptors may also have the dual role of being a faculty member at a university or a nursing professional development specialist within their facility.

Matching the Preceptor and Learner

Faculty and nursing organization leadership work to carefully match preceptors with the individual and specific needs of learners. The clinical practicum assignment should be based on the orientee's educational progress and previous experience, and then built upon in logical steps (Grealish et al., 2018). Best practice indicates that the learner gradually assumes increased responsibilities based on advancement from simple to complex experiences (Joswiak, 2018). This process is referred to as "scaffolding," as skill complexity and clinical decision-making develops over time.

Nurse Residency Programs and Preceptors

Within many healthcare centers, nurse residency programs have emerged as a preferred method of orienting nurse trainees. Preceptors role model the application of skills in clinical practice within residency programs. The curriculum for a successful nurse residency program includes a didactic component that focuses on evidence-based care and patient outcomes, clinical immersion facilitated by trained preceptors, and dedicated mentoring to model professionalism and build confidence (Walsh, 2018; Chant & Westendorf, 2019). These programs are designed to improve job satisfaction and nurse retention.

The focus of residency programs is on assessing competencies, developing skills, and assisting in role transition. Time is devoted to the development of communication, clinical judgment, organization, and stress management skills, taught by those who work in and know the organization. There is no standard for how long a nursing orientation may last in the hospital setting. Nurse residency programs may last between 6 and 24 months, with an average of 12 months.

Maintaining Boundaries

The preceptor–learner relationship may feel personal at times, yet personal boundaries must be maintained. While the preceptor is the "expert" in the relationship with the student or orientee, they may also feel vulnerable to criticism (see Chapter 18, *Imposter Syndrome*). Some clinicians are recruited to precept based on the readiness for the role that others have recognized, even though clinicians may not perceive themselves as ready. They are often concerned that they lack qualifications and experience, thereby making them vulnerable and hesitant to set boundaries. Adding to the sense of vulnerability, the preceptor may be formally or informally evaluated by the orientee for their teaching effectiveness (Law et al., 2014). With time and experience, navigating preceptor–learner boundaries becomes easier and more comfortable.

The Role of the Preceptor in Onboarding New Colleagues

Onboarding and orientation are terms that are often used interchangeably but have different meanings and goals. Onboarding is an ongoing, formal process where employees new to an organization are supported and provided with information on organizational beliefs and values, standardized processes, and the expectations for their role (Thrasher & Walker, 2018). Onboarding further includes socializing the employee to the structure of the organization, unit, clinic, or other specialized healthcare setting (Cappiello & Boardman, 2022). Successful onboarding can lead to improved confidence and job satisfaction, professional development, and socialization (Loughran & Koharchik, 2019).

Orientation, which can be both formal and informal, is part of the onboarding process. Orientation occurs at the beginning of the onboarding process and formally familiarizes new employees with policies and procedures specifically related to the role (Thrasher & Walker, 2018). This includes learning specific institutional policies and procedures for patient care. The orientee expands their previous knowledge and experience, adjusting their mindset to meet the expectations of the new work environment. Orientee comments such as "at my old job, we used to…" and "my clinical instructor told me that I have to…." may need to be reframed by the preceptor. The transition to a new practice environment or role can be stressful and demanding. The preceptor facilitates the transition to clinical practice and ensures clinical competence and patient safety.

Setting-Specific Orientations

In inpatient unit settings, the preceptor helps socialize the orientee to how, when, and by whom patient assignments are made, time-specific priorities (e.g., patient rounding), management of report and bedside hand-offs, and typical schedules for patient care activities (e.g., phlebotomy, therapies, or procedures). In outpatient clinic settings, orientation specifics might include review of processes such as scheduling templates and the flow of the clinic day, admitting patients, obtaining patient information, ordering tests, and referring, discharging, and following up with patients.

UNDERSTANDING PRECEPTOR QUALIFICATIONS

Skills and Attributes of the Preceptor

Attributes are qualities that an individual is born with, and skills are abilities that are learned and develop with practice. Both qualities are complementary. For example, the attribute of "being confident" can inform the degree of success in *completing* various skills or competencies such as inserting a nasogastric tube or conducting a comprehensive physical exam. Nurses and APRNs need to have the appropriate skill sets in order to function successfully as preceptors, as well as personal attributes that help them successfully share those skills with students. Cotter et al. (2018) developed a consistent and measurable process for selecting preceptors based on several skills and attributes: clinical competence, use of the nursing process, transformational leadership skills, collaboration/communication skills, professional development, conflict resolution, commitment, flexibility, empowerment, and values. When rating a preceptor candidate using this tool, a score ≥35 indicates that the candidate has the appropriate skill set and attributes to succeed in this role (Table 2.1). The results from this self-evaluation can verify or provide reassurance of a nurse's readiness to take on the precepting role.

Two additional skills for the preceptor to hone are emotional intelligence and self-awareness, as these effect both the preceptor and the orientee. Emotional intelligence is defined as the ability to understand your own feelings and those of other people, to make choices that reflect this understanding, and then to apply this knowledge in actions (Şenyuva et al., 2014). Emotional intelligence can impact the preceptor's and educator's teaching self-efficacy, interpersonal relationships, and performance (Allen et al., 2012; Lalonde & Hall, 2016). Self-awareness, a critical component of emotional intelligence, is differentiated by internal and external perspectives. *Internal* self-awareness refers to how clearly an individual sees their own reactions (including thoughts, feelings, and behaviors), strengths, weaknesses, values, and aspirations in the context of how others are affected. In other words, internal self-awareness is "how we see ourselves." *External* self-awareness involves understanding how others view an individual in terms of these same factors (Eurich, 2018) or may be referred to as "how others view us."

Developing self-awareness as a preceptor means understanding how to communicate *and* how the student or orientee hears your words and tone. It is important to recognize how to tailor communication as a means to prevent stress for both yourself and the student (Shealy et al., 2019) (See Chapter 6). Self-awareness can be built by seeking honest feedback about the words, tone, and behavior used and by focusing on what meaningful changes can be made.

Qualities of Exceptional Preceptors

Educators, researchers, clinicians, and students describe effective professional and personal qualities of exceptional preceptors. The qualities presented are not all inclusive. Preceptors can develop these qualities as they gain experience and engage in on-going self-reflection and self-evaluation (Box 2.1) (Lalonde & McGillis-Hall, 2016; Newman et al., 2015).

Roles of the Preceptor

It is essential that preceptors seek clarity on the role that is being asked of them from their places of employment, from the schools of nursing that send students to the clinical site, and from students themselves. Preceptors describe themselves as educators, tutors, supervisors, advisors, mentors, and role models to students and other professionals within the clinical setting (Girotto et al., 2019). *Educators* expand the student's or orientee's knowledge while providing real-time patient care. *Tutors* provide a personalized

TABLE 2.1   Cotter Preceptor Selection Instrument

Please rate_____, who is a candidate for preceptor on the attributes listed below. Each attribute is worth up to three (3) points: A score of 35 or higher is needed to be accepted as a preceptor by the unit-based council. *1 = Needs Improvement; 2 = Meets Expectations; 3 = Exceeds Expectations*

Score	Attribute
	Clinical competence
	1. Provides nursing care according to established nursing standards.
	Nursing process
	2. Documentation is appropriate and complete.
	3. Sets priorities and demonstrates time management skills.
	Transformational leadership
	4. Sets priorities and demonstrates clinical judgment skills.
	5. Delegates appropriately and effectively to nursing support staff.
	Collaboration/communication skills
	6. Promotes effective/skilled communication through the use of tactful, direct, and sensitive interaction.
	7. Narrates patient care and explains the purpose behind his/her actions to others.
	Professional development
	8. Participates in learning activities, committees, and/or staff meetings.
	9. Provides "learning moments" to develop peers.
	Conflict resolution
	10. Demonstrates problem-solving skills and minimizes escalation of situations to assure safe patient care.
	Commitment
	11. Works to provide feedback to new employees. Welcomes and provides feedback to new employees.
	Flexibility
	12. Demonstrates willingness to vary work assignment/schedule to meet unit needs and needs of new orientees.
	Empowerment
	13. Objectively identifies strengths and weaknesses of self and others. Provides constructive feedback in a manner that allows for progression and growth.
	Values
	14. Projects positive attitudes as they relate to work environment.
Total Score	

Cotter, E., Eckardt, P., & Moylan, L. (2018). Instrument development and testing for selection of nursing preceptors. *Journal for Nurses in Professional Development*, 34(4), 185–193. https://doi.org/10.1097/nnd.0000000000000464

learning experience to share specialized knowledge and to hone the orientee's skills. *Supervisors* monitor the learner's skills and patient care. *Advisors*, using a formal or informal approach, provide guidance or recommendations for learner success. *Mentors* guide and support the learner in developing competence (See Chapter 4). *Role models* exemplify what it is like to know the job and do the job well. Preceptors serve as *socializers* to help build upon the learner's professional identity and provide introduction into the

BOX 2.1   Qualities of Exceptional Preceptors

Professional qualities exemplified by
- Maintaining clinical competence
- Role modeling of professionalism
- Providing constructive, meaningful feedback
- Collaborating interprofessionally and intra-professionally
- Creating a safe learning environment
- Sharing responsibility and moving learner toward autonomy
- Asking questions of the learner effectively

Personal qualities include
- Warm
- Respectful
- Enthusiastic
- Empathetic
- Nonjudgmental
- Fair
- Dependable
- Consistent
- Humorous
- Flexible

Newman LR, Tibbles CD, Atkins KM, Burgin S., Fisher LJ, Kent TS, Smith CC, Aluko A, Ricciotti HA (2015). Resident-as-teacher DVD series. *MedEdPORTAL*, https://doi.org/10.15766/mep_2374-8265.10152

specific clinical culture. Other critical roles can be to serve as a *protector* and *champion* for the learner, thereby creating a safe, supportive, and welcoming environment (Trede et al., 2016).

Awareness and Management of Horizontal Violence and Microaggression

The healthcare culture can be complex and daunting. As *protectors*, preceptors advocate for students and novice RNs who are learning a new role within the clinical environment (Harper et al., 2021). Thus, it is important to acknowledge and discuss the presence of horizontal violence and microaggression within the healthcare profession. "Horizontal violence" is a term referring to aggression between colleagues that ranges from written or verbal threats to physical or verbal harassment and assault. Incivility can range from gossip to rudeness to refusal to help a coworker. Further, the American Nurses Association (ANA) describes bullying as "repeated, unwanted harmful actions intended to humiliate, offend, and cause distress in the recipient," with

behaviors including hostile comments, verbal attacks, and intimidation (ANA, 2015, p. 3). Preceptors must be consciously aware of their own emotions and responses as they lay the framework for a culture of civility and respect. Emotions and responses range from satisfaction and pride to frustration depending on the performance of the orientee. The mix of emotions, particularly those of frustration, can lead to the preceptor exhibiting unintentional microaggressive behaviors.

"Self-justified" bullying, where the preceptor adopts a "tough-love" attitude that criticizes or berates the orientee, must be avoided (Taylor & Taylor, 2017). Many students and nurses recall bad memories of how they were treated terribly or made to feel inadequate by an experienced nurse or preceptor. Preceptors sometimes adopt this type of bullying behavior because they believe it provides motivation or because they feel enthusiastic about the job and "demand" excellence. No matter the reason, scolding criticism is a form of verbal abuse.

Diversity, Equity, Inclusion, and Belonging

Racial and ethnic disparities in healthcare delivery persist, and there remains limited racial and ethnic diversity within the professional nursing workforce (National Organization of Nurse Practitioner Faculties [NONPF], 2018). Within the workplace, Black, Indigenous, and People of Color (BIPOC), immigrants, and other minority populations continue to experience microaggressions, which include insults or offensive actions meant to demean or marginalize one's identity (Pusey-Reid & Blackman-Richards, 2022). Healthcare continues to focus on improving diversity, inclusion, and equity in education, practice, and scholarship. Policies on diversity and inclusion in nursing have been adopted by nursing education organizations including the American Association of Colleges of Nursing (AACN) (2017) and the National League for Nursing (NLN) (2016).

Diversity, equity, inclusiveness, and belonging (DEIB) through the lens of precepting warrants attention. Preceptors must understand and implement initiatives that promote a vibrant workforce and enhance DEIB for patients, students, and colleagues. The terms "diversity" and "inclusion" are often used simultaneously, yet it is essential to understand that these terms have different meanings. "Diversity" embraces an individual's unique qualities and recognizes individual differences (NLN, 2016). These differences may include, but are not limited to race, ethnicity, gender, sexual orientation and gender identity, socioeconomic status, age, physical abilities,

---

Exemplar: Qualities of Good Preceptors

Rosie Zeno

Throughout my tenure of clinical teaching, I have reviewed hundreds of preceptor evaluations that students have completed over the years. The preceptor evaluation scores are informative, but the students' narrative comments have provided meaningful insight into the preceptor qualities that are most conducive to a student's learning. One preceptor, who was recognized with an *Excellence in Precepting Award*, embodied the qualities that students and clinical faculty desire in a preceptor. Beyond the time, knowledge, and expertise that many valued preceptors share with students, this preceptor exhibited several key attributes that truly set him apart. He was often recognized for his willingness to engage in questioning without becoming defensive. He genuinely fostered a spirit of inquiry in students by urging them to be curious, to ask questions, and to respectfully challenge his clinical decision-making using evidence to support an alternate approach. In addition, he cultivated their clinical judgment by regularly seeking their input to clinical management and engaging in professional discourse. This preceptor recognized students as budding colleagues rather than imposing a hierarchical preceptor-student dynamic.

Students voiced appreciation for the opportunity to learn in a safe space and frequently commented that the preceptor helped them to overcome a fear of "being wrong" or making a mistake. He often reminded them that making mistakes is an essential aspect of the learning process.

Without fears of criticism or embarrassment, the students expressed feeling less inhibited and more engaged in clinical learning. Perhaps the most impactful takeaway is that students departed the rotation with a remarkable ability to readily discern their own areas for potential growth. They also had greater confidence in their aptitude for effectively using point-of-care resources to support their clinical decision-making. Students realized that a well-regarded provider does "not always know the answer" and can be adept at seeking consultation and navigating appropriate clinical resources to guide clinical decision-making. The preceptor's inclination for transparency and willingness to readily acknowledge his own limitations contributed to his professionalism as a role model who demonstrates genuine integrity and life-long learning.

As a clinical educator, I have been impressed by this preceptor's ability to engage with students. Prior to the start of each clinical rotation, he routinely made time to meet with students to provide orientation to the clinic and set expectations. More importantly, he learns about the student's past experiences, self-perceived strengths and weaknesses, and current learning goals. By connecting with the students as individuals, he builds trust in the preceptor-student relationship, which is reflected in the students' sincere expression of the value of his feedback. Overall, the students leave this clinical rotation with greater clarity for embracing their own professional identity.

---

religious beliefs, political beliefs, or other attributes. "Inclusion" refers to the environmental or organizational culture that embraces difference or respect for all and results in the ability to thrive (AACN, 2017; NLN, 2016). Diversity may be considered the "what" or various characteristics of the individual. Inclusion is about "how" the individual is embraced within the culture. Interconnected with diversity and inclusion is equity. "Equity" reflects the ability to recognize and acknowledge differences so that all individuals are treated fairly without barriers (AACN, 2017). Finally, "belonging" conveys a sense of security. Individuals feel included and supported, knowing their voice is both welcomed and heard, and their work is valued.

Cultural intelligence (also known as "cultural quotient" or "CQ") refers to a person's ability to function efficiently within a culturally diverse environment (Richard-Eaglin, 2021). Personal attributes associated with intercultural success include cultural empathy, flexibility, social initiative, emotional stability, and open-mindedness (Wang et al., 2021). Cultural exposure can promote understanding and appreciation of diverse cultures and reduce implicit (unconscious) bias, which refers to the tendency to judge without consciously thinking or questioning. Unconscious bias occurs outside of one's awareness and may present as a contradiction between beliefs and values (Durkin et al., 2022; Nordell, 2021). Unconscious bias influences how an individual processes information about others, leading to unintended disparities (Stamps, 2021).

It is the responsibility of the preceptor to develop and maintain an equitable practice in a reciprocal, supportive learning environment with students or orientees. Those who are new to a clinical setting have the opportunity to develop cultural humility by observing and modeling the words and actions of their preceptor (Killick, 2018; Robinson et al., 2021). Understanding implicit biases means challenging assumptions, broadening perspectives, and enhancing socialization between students and patients. Most importantly, preceptors can

BOX 2.2 Examples of Conduct that Embraces Diversity and Inclusiveness

Behaviors toward patients
- Avoids stereotypes, discrimination, prejudice
  - Holds oneself and others accountable (e.g., identifies microaggressions and models an inclusive, respectful response)
    - Note: Choosing to *not* respond to microaggressions can be viewed as agreeing with or validating the offense
- Expresses willingness to learn from others
  - Recognizes all are responsible for addressing implicit biases and creating a safe space for discussion and growth
- Acknowledges and respects different beliefs

Behaviors toward colleagues
- Handles conflict respectfully
- Advocates for self and for those who are disempowered

Behaviors within the profession
- Communicates and collaborates with interdisciplinary colleagues
- Contributes to the professional development of students and other nurses

Behaviors within society
- Advocates for underrepresented populations
  - Commits to changing culture by speaking up in defense of recipients of microaggressive comments and racialized behaviors
- Demonstrates fair allocation of resources

Adapted from Pusey-Reid, E., & Blackman-Richards, N. (2022). The importance of addressing racial microaggression in nursing education. *Nurse Education Today*, 105390.

promote diversity and inclusivity by attending diversity training to confront and reduce their own unconscious biases, commit to culture change, and champion diversity and inclusion in learning and clinical environments (Johnson et al., 2021) (Box 2.2).

UNDERSTANDING CLINICAL EDUCATION REGULATIONS

State Board Rules and Regulations

There is variability among individual state boards of nursing when it comes to the qualifications to precept student nurses, just as there is variability between hospitals and institutions regarding when a nurse is considered to be "qualified" to begin precepting new orientees. The National Council of State Boards of Nursing (NCSBN) (2021) mandates that anyone providing clinical education to a student in an RN program holds a current, active RN license (or privilege to practice) that is unencumbered and meets requirements in the state where the school program is approved. Some states require preceptors to hold a minimum of a BSN degree, while others specify that the preceptor must hold comparable or greater education than the student that they precept. It is the preceptor's responsibility to know the qualifications to precept in their state and facility before agreeing to provide clinical education opportunities (NCSBN, 2023).

Undergraduate Student Orientation: Clinical Hour Requirements

There is no current consensus about the type, quantity, and quality of clinical experiences needed to produce a competent graduate RN (Cipher et al., 2020). The two bodies that accredit schools of nursing are the Commission on Collegiate Nursing Education (CCNE) and the Accreditation Commission for Education in Nursing (ACEN). Neither of these commissions identifies a specific *number* of clinical hours required for degree completion. Instead, the focus remains on clinical learning activities reflecting evidence-based practice while supporting patient safety and health (Cipher et al., 2020). These activities can include skills labs and simulation experiences, along with direct patient care facilitated by instructors and preceptors.

The requirements regarding time spent in clinical experiences by graduating nurses are stipulated by individual state boards of nursing. Some states only define the *nature* of required clinical experiences, which can include simulation practice. A relatively small number of state boards of nursing currently require that students complete a specific *number* of direct clinical hours in prelicensure programs. As a preceptor, it is important to know the amount of time students have spent in direct patient care *prior* to coming to the clinical site, as well as the amount of time the learner needs to spend and the types of direct experiences they need to acquire.

Exemplar: Addressing Racism in the Clinical Setting

Lauren Gabrielle Johnson

One of the key roles as a preceptor is ensuring a safe environment for students while in the clinical setting. Often, we focus solely on their physical safety (e.g., proper PPE use, injury prevention). However, it is also imperative to protect the student's emotional and psychological well-being.

As a preceptor, I once experienced a challenging situation when a patient exhibited racist behavior towards a student. The student and I had received morning report together for our patient assignment. We reviewed charts and orders to ensure the student felt confident and prepared to assess the patients and provide care. Having progressed tremendously in her orientation, I was confident in allowing her to independently begin patient care but made sure that she knew I was available for any questions or concerns. Shortly thereafter, the student returned to the nursing station with tears in her eyes and trembling hands. She was visibly shaken, and I led her away from the nurse's station to inquire about what had occurred.

The student explained how she began to assess her first patient and noted that the patient was visibly uncomfortable. She asked if something was wrong or if the patient was in pain. The patient denied that anything was wrong, so the student continued with her assessment. The patient was minimally responsive to the questions that the student asked and seemed to convey a sense of annoyance. At the conclusion of the assessment, the patient expressed that they no longer wished for the student to serve as their nurse. The student self-consciously assumed that the patient was concerned that she was a novice and tried to defend her competence. The patient stated that she would rather have a White nurse take care of her and asked if she could speak with someone to have a new nurse assigned.

Addressing racism can be an uncomfortable situation and requires having difficult conversations. As preceptor, I followed up with the patient and made sure they understood that their request reflected an attitude of racism. I explained that our institution never tolerates such behavior toward anyone in our facility. I did not want to honor the patient's request to change nurses, because I believed that would reward and affirm their racist attitude. However, I also wanted to protect the student. Although the student might not have felt physically threatened, I did not think it would be fair to force her to continue caring for the patient if she did not feel psychologically safe. Ultimately, the student decided that she wanted to continue caring for the patient. Before the student was allowed to re-enter the room, a patient relations supervisor spoke to the patient to explain why their request would not be fulfilled and to inform them of the consequences that would ensue if their racist demeanor continued. I checked in with the student frequently throughout the shift and we debriefed at the end of the day.

APRN Student Orientation: Clinical Hour Requirements

In nurse practitioner (NP) population-focused education tracks, the *minimum* requirement for direct patient care clinical hours is 750 hours to prepare the graduate with competencies for full scope of practice (National Quality Forum Standards for Quality Nurse Practitioner Education, 2022). It is the student's responsibility to meet the appropriate requirements for graduation, national certification, and licensure. Clinical hours must include a variety of experiences to help students become competent in basic NP skills. However, the number of hours spent in a clinical practice setting is not predictive of achievement of core clinical competencies (Bargagliotti & Davenport, 2017; AACN, 2021). For example, a student may have many hours of experience collaborating with patients with diabetes, yet they still may not be able to meet the necessary competencies in this area.

Typically, students in certified registered nurse anesthesia (CRNA) educational programs obtain around 2600 hours of clinical experience during their training (American Association of Nurse Anesthesiology, 2019). Students in certified nurse midwife (CNM) programs obtain between 600 and 1200 hours of clinical experience (NurseMidwifery.org, n.d.). Finally, students in clinical nurse specialist (CNS) programs obtain between 500 hours (for master's and post-graduate certificate students) and 1000 hours (for post-baccalaureate DNP students) for their clinical experience prior to graduation (National Task Force on the Guidelines for Clinical Nurse Specialist Education, 2011). All of these students require supervised clinical hours and expertise by the preceptor who trains and welcomes new colleagues to the advanced practice roles.

REFERENCES

Allen, D. E., Ploeg, J., & Kaasalainen, S. (2012). The relationship between emotional intelligence and clinical teaching effectiveness in nursing faculty. *Journal of Professional Nursing, 28*(4), 231–240. https://doi.org/10.1016/j.profnurs.2011.11.018

American Association of Colleges of Nursing. (2017). *Diversity, equity, and inclusion in academic nursing.* https://www.aacnnursing.org/Portals/42/News/Position-Statements/Diversity-Inclusion.pdf

American Association of Colleges of Nursing. (2021). *The essentials: Core competencies for professional nursing education.* American Association of Colleges of Nursing. https://www.aacnnursing.org/Portals/42/AcademicNursing/pdf/Essentials-2021.pdf

American Association of Nurse Anesthesiology. (2019). *CRNA fact sheet.* AANA. https://www.aana.com/membership/become-a-crna/crna-fact-sheet

American Nurses Association (2015). *American Nurses Association position statement on incivility, bullying, and workplace violence.* https://www.nursingworld.org/~49d6e3/globalassets/practiceandpolicy/nursing-excellence/incivility-bullying-and-workplace-violence--ana-position-statement.pdf

Bargagliotti, L. A., & Davenport, D. (2017). Entrustables and entrustment: Through the looking glass at the clinical making of a nurse practitioner. *The Journal for Nurse Practitioners, 13*(8), e367–e374. https://doi.org/10.1016/j.nurpra.2017.05.018

Cappiello, J. D., & Boardman, M. B. (2022). The key to successful NP transition to practice. *The Nurse Practitioner, 47*(2), 33–39. https://doi.org/10.1097/01.npr.0000802992.36571.2b

Chant, K. J., & Westendorf, D. S. (2019). Nurse residency programs. *Journal for Nurses in Professional Development, 35*(4), 185–192. https://doi.org/10.1097/nnd.0000000000000560

Cipher, D. J., LeFlore, J. L., Urban, R. W., & Mancini, M. E. (2020). Variability of clinical hours in prelicensure nursing programs: Time for a reevaluation? *Teaching and Learning in Nursing, 16*(1), 43–47. https://doi.org/10.1016/j.teln.2020.05.005

Cotter, E., Eckardt, P., & Moylan, L. (2018). Instrument development and testing for selection of nursing preceptors. *Journal for Nurses in Professional Development, 34*(4), 185–193. https://doi.org/10.1097/nnd.0000000000000464

Durkin, G. J., Cosetta, M. A., Mara, C., Memmolo, S., Nixon, C., Rogan, M. L., & Pignataro, S. (2022). A multimodal project to assess preceptor burnout. *Journal for Nurses in Professional Development*, Published ahead of print. https://doi.org/10.1097/nnd.0000000000000820

Eurich, T. (2018, January 4). What self-awareness really is (and how to cultivate it). *Harvard Business Review.* https://hbr.org/2018/01/what-self-awareness-really-is-and-how-to-cultivate-it

Girotto, L. C., Enns, S. C., de Oliveira, M. S., Mayer, F. B., Perotta, B., Santos, I. S., & Tempski, P. (2019). Preceptors' perception of their role as educators and professionals in a health system. *BMC Medical Education, 19*(1). https://doi.org/10.1186/s12909-019-1642-7

Grealish, L., van de Mortel, T., Brown, C., Frommolt, V., Grafton, E., Havell, M., Needham, J., Shaw, J., Henderson, A., & Armit, L. (2018). Redesigning clinical education for nursing students and newly qualified nurses: A quality improvement study. *Nurse Education in Practice, 33*, 84–89. https://doi.org/10.1016/j.nepr.2018.09.005

Harper, M. G., Ulrich, B., Whiteside, D., Warren, J. I., & MacDonald, R. (2021). Preceptor practice: Initial results of a National Association for Nursing Professional Development study. *Journal for Nurses in Professional Development, 37*(3), 154–162. https://doi.org/10.1097/NND.0000000000000748

Johnson, R., Browning, K., & DeClerk, L. (2021). Strategies to reduce bias and racism in nursing precepted clinical experiences. *Journal of Nursing Education, 60*(12), 697–702. https://doi.org/10.3928/01484834-20211103-01

Joswiak, M. E. (2018). Transforming orientation through a tiered skills acquisition model. *Journal for Nurses in Professional Development, 34*(3), 118–122. https://doi.org/10.1097/nnd.0000000000000439

Kantar, L. (2021). Teaching domains of clinical instruction from the experiences of preceptors. *Nurse Education in Practice, 52*, 103010. https://doi.org/10.1016/j.nepr.2021.103010

Ke, Y. T., Kuo, C. C., & Hung, C. H. (2017). The effects of nursing preceptorship on new nurses' competence, professional socialization, job satisfaction and retention: A systematic review. *Journal of Advanced Nursing, 73*(10), 2296–2305. https://doi.org/10.1111/jan.13317

Killick, D. (2018). Critical intercultural practice: Learning in and for a multicultural globalizing world. *Journal of International Students, 8*(3), 1422–1439. https://doi.org/10.32674/jis.v8i3.64

Lalonde, M., & McGillis Hall, L. (2016). Preceptor characteristics and the socialization outcomes of new graduate nurses during a preceptorship programme. *Nursing Open, 4*(1), 24–31. https://doi.org/10.1002/nop2.58

Law, M., Baker, L., Leslie, K., Shamji, A., Eng, L., Fung, H. H. T., Lindzon, G., Tannenbaum, E., Mccaffrey, J., & Yeung, E. (2014). Negotiating learner–teacher boundaries in medical education. *Medical Teacher, 37*(5), 490–491. https://doi.org/10.3109/0142159x.2014.947944

Loughran, M. C., & Koharchik, L. (2019). Ensuring a successful preceptorship. *AJN, American Journal of*

Nursing, 119(5), 61–65. https://doi.org/10.1097/01. naj.0000557917.73516.00

National Council of State Boards of Nursing (2021). *NCSBN Model Act*. National Council of State Boards of Nursing. https://www.ncsbn.org/21_Model_Act.pdf

National Council of State Boards of Nursing (2023). www. ncsbn.org

National League for Nursing (2016). Achieving diversity and meaningful inclusion in nursing education: A living document from the National League for Nursing. Retrieved from: vision-statement-achieving-diversity. pdf (nln.org)

National Organization of Nurse Practitioner Faculties (2018). *NONPF calls for greater racial and ethnic diversity in nurse practitioner education*. https://cdn.ymaws.com/www.nonpf.org/resource/resmgr/docs/20180807_diversity_statement.pdf

National Task Force on the Guidelines for Clinical Nurse Specialist Education (2011). Criteria for the evaluation of Clinical Nurse Specialist Master's, Practice Doctorate, and Post-Graduate certificate educational programs. https://nacns.org/wp-content/uploads/2016/11/CNSEducation-Criteria.pdf

National Task Force on Quality Nurse Practitioner Education (2022). *Standards for quality nurse practitioner education* (6th ed.). American Association of Colleges of Nursing; National Organization of Nurse Practitioner Faculties. https://cdn.ymaws.com/www.nonpf.org/resource/resmgr/2022/ntfs_/ntfs_final.pdf

Newman, L., Tibbles, C. D., Atkins, K. M., Burgin, S., Fisher, L. J., Kent, T. S., & Aluko, A. (2015). Resident-as-teacher DVD series. *MedEdPORTAL, 11*, 10152.

Nordell, J. (2021). *The end of bias: A beginning: the science and practice of overcoming unconscious bias*. Metropolitan Books.

NurseMidwifery.org (n.d.). *Online Nurse Midwife Programs | Certified Nurse Midwife*. from https://www.nursemidwifery.org/program/online-cnm

Pusey-Reid, E., & Blackman-Richards, N. (2022). The importance of addressing racial microaggression in nursing education. *Nurse Education Today*, 105390. https://doi.org/10.1016/j.nedt.2022.105390

Richard-Eaglin, A. (2021). The significance of cultural intelligence in nurse leadership. *Nurse Leader, 19*(1), 90–94. https://doi.org/10.1016/j.mnl.2020.07.009

Robinson, D., Masters, C., & Ansari, A. (2021). The 5 Rs of cultural humility: A conceptual model for health care leaders. *The American Journal of Medicine, 134*(2), 161–163. https://doi.org/10.1016/j.amjmed.2020.09.029

Şenyuva, E., Kaya, H., Işik, B., & Bodur, G. (2014). Relationship between self-compassion and emotional intelligence in nursing students. *International Journal of Nursing Practice, 20*(6), 588–596. https://doi.org/10.1111/ijn.12204

Shealy, S. C., Worrall, C. L., Baker, J. L., Grant, A. D., Fabel, P. H., Walker, C. M., Ziegler, B., & Maxwell, W. D. (2019). Assessment of a faculty and preceptor development intervention to foster self-awareness and self-confidence. *American Journal of Pharmaceutical Education, 83*(7). https://doi.org/10.5688/ajpe6920

Stamps, D. (2021). Nursing leadership must confront implicit bias as a barrier to diversity in health care today. *Nurse Leader, 19*(6), 630–638. https://doi.org/10.1016/j.mnl.2021.02.004

Taylor, R., & Taylor, S. (2017). Enactors of horizontal violence: The pathological bully, the self-justified bully and the unprofessional co-worker. *Journal of Advanced Nursing, 73*(12), 3111–3118. https://doi.org/10.1111/jan.13382

Thrasher, A. B., & Walker, S. E. (2018). Orientation process for newly credentialed athletic trainers in the transition to practice. *Journal of Athletic Training, 53*(3), 292–302. https://doi.org/10.4085/1062-6050-531-16

Trede, F., Sutton, K., & Bernoth, M. (2016). Conceptualisations and perceptions of the nurse preceptor's role: A scoping review. *Nurse Education Today, 36*, 268–274. https://doi.org/10.1016/j.nedt.2015.07.032

Walsh, A. (2018). Nursing residency programs and the benefits for new graduate nurses. *Pediatric Nursing, 44*(6), 275–279.

Wang, C., Shakespeare-Finch, J., Dunne, M., Hou, X., & Khawaja, N. (2021). How much can our universities do in the development of cultural intelligence? A cross-sectional study among health care students. *Nurse Education Today, 103*, 104956. https://doi.org/10.1016/j.nedt.2021.104956

3

Why Precept?

Beth Heuer, Imelda Reyes, and Cynthia A. Danford

CHAPTER OBJECTIVES

- Examine the personal and professional benefits related to precepting
- Describe the influence of preceptors in the academic and institutional setting
- Review the benefits of educational preparation to promote precepting excellence

The decision to precept may be personal or may be a result of professional expectations and obligations. No matter the impetus, many nurses find value in the precepting experience and participate because they have an affinity to educate others and recognize their own potential as a clinical educator (Morgan et al., 2018). Other nurses choose to precept students or novice nurses as they are committed to strengthening the workforce and building nursing as a respectable profession. Precepting inspires others toward excellence in nursing practice and opens doors for personal and professional growth. Dedicated preceptors who are passionate about nursing and improving the health and well-being of patients, families, and communities are in a prime position to strengthen the nursing workforce and advance the contribution of the nursing profession. This chapter highlights many benefits of precepting.

SHARING EXPERTISE

Preceptors are called upon to share their expertise and specialized knowledge. Guided by skilled clinicians, learners are able to apply new knowledge in clinical settings in real-time (DeClerk et al., 2022). Precepting provides a "gateway to true clinical practice" (Gassas, 2021),

and preceptors provide the means to pass through the gateway. With guided opportunities and gradual movement toward independence, learners are able to develop and master physical exam and diagnostic skills, synthesize didactic content, and become socialized into the role of the nurse and APRN in a variety of settings (Lafrance, 2018). The preceptor role models the realities of nursing practice related to safe and effective patient care and management (DeClerk et al., 2022).

PAYING IT FORWARD

Precepting is a way to honor nurses and preceptors who have been instrumental in teaching in clinical practice and academic settings. "Giving back" to the profession is an optimal way to support nursing and build an effective workforce, while also gaining personal and professional satisfaction (Roberts et al., 2020). Nurses are invited or selected to precept based on exceptional skills, abilities, and attributes recognized during patient care and clinical practice. Top reasons for precepting are: 1) a passion for teaching students, 2) a sense of professional obligation, and 3) fulfillment of a "social contract" that assures an adequate workforce pipeline (Heard, 2017; Onieal, 2016; Renda et al., 2022).

Paid Preceptorships

Jennifer Sonney

Clinical training site availability is an important determinant of the enrollment capacity in professional health educational programs. Growing demands for health professionals coupled with clinical training site shortages have resulted in intense competition for clinical preceptors (Erikson et al., 2014). This is especially true in nursing, where over 90,000 qualified applicants to undergraduate and graduate nursing programs were turned away in 2021 due to insufficient training capacity (American Association of Colleges of Nursing AACN, 2022). The COVID-19 pandemic further exacerbated nursing preceptor shortages due to the devastating effects of burnout and nurses leaving the profession entirely (National Advisory Council on Nurse Education & Practice (NACNEP), 2021; Office of the Surgeon General, 2022). Creative and sustainable solutions are needed to promote immediate and long-term precepting capacity, especially in graduate nursing education. Fee-based services that arrange clinical placements have been suggested as a possible solution, yet their use is controversial and warrants careful consideration.

Fee-based preceptorship models vary, but typically entail a third-party agency with whom an academic institution or a student contracts. The agency seeks a preceptor match that meets the students' learning needs in exchange for an honorarium paid to the preceptor or preceptor's clinical agency. Payment models also vary, including hourly, preceptor-determined fee, and a lump sum, which is paid by the student or the student's academic program. The AACN and American Organization for Nursing Leadership (2020) identified that 10% of graduate nursing programs are paying for preceptors. The primary benefit of fee-based preceptorship models is to reduce the burden on faculty or students in need of identifying clinical sites willing to train students. From the preceptor perspective, honoraria are thought to offset the increased responsibility that comes with training a student, including potential reductions in clinical productivity.

While there are benefits to fee-based preceptorship models, there are important disadvantages to consider.

Regardless of the payment model, the cost of paid preceptorships will invariably be shifted to the student, whether through direct payment or fee adjustments by the educational program. Tuition increases are a known deterrent for pursuing higher education, especially for low-income students and students of color (Mitchell et al., 2019). Amidst national calls for nursing workforce diversification (Wakefield et al., 2021), the additional financial hardship of paying preceptors will further disadvantage students of marginalized communities who may not have the ability to assume such costs. Higher student debt trickles down, subsequently influencing healthcare availability in communities. Students with large loans may seek higher paying jobs, which further perpetuates healthcare provider shortages in rural and medically underserved communities.

Academic programs may provide evidence-based incentives for preceptors, including free continuing education, access to resources, formalized feedback, credit hours for national recertification, and meaningful recognition (Durkin et al., 2022; Gaynor & Barnes, 2022). Another alternative that has been effective in other states is provision of tax incentives for preceptors (Carelli et al., 2019). Additionally, there is a need for expanded federal investment in graduate nursing education. Models such as those used in graduate medical education (GME) would provide federal funding support to clinical agencies who commit to training graduate nursing students. The result could be a substantial increase in clinical training site availability without additional financial burden to students.

The national shortage in clinical training capacity is an alarming threat to graduate nursing education. While fee-based preceptorships may represent a short-term solution for some, this is not a sustainable or equitable model to address the critical shortage of preceptors. Instead, multi-level solutions are needed to incentivize precepting across educational programs, state, and federal entities.

BRIDGING THE THEORY-PRACTICE GAP

When preceptors role-model evidence-based practices, they influence learners who are navigating the process of understanding and applying theoretical principles to practice (Lam et al., 2020). By sharing observations of student clinical performance, preceptors become change agents for educational curricula. Sharing patterns among students from the same program, such as gaps in knowledge or skills, may help strengthen the school's nursing curriculum (Roberts et al., 2020). Programs value feedback from preceptors about how content is delivered and how students are comprehending and applying new and existing knowledge to evidence-based practice decisions with patients. When preceptors offer valuable input, they may be asked to serve on advisory panels for local schools or programs (Webb et al., 2015).

STAYING UP-TO-DATE

Precepting provides a means for the nurse to learn new knowledge and stay abreast of the latest evidence and practice changes. Additionally, students add an interesting and new perspective to patient care and provide challenging, well-formulated questions (Macey et al., 2021). Some questions may be complex and prompt the preceptor to explore the evidence deeply themselves or direct the student back to the evidence for later discussion of findings. Other questions may lead preceptors to pause and reflect on their own practice. Either way, the exploration, validation, and application of new and existing knowledge contributes to a cycle of continuous learning, thereby keeping the preceptor updated (Roberts et al., 2020). When learning is interactional, it maintains a stimulating environment and fosters a sense of enrichment and renewal (DeClerk et al., 2022).

ENTERING ACADEMIA

Serving as a preceptor can open doors for new opportunities, such as presenting guest lectures, acquiring academic appointments, and advancing into leadership roles. Prospective employers value precepting experiences as reflective of clinical excellence, leadership abilities, and professional commitment (Gatewood & De Gagne, 2019). Some schools grant adjunct faculty status to clinicians who have precepted for a few semesters. Being an adjunct faculty member often comes with perks, such as the use of a formal academic title (e.g., Adjunct Assistant Professor); access to university resources, such as the library; or faculty discounts (Roberts et al., 2020; Fraino & Selix, 2021). Library resources may include online clinical resources, such as UpToDate and research databases such as PubMed or CINAHL (DeClerk et al., 2022). In a 2015 survey, over 400 nurse practitioners ranked the benefits of precepting from most to least valued. The most valued benefits included: learning about clinical guidelines and new medications, having access to online clinical materials and continuing education programs, and developing relationships with faculty (Roberts et al., 2017).

NETWORKING

Networking between preceptors, faculty members, and other healthcare colleagues provides additional opportunities for growth. Ongoing collaboration helps with the development and dissemination of scholarly works, such as research or quality improvement projects. Faculty and other leaders are often willing to provide support through networking and mentoring for preceptors who are enrolled in or beginning to advance their education in Doctor of Nursing Practice (DNP) or Doctor of Philosophy (PhD) programs. Peer interaction with faculty can provide support and a sense of connectedness (Gholizadeh et al., 2022).

Preceptor appreciation events or awards may be sponsored by universities or healthcare institutions and not only provide recognition, but open doors for networking. Academic-practice partnerships, which are mutually cooperative agreements between universities and clinical institutions, further enhance preceptor support and appreciation (Yi et al., 2020).

ADVANCING RANK AND MAINTAINING PROFICIENCY

Precepting is a highly regarded endeavor and contributes to maintaining and advancing competencies in nursing practice. It is often an optional contribution, but in some cases may be a requirement dependent on the preceptor's situation. Some employers require precepting as criteria for promotion or clinical ladder advancement (Kauffman et al., 2021). Many preceptors utilize precepting hours for recertification credit (Lofgren et al., 2021; DeClerk et al., 2022). Certification bodies that accept APRN precepting hours for credit are the American Association of Nurse Practitioners (AANP), the American Nurses Credentialing Center (ANCC), and the Pediatric Nurse Certification Board (PNCB). Other specialty organizations and individual certification agencies can be explored for details on how precepting experiences can be applied.

GAINING EXTERNAL RECOGNITION

The altruistic nature of nurses often means *giving* to others and giving back to the nursing profession. However, *receiving* recognition external to the clinical institution and academic setting is reaffirming, both personally and professionally. In addition to recognition in the clinical or university setting, precepting excellence may also be recognized at the national level. Preceptor awards are available through professional organizations, including the National Association of Clinical Nurse Specialists, the Association of Faculties of Pediatric Nurse Practitioners, the American College of Nurse Midwives, and the National Organization of Nurse Practitioner Faculties. Educational and healthcare institutions are also notable for awarding precepting excellence (e.g., DAISY award). Preceptors are encouraged to nominate themselves and other colleagues for recognition.

THE PATHWAY TO REAPING BENEFITS

Precepting can be done without formal training. Yet, to ease the experience, preceptors should seek support, resources, appropriate guidance, or training from the clinical site before clinical teaching or orientation begins (Bodine, 2022). Precepting knowledge and expertise are enhanced through understanding adult learning concepts, effective communication practices, clinical teaching techniques, and evaluation methods (Ward & McComb, 2017; Barba et al., 2019; Good, 2021). There is a learning continuum for preceptors as they move from novice to expert in the precepting role (See Chapter 7). This educational process typically will not happen in the classroom, but comes from experience in a real-life clinical environment. However, educational modules on precepting or learning how to be a more effective preceptor are available and can often apply towards required continuing education units (CEUs). Online training tends to be most convenient and favored by many nurse preceptors (Good, 2021). Other options can include preceptor training workshops through universities or professional organizations (Fraino & Selix, 2021; Boyce et al., 2022). Within hospital settings, nursing professional development staff may offer clinical teaching programs to enhance preceptor competency and support preceptor management (Gholizadeh et al., 2022). The opportunity to practice the role of preceptor in a simulated manner using vignettes and role play can be an effective way to learn (Good, 2021; Hong & Yoon, 2021).

Being a preceptor for a prelicensure student, new registered nurse (RN) or APRN, or a new orientee can be a rich and insightful experience. Reflecting on principles

of adult learning and personal experiences with preceptors during days as a novice nurse will help to maintain a sensitive, empathetic, and realistic perspective. The outcome is personal and professional growth for preceptors and the satisfaction of being a part of contributing to the growing nursing workforce.

REFERENCES

American Association of Colleges of Nursing (AACN). (2022). *Highlights from AACN's 2021 annual survey.* https://www.aacnnursing.org/Portals/42/Data/Survey-Data-Highlights-2021.pdf

American Association of Colleges of Nursing and American Organization for Nursing Leadership (2020). *AACN-AONL clinical preceptor survey summary report.* https://www.aacnnursing.org/Portals/42/Data/AACN-AONL-Clinical-Preceptor-Survey-May-2020.pdf

Barba, M., Valdez-Delgado, K., VanFosson, C. A., Caldwell, N. W., Boyer, S., Robbins, J., & Mann-Salinas, E. A. (2019). An evidence-based approach to precepting new nurses. *AJN, American Journal of Nursing, 119*(3), 62–67. https://doi.org/10.1097/01.naj.0000554036.68497.61

Bodine, J. (2022). Supporting preceptors through the nursing shortage. *Journal for Nurses in Professional Development, 38*(5), 316–318. https://doi.org/10.1097/NND.0000000000000928

Boyce, D. J., Shifrin, M. M., Moses, S. R., & Moss, C. R. (2022). Perceptions of motivating factors and barriers to precepting. *Journal of the American Association of Nurse Practitioners, 34*(11), 1225–1234. https://doi.org/10.1097/jxx.0000000000000788

Carelli, K. V., Gatiba, P. N., & Thompson, L. S. (2019). Tax incentives for preceptors of nurse practitioner students in Massachusetts: A potential solution. *Journal of the American Association of Nurse Practitioners, 31*(8), 462–467. https://doi.org/10.1097/JXX.0000000000000257

DeClerk, L., Lefler, L., Nagel, C., Mitchell, A., Rojo, M., & Sparbel, K. (2022). Why don't all nurse practitioners precept? A comparative study. *Journal of the American Association of Nurse Practitioners, 34*(4), 668–682. https://doi.org/10.1097/JXX.0000000000000680

Durkin, G. J., Cosetta, M. A., Mara, C., Memmolo, S., Nixon, C., Rogan, M. L., & Pignataro, S. (2022). A multimodal project to assess preceptor burnout: Implications for professional development practitioners. *Journal for Nurses in Professional Development.* https://doi.org/10.1097/NND.0000000000000820

Erikson, C., Hamann, R., Levitan, T., Pankow, S., Stanley, J., & Whatley, M. (2014). *Recruiting and maintaining US clinical training sites: Joint report of the 2013 multi-discipline clerkship/clinical training site survey.* Washington, DC: Association of American Medical Colleges. 2019-2007.

Fraino, J., & Selix, N. (2021). Facilitating well-rounded clinical experience for psychiatric nurse practitioner students. *The Journal for Nurse Practitioners, 17*(8), 1004–1009. https://doi.org/10.1016/j.nurpra.2021.05.015

Gassas, R. (2021). Sources of the knowledge-practice gap in nursing: Lessons from an integrative review. *Nurse Education Today, 106,* 105095. https://doi.org/10.1016/j.nedt.2021.105095

Gatewood, E., & De Gagne, J. C. (2019). The One-Minute Preceptor model: A systematic review. *Journal of the American Association of Nurse Practitioners, 31*(1), 46–57. https://doi.org/10.1097/jxx.0000000000000187

Gaynor, B., & Barnes, H. (2022). Nurse practitioner preceptor plan: A focus on preceptor rewards and preferences. *Nursing Education Perspectives, 43*(1), 35–37. https://doi.org/10.1097/01.NEP.0000000000000773

Gholizadeh, L., Shahbazi, S., Valizadeh, S., Mohammadzad, M., Ghahramanian, A., & Shohani, M. (2022). Nurse preceptors' perceptions of benefits, rewards, support, and commitment to the preceptor role in a new preceptorship program. *BMC Medical Education, 22*(1). https://doi.org/10.1186/s12909-022-03534-0

Good, B. (2021). Improving nurse preceptor competence with clinical teaching on a dedicated education unit. *The Journal of Continuing Education in Nursing, 52*(5), 226–231. https://doi.org/10.3928/00220124-20210414-06

Heard, C. (2017). 20,000 hours: Why I precept. *Occupational Therapy Now, 19*(1), 19–20.

Hong, K. J., & Yoon, H. -J. (2021). Effect of nurses' preceptorship experience in educating new graduate nurses and preceptor training courses on clinical teaching behavior. *International Journal of Environmental Research and Public Health, 18*(3), 975. https://doi.org/10.3390/ijerph18030975

Kauffman, K. R., Cline, G. J., & Hays, S. M. (2021). A ladder that matters. *Journal of the American Association of Nurse Practitioners,* Publish Ahead of Print. https://doi.org/10.1097/jxx.0000000000000662

Lafrance, T. (2018). Exploring the intrinsic benefits of nursing preceptorship: A personal perspective. *Nurse Education in Practice, 33,* 1–3. https://doi.org/10.1016/j.nepr.2018.08.018.

Lam, C. K., Schubert, C. F., & Herron, E. K. (2020). Evidence-based practice competence in nursing students preparing to transition to practice. *Worldviews on Evidence-Based Nursing, 17*(6). https://doi.org/10.1111/wvn.12479

Lofgren, M., Dunn, H., Dirks, M., & Reyes, J. (2021). Perspectives, experiences, and opinions precepting advanced practice registered nurse students. *Nursing Outlook, 69*(5), 913–926. https://doi.org/10.1016/j.outlook.2021.03.018

Macey, A., Green, C., & Jarden, R. J. (2021). ICU nurse preceptors' perceptions of benefits, rewards, supports and commitment to the preceptor role: A mixed-methods study. *Nurse Education in Practice, 51,* 102995. https://doi.org/10.1016/j.nepr.2021.102995

Mitchell, M., Leachman, M., & Saenz, M. (2019). State higher education funding cuts have pushed costs to students, worsened inequality. *Center on Budget and Policy Priorities, 24,* 9–15.https://www.cbpp.org/sites/default/files/atoms/files/10-24-19sfp.pdf

Morgan, M., Brewer, M., Buchhalter, F., Collette, C., & Parrott, D. (2018). Sustaining regional preceptor partnerships: Preceptor incentive survey. *The Journal for Nurse Practitioners, 14,* e1–e4. https://doi.org/10.1016/j.nurpra.2017.08.013

National Advisory Council on Nurse Education, & Practice (NACNEP) (2021). *Preparing nurse faculty and addressing the shortage of nurse faculty and clinical preceptors.* https://www.hrsa.gov/sites/default/files/hrsa/advisory-committees/nursing/reports/nacnep-17report-2021.pdf

Office of the Surgeon General (2022). Addressing health worker burnout: The US Surgeon General's advisory on building a thriving health workforce. https://www.hhs.gov/surgeongeneral/priorities/health-worker-burnout/index.html

Onieal, M. E. (2016). Precepting: Holding students and programs accountable. *Clinician Reviews, 26*(7), 11–16.

Renda, S., Fingerhood, M., Kverno, K., Slater, T., Gleason, K., & Goodwin, M. (2022). What motivates our practice colleagues to precept the next generation? *The Journal for Nurse Practitioners, 18*(1), 76–80. https://doi.org/10.1016/j.nurpra.2021.09.008

Roberts, L. R., Champlin, A., Saunders, J. S., Pueschel, R. D., & Huerta, G. M. (2020). Meeting preceptor expectations to facilitate optimal nurse practitioner student clinical rotations. *Journal of the American Association of Nurse Practitioners, 32*(5), 400–407.

Roberts, M. E., Wheeler, K. J., Tyler, D. O., & Padden, D. L. (2017). Precepting nurse practitioner students: A new view—results of two national surveys of nurse practitioner preceptors. *Journal of the American Association of Nurse Practitioners, 29*(8), 484–491. https://doi.org/10.1002/2327-6924.12482

United States Government Accountability Office (2019). Health care workforce: Views on expanding Medicare Graduate Medical Education funding to nurse practitioners and physicians assistants. https://www.gao.gov/products/gao-20-162

Wakefield, M., Williams, D. R., & Le Menestrel, S. (2021). *The future of nursing 2020-2030: Charting a path to achieve health equity*. National Academy of Sciences. https://doi.org/10.17226/25982

Ward, A., & McComb, S. (2017). Precepting: A literature review. *Journal of Professional Nursing*, *33*(5), 314–325. https://doi.org/10.1016/j.profnurs.2017.07.007

Yi, Y. J., Lee, H., & Park, K. (2020). The role of academic-practice partnerships from perspectives of nursing students: A cross -sectional study. *Nurse Education Today*, *89*, 104419. https://doi.org/10.1016/j.nedt.2020.104419

4

Coaching and Mentoring

Nancy M. Albert

CHAPTER OBJECTIVES

- Describe differences between coaching and mentoring roles
- Identify characteristics and behaviors of preceptor coaches and mentors
- Discuss benefits of coaching and mentoring from the learner and leader perspectives
- Explore potential challenges of preceptor coaching and mentoring

The preceptor role spans many work settings or areas including, but not limited to, hospital clinical units, ambulatory care settings, or specialty areas (e.g., quality improvement, infection prevention, employee/occupational health, and research). The preceptor engages with nurses in multiple job functions, including newly hired nurses, advanced practice nurses, and leaders. Being holistically in-tune to the learning needs of the orientee means that the preceptor may also serve as a coach and mentor. Understanding the differences between coaching and mentoring can enhance the precepting process.

COACHING VERSUS MENTORING

Before delving into the unique characteristics of coaching and mentoring, preceptors should understand that each term has a unique definition. "Coaching" is derived from the social sciences. Simply put, it is an experiential process that guides learners toward performance improvement (Landreville et al., 2019). As a process, it is interactive and interpersonal, with a focus on skill acquisition. Coaching offers personal and professional support as the learner acquires knowledge, skills, and

fundamental actions used in clinical practice (Sarroeira et al., 2020). Coaching reflects the *how* and *when* to use a skill and *how to use it most effectively*. It is more than simply giving feedback to improve performance. Coaching involves bi-directional one-on-one conversations between the preceptor/coach and learner that are meant to lead to meaningful feedback and practice suggestions. In addition, coaching should enhance learning and development, increase self-awareness, and strengthen a sense of personal responsibility. To achieve outcomes, the coach questions, listens actively, and provides appropriate challenges in an encouraging climate. Coaching practices can occur in the moment or later and on an ongoing basis (Landreville et al., 2019). The coach–learner dyad involves a one-on-one, nonhierarchical, collaborative relationship, where together they set individualized goals aimed at refining learner skills. The coach is responsible for providing learner-centered, action-oriented, and objective feedback (Toh et al., 2022). As a rule, preceptors who use coaching techniques should not have formal supervisor authority over learners.

When preceptors act as mentors to nurses, they are engaging in *formal* or *informal, general* or *specific,* and *time-limited* or *long-term* learning partnership processes that serve a functional purpose of general or specific career success. The mentoring relationship should be structured and trusting, bringing people together for guidance, support, and encouragement, while developing competence and character. Mentorship processes can be strengthened when the mentee chooses the mentor, but can be successful regardless of the mentee's previous knowledge of the mentor. The preceptor mentor shares in-depth knowledge and nursing expertise and promotes a supportive environment that increases mentee confidence and competency (Yarbrough & Phillips, 2022).

To achieve outcomes, preceptor mentors need to demonstrate behaviors such as emotional intelligence, including sensitivity to cultural and individual differences. Preceptors need to *want* to spend time and energy with the goal of developing, motivating, and encouraging the novice toward a successful personal career path (Ward et al., 2024). Listening to the needs of the novice is important, as the goal is not to provide advice that creates a "mini-me." Mentoring differs from coaching, in that a coach facilitates safe passage of a learner into a new role, whereas a mentor acts as a career guide. The mentoring process explores (but may not facilitate) mentee growth and career development.

BEHAVIORS OF COACHES AND MENTORS

The overarching goal of coaching and mentoring is to provide learners with confidence in developing their own knowledge and skills to grow professionally. Coaches use their technical and interpersonal competence in their clinical field to guide the learner in strategizing processes to build skills. Using a solutions-focused approach, coaches help strengthen the learner's performance and ability to see the "big picture" related to patient outcomes (Table 4.1).

Qualities of exceptional mentors include being available, approachable, supportive, enthusiastic, and encouraging (Cho et al., 2011; Hill et al., 2022). The seasoned mentor provides experience and knowledge, imparts wisdom, guidance, moral support, and encouragement, and facilitates collaborative goal-setting (Hill et al., 2022). Guiding mentees in self-reflection and growth is more important than simply providing advice and challenging decisions and rote thinking. Table 4.2 includes qualities of admired mentors. Behaviors that promote the healthiest mentor-mentee relationships

TABLE 4.1 Learner Needs and Coaching Interventions

Learner Needs	Coaching Interventions
Improve technical skill performance	• Demonstrate with return demonstration • Discuss pertinent policies and procedures • In-person audit and feedback
Improve nontechnical skills • Patient related • Personnel (team) related • Interpersonal	• Train on episodic team processes (admissions, discharges, transfers, shift changes, patient acuity changes, responses to actions) • Discuss alternate methods to achieve goals • Discuss interpersonal skills and their influence on outcomes • Observe collaboration skills
Enhance interpersonal skills	• Observe and discuss empathetic communication skills • Communicate team expectations regarding innovation, change, and clinical excellence
Enhance well-being	• Observe and discuss work time management, schedule planning, and time off • Discuss available resources to reduce stress and burnout and improve resilience to enhance workplace satisfaction • Discuss workplace violence and prevention strategies

are 1) demonstrating active listening, 2) role-modeling professional behavior, 3) asking thought-provoking questions, 4) offering specific and intentional praise and reinforcement, 5) role-playing communication strategies, and 6) providing constructive criticism (Ward et al., 2024).

TABLE 4.2   Attributes of Outstanding Mentors

Qualities	Details
Admirable characteristics of mentors	• Kindness • Justness • Outgoing and interactive personality • Selflessness
Support and guidance of the mentees' career	• Setting high standards and realizing the mentee's potential • Tailoring/individualizing the support provided • Offering numerous opportunities for recognition and promotion • Engaging in concrete activities to foster career development
Strength of time commitment	• Frequent contact with the mentee • Contact viewed as high in quality • Mentors were viewed as available • Mentors provided guidance over long periods (even decades)
Support of personal/professional life balance	• Providing guidance on leading a full, balanced home life • Offering support during times of stress in mentees' lives
Legacy of mentorship	• Providing guidance as mentees move into the mentor role themselves
Use of a narrative science framework in decision-making processes (uses techniques associated with the "art" of science)	• Helping to 1) describe the situation using narrative thinking, 2) provide meaning for clinical impressions using observation and other qualitative techniques, and 3) talk through each decision-making process based on understanding and stories, knowledge and experience

Adapted from Cho, C. S., Ramanan, R. A., & Feldman, M. D. (2011). Defining the ideal qualities of mentorship: A qualitative analysis of the characteristics of outstanding mentors. *The American Journal of Medicine, 124*(5), 453–458; and de Leon J. (2018). Teaching medical students how to think: Narrative, mechanistic and mathematical thinking. *Actas Espanolas De Psiquiatria, 46*(4), 133–145.

In the words of Maya Angelou:

In order to be a mentor, and an effective one, one must care. You must care. You don't have to know how many square miles are in Idaho, you don't need to know the chemical make-up or chemistry of blood or water. Know what you know and care about the person, care about what you know, and care about the person you're sharing with.

BENEFITS OF COACHING AND MENTORING

Coaching provides broad-reaching benefits influencing the individual, the learner, the team, and the institution. Nurses who coach exhibit higher training motivation, self-efficacy, and behavior transfer in multiple nursing skills compared with nurses without coaching skills (Kushnir et al., 2008). In addition, preceptors who coach nurses are less likely to have deterioration in some skills, especially related to medication management and communication (Kushnir et al., 2008). Coaching in clinical settings also benefits others by developing communication skills, promoting a positive workplace culture, facilitating demonstration of competencies that optimize clinical performance, and improving social support and team cohesion (Costeira et al., 2022; Skinner et al., 2022). In addition, the skills learned or honed by nursing peers also enhance positive communication and may promote retention over time. All members of the healthcare team, including coaches and interprofessional team members, benefit when nurses are successfully skilled in problem-solving, decision-making, and optimizing patient care.

In mentorship practices, mentors have an opportunity to positively influence future nurses. Mentors may obtain new or more contemporary insights and perspectives that lead to personal and professional growth (Ward, Love, & Williams, 2024). The mentoring experience creates a break from everyday work life and allows nurses to "pay it forward" or give back to their professional community. Mentors also gain personal benefits such as increasing patience, feeling like a "better" person, and developing new friendships. Mentoring provides a sense of fulfillment and satisfaction. In an integrated review, Kakyo et al. (2022) found other benefits to mentors that included developing and demonstrating leadership, networking with others, and updating knowledge based on self-reflection. Further, mentors believed they had a heightened reputation and influence among colleagues and identified that mentoring had a positive effect on job satisfaction.

CHALLENGES OF COACHING AND MENTORING

Although there are multiple benefits to coaching, there are also challenges. Appropriate teaching methods may vary based on nurses' preferred learning styles. Coaches may not use the best teaching methods to keep learners engaged and focused, especially if they are newer nurses themselves or have poor coaching skills. A facilitative approach encourages deep-level learning. Two methods that faciliate engagement are using vivid examples when presenting material (e.g., case studies) and encouraging learners to ask "what-if" questions that promote development of clinical judgment (Noble, 2009). (Refer to Chapter 8 for additional ways to promote clinical judgment skills). Further, to remain current in evidence-based clinical practices, coaches may need to review and synthesize the literature on key topics. The process of literature review is time-consuming and coaches may not be adequately trained to perform a literature synthesis. Reference librarians and nurse scientists can be instrumental in facilitating efficient literature review.

Common mentoring challenges include: 1) difficulties in aligning schedules for meetings, 2) poor communication, 3) unrealistic or incongruent expectations between mentor and mentee, 4) poor mentorship skills, and 5) breaches in confidentiality that reduce trust in the relationship. Conversations early in the mentoring process clarify roles, goals, and timelines, and lay the groundwork for deeper work and trust-building (Ward et al., 2024). Other challenges are lack of mentoring resources, limited training in the mentoring process, lack of incentives, and inadequate time to accomplish all expected professional responsibilities (Kakyo et al., 2022). Limited organizational support for mentors can have long-term repercussions. Without adequate time for mentoring, a snowball effect may result. For

example, less mentoring leads to decreased professional growth, potentially creating increased nursing turnover (Rohatinsky et al., 2018) and reduction in the nursing workforce. The end result is an adverse effect on patient care.

Ultimately, coaching and mentoring of nurses involves interpersonal relationships that can be a source of challenges. There could be disagreements, arguments, or an unwillingness of coaches or mentors to admit to lack of knowledge about a topic. Further, learners and mentees could be manipulative in an attempt to meet their own needs. There may also be a mismatch in preceptor and learner personality or temperament that could minimize the ability to develop reciprocal relationships (Merga et al., 2020). The coach or mentor needs to be aware of the learner's behaviors and intrinsic/extrinsic motivation and, at the same time, try to foster a trusting, meaningful relationship.

The preceptor has perceived power in the relationship, and thus, must maintain strong ethical standards. For example, a coach or mentor should not take credit for learner work and should not exclude a learner from growth opportunities. The preceptor must remain self-aware in order to clearly recognize and acknowledge the contributions of the learner. Preceptors also need to be aware of personal behaviors and motivations when agreeing to coach or mentor. Professional integrity is essential, especially since the learner may be eager to please and might be unduly influenced by the preceptor. Ultimately, the preceptor has an ethical responsibility to not take advantage of their real (and perceived) power within the relationship. Table 4.3 describes five types of dysfunctional coaches or mentors based on relationships (Green & Jackson, 2014).

PREPARING THE COACH AND MENTOR FOR SUCCESS

In healthcare centers, administrative leadership must support preceptors as coaches and mentors. Preceptors may be willing to volunteer to assume coaching and mentoring roles, but may feel unprepared to take on added responsibilities, especially if they have never received formal training. Nursing professional development staff can provide written or online coaching resources or implement a structured preceptor coach training program with performance feedback. A positive coaching

TABLE 4.3   Five Types of Dysfunctional Coach and Mentor Behaviors

Dysfunctional Behaviors	Coaching Examples	Mentor Examples
Avoider	Coach is not available when critical patient decisions need to be made during hemodynamic compromise.	Mentee contacts the mentor via text for a meeting within the next 2 weeks to provide "news." The mentor fails to respond to the message.
Dumper	Coach identifies the learner needs to become less dependent. Without prior communication, the learner is told to work independently that shift.	The mentee identifies a goal of improving communication with "difficult people." Although having expertise in communication techniques to offset difficult situation, the mentor chooses to not give advice or discuss communication strategies. The mentee is forced into a sink or swim situation.
Blocker	The learner quickly demonstrates proficiency in completing care of four patients on day shift and communicates the desire to be challenged. The coach insists that the learner needs 2 more weeks of similar assignments to reinforce learned skills.	The mentee has been invited to present on a clinical topic at the next shared governance meeting. The mentor feels the mentee is becoming too successful too quickly and contacts the meeting planner to suggest that another presenter be invited to present.
Destroyer/ Criticizer	The learner competently completes simple procedures (IV access and urinary catheter insertion) independently per protocol. The coach hovers and criticizes the learner's performance.	The mentee proficiently meets individualized goals. Rather than acknowledging and affirming, the mentor unnecessarily criticizes the mentee's work outcomes.
Smotherer	The coach repeatedly requires the learner to change the plan of care to match that of the coach, despite the learner exhibiting proficiency in providing care.	The mentor expects the mentee to use the mentor's preferred communication style without allowing the mentee to develop their own comfortable and preferred style.

Adapted from Green, J., & Jackson, D. (2014). Mentoring: Some cautionary notes for the nursing profession. *Contemporary Nurse, 47*(1–2), 79–87.

experience relies on a balance between supportive leadership and engaged learners.

For mentors to succeed in giving career advice, there needs to be a good match between mentor and mentee. Mentors must stay true to their areas of strength and knowledge so that the time spent with mentees is of the greatest value possible. In some situations, mentors with similar expertise may share the work of mentoring to balance workload and provide the mentee with diverse perspectives. Each mentor has their own mentoring style, previous experiences, and knowledge base, which can add depth of learning for the mentee. Similar to coaches, mentors refer learners to appropriate resources outside their areas of expertise. For example, if the mentee asks to learn more about organization leadership, the mentor can provide appropriate resources and facilitate networking with an expert. Table 4.4 presents responsibilities of the mentor at various phases of the mentoring experience.

CONCLUSION

Coaching and mentoring are distinct roles, as their purposes and expected outcomes are unique. Coaches and mentors work in diverse ways to assure that learners are exposed to clinical experiences and knowledge that creates readiness for independent practice or expansion of current practice. Each role has personal and professional benefits and challenges. To better understand the uniqueness of each role and the

TABLE 4.4	Responsibilities of the Mentor at Various Phases of the Experience
Phase	**Responsibilities**
At initiation	• Communicates availability for meetings • Mutually agrees on appropriate meeting interval • Communicates that meeting content is confidential • Facilitates sharing of role, experience, career development, and goals
Early start-up	• Clarifies the needs and expectations of mentees • Uses mentee needs and expectations to guide mentoring • Discusses mentee priorities and focus for career development • Encourages the mentee to use the mentor as a sounding board for ideas or plans
Anytime during the mentoring process	• Makes the time to meet • Seeks understanding without making assumptions • Provides honest and timely feedback • Assesses mentee needs and redirects mentoring as needed • Debriefs regularly • Recognizes own limits, based on areas of expertise • Helps mentees establish new connections/expand their network • Supports in a direct way to minimize mentee's feelings of intimidation, humiliation or embarrassment • Encourages open discussion of failures by mentee to promote growth • Celebrates successes

work involved, it is helpful for coaches and mentors to receive resources and training, especially in relation to fostering interpersonal relationships and providing effective feedback.

REFERENCES

Cho, C. S., Ramanan, R. A., & Feldman, M. D. (2011). Defining the ideal qualities of mentorship: A qualitative analysis of the characteristics of outstanding mentors. *The American Journal of Medicine, 124*(5), 453–458. https://doi.org/10.1016/j.amjmed.2010.12.007

Costeira, C., Dixe, M. A., Querido, A., Vitorino, J., & Laranjeira, C. (2022). Coaching as a model for facilitating the performance, learning, and development of palliative care nurses. *SAGE Open Nursing, 8,* 23779608221113864. https://doi.org/10.1177/23779608221113864

de Leon, J. (2018). Teaching medical students how to think: Narrative, mechanistic and mathematical thinking. *Actas Espanolas De Psiquiatria, 46*(4), 133–145.

Green, J., & Jackson, D. (2014). Mentoring: Some cautionary notes for the nursing profession. *Contemporary Nurse, 47*(1–2), 79–87. https://doi.org/10.1080/10376178.2014.11081909

Hill, S. E. M., Ward, W. L., Seay, A., & Buzenski, J. (2022). The nature and evolution of the mentoring relationship in academic health centers. *Journal of Clinical Psychology in Medical Settings, 29*(3), 557–569. https://doi.org/10.1007/s10880-022-09893-6

Kakyo, T. A., Xiao, L. D., & Chamberlain, D. (2022). Benefits and challenges for hospital nurses engaged in formal mentoring programs: A systematic integrated review. *International Nursing Review, 69*(2), 229–238. https://doi.org/10.1111/inr.12730

Kushnir, T., Ehrenfeld, M., & Shalish, Y. (2008). The effects of a coaching project in nursing on the coaches' training motivation, training outcomes, and job performance: An experimental study. *International Journal of Nursing Studies, 45*(6), 837–845. https://doi.org/10.1016/j.ijnurstu.2006.12.010

Landreville, J., Cheung, W., Frank, J., & Richardson, D. (2019). A definition for coaching in medical education. *Canadian Medical Education Journal, 10*(4), e109–e110. https://doi.org/10.36834/cmej.68713

Merga, M. K., Hays, A. M., & Coventry, T. (2020). Nurse managers' perceptions of barriers to the mentoring of early career nurses. *Mentoring & Tutoring, 28*(1), 60–77. https://doi.org/10.1080/13611267.2020.1737778

Noble, H. (2009). The challenges of setting up a teaching event for health-care staff. *British Journal of Nursing, 18*(6), 374–377. https://doi.org/10.12968/bjon.2009.18.6.40771

Rohatinsky, N., Udod, S., Anonson, J., Rennie, D., & Jenkins, M. (2018). Rural mentorships in health care: Factors influencing their development and sustainability.

The Journal of Continuing Education in Nursing, 49(7), 322–328. https://doi.org/10.3928/00220124-2018 0613-08

Skinner, S. C., Mazza, S., Carty, M. J., Lifante, J. C., & Duclos, A. (2022). Coaching for surgeons: A scoping review of the quantitative evidence. *Annals of Surgery Open, 3*(3), e179. https://doi.org/10.1097/AS9.0000000000000179

Toh, R. Q. E., Koh, K. K., Lua, J. K., Wong, R. S. M., Quah, E. L. Y., Panda, A., Ho, C. Y., Lim, N. A., Ong, Y. T., Chua, K. Z. Y., Ng, V. W. W., Wong, S. L. C. H., Yeo, L. Y. X., See, S. Y., Teo, J. J. Y., Renganathan, Y., Chin, A. M. C., & Krishna, L. K. R. (2022). The role of mentoring, supervision, coaching, teaching and instruction on professional identity formation: A systematic scoping review. *BMC Medical Education, 22*(1), 531. https://doi.org/10.1186/s12909-022-03589-z

Ward, W., Love, J., & Williams, V. (2024). *Mentoring.* https://www.aamc.org/professional-development/affinity-groups/gfa/mentoring

Yarbrough, A., & Phillips, L. K. (2022). Peer mentoring in nursing education: A concept analysis. *Nursing Forum, 57*(6), 1545–1550. https://doi.org/10.1111/nuf.12832

5

Understanding the Learner and the Learning Process

Mary Frances Terhaar

CHAPTER OBJECTIVES

- Describe the learning process and its importance
- Explore special considerations related to learning in a practice setting
- Identify learner characteristics relevant for success
- Discuss characteristics of an effective and supportive learning environment

Every practicing nurse and advanced practice registered nurse (APRN) has had the benefit of learning from remarkable clinical preceptors. These masters left indelible marks on our careers and we owe them a debt of gratitude. They helped us exceed our expectations and, in so doing, helped to move our practice and the profession forward. Similarly, we as preceptors owe future nurses positive, inspirational, and transformative experiences as they progress along their professional journies.

Unfortunately, many of us have also had the experience of learning from nurses who just did not "show up" for us as learners in the way we needed. Perhaps they did not take the responsibility of instruction seriously or did not have a foundation for the important work they were asked to take on. Perhaps they were disrespectful or "ate their young." Preceptors and educators who did a poor job may have been reluctant recruits, may have been overwhelmed, may not have had grounding in learning theory, or may not have had the benefit of good clinical educators and preceptors (role models) themselves.

Preceptors have an effect by helping novices develop a strong foundation to launch their nursing careers. They also rise to the challenge of expanding the nursing workforce and moving the profession ahead. Preceptors are in a position of tremendous significance and influence. They have the potential to transform didactic content covered in the classroom into well understood, contextually situated, critically applied, and memorable clinical learning experiences. Witnessing the learner's application of knowledge in a real-life setting, or that "a-ha" moment, is an exciting outcome for which all educators strive.

This chapter is written to help the preceptor understand the learner and learning environment by setting a solid, theoretically grounded, evidence-based foundation.

THE PROCESS OF LEARNING

There's more to see than can ever be seen
More to do than can ever be done
There's far too much to take in here
More to find than can ever be found
       "The Circle of Life" (John & Rice, 1994)

The wonder and awe expressed in the opening of *The Lion King* parallels the feeling of the learner new to clinical practice. The role of the preceptor is to help the learner make sense of all that they discover during their interactions with those in their care.

Expert clinical preceptors have learned to naturally integrate knowledge of physiology, pathophysiology, human behavior and development, pharmacology, genetics, and public health into their practice. Learners need the expert guidance of the preceptor in translating and applying didactic knowledge. However, few preceptors have had education about the principles of learning essential to their clinical teaching roles. When clinical experts understand principles of learning, they become effective preceptors.

There are several ways of understanding the learning process. Four common theories include: adult learning theory, social learning theory, metacognition, and Socratic inquiry. Whether consciously or unconsciously, educators tend to incorporate theoretical principles of learning, dependent on the situation and the learner. Table 5.1 provides a guide to terminology and principles common to discussion of the learning process.

TABLE 5.1	**Examples of Application of Theoretical Concepts to Preceptor Instruction**	
Framework	**Concept**	**Example of Application**
Socratic inquiry	Elenchus	Preceptor conducts clinical rounds where students present patient conditions, assessments, problems, plans, and proposed metrics for evaluation based on evidence
		Preceptor challenges the plan and the evidence upon which it is based
		Preceptor proposes alternative interventions and seeks rationale for selecting the approach backed by strongest evidence
Pedagogy	Set clear expectations for performance for all learners	Faculty and preceptor articulate clear and measurable learning objectives
		Faculty and preceptor identify key literature to review in preparation for clinical experience
Andragogy	Build on existing knowledge	Preceptor assesses baseline knowledge and experience of each learner
	Learner sets personal goals	Preceptor invites learner to refine expected outcomes in ways that meet their personal developmental goals
Heutagogy	Student-designed learning experiences	Learner sets personal goals and plans assignments to demonstrate mastery; these may include team projects or very individualized efforts
Social learning	Reinforcement	Preceptor observes target behaviors and makes explicit connections to favorable outcomes
	Constructive feedback	Preceptor, especially when new to the role, may find it challenging to provide constructive feedback; they may be more comfortable with positive feedback and may avoid providing correction; working with faculty can help facilitate skills to provide constructive feedback
Metacognition	Reflective practice	Learner integrates content from classroom into clinical learning by reflecting on clinical experiences, their own readiness and accountability, and the outcomes achieved
	Thinking about thinking	Learner reflects on their own learning practices and creates plans to increase their success
	Muddiest points	Learner may struggle with integrating particular content into practice; the preceptor consistently invites the learner to identify knowledge needs and engages in discussion or additional learning experiences to increase comprehension, judgment, discernment, or abilities
	Johari windows	Preceptor invites the learner to reflect on their performance, knowledge, confidence, and clinical practice outcomes in order to help the learner recognize "blind-spots" and focus learning experiences

(Continued)

TABLE 5.1 **Examples of Application of Theoretical Concepts to Preceptor Instruction—Cont'd**

Framework	Concept	Example of Application
Novice to expert	Novice thinking	Preceptor explains the basic rules and guidelines to support safe practice
		Learners develop a practice of seeking reliable information to promote safe practice
	Advanced beginner	Preceptor provides numerous experiences that enable the learner to build a detailed understanding of clinical phenomena across multiple patients
	Competent	Preceptor decreases support and offers consultation to enable the learner to build a detailed understanding of clinical phenomena across multiple patients
	Proficient	Patient assignments enable the learner to increase confidence in their abilities and seek experiences to expand understanding and abilities
	Expert	Expert clinicians who serve as preceptors may have difficulty breaking down their highly integrated understanding of select clinical situations; it is useful to be intentional about providing detailed descriptions of clinical situations including antecedents to events; it is helpful to explain which data were relevant, which were contextual, and which were irrelevant in the particular situation
Synergy	Nurse competencies	Preceptor provides experiences and guidance to assist the nurse in developing competencies related to patient needs
	Systems thinking	Preceptor guides the learner to consider conditions in the practice setting that impact care, the family, the patient, and the outcomes
	Moral agency	Preceptor guides the learner to reflect on their moral responsibility as they provide care to a vulnerable patient
	Advocacy	Preceptor coaches the learner in ways to effectively speak up on behalf of the family and patient to ensure their needs and preferences are made explicit and carefully addressed
	Responsiveness to diversity	Preceptor challenges the student to recognize the contribution of social determinants of health to the condition and needs of the patient and family

Adult Learning Theory

Education has evolved over time from its origin as pedagogy to andragogy and, most recently, to heutagogy. Each of these terms has a Greek word at its root, learning at its center, and has described and expanded our understanding of the learner, instructor, methods, resources, context, and beliefs of those who practice in education. It is worthwhile to understand the distinctions between these terms and the context to which they are best suited.

Pedagogy is the most familiar. Well represented in common language and defined in the Oxford dictionary, pedagogy refers to the conventional approach where the teacher has knowledge and conveys it to the learner.

Sometimes referred to as the "sage on the stage" model, the approach was designed for young learners, who historically played a passive role.

> *Pedagogy: "the method and practice of teaching, especially as an academic subject or theoretical concept." It also connotes "the study of teaching methods."*
>
> *Pedagogue: "a teacher; a person who likes to teach people things, especially because they think they know more than other people."*
>
> https://www.oxfordlearnersdictionaries.com/definition/english/pedagogy?q=pedagogy

Learners were recipients of wisdom shared by teachers who determined the educational goals. Retention and understanding of the content were the focus. Evaluation of learning relied heavily on testing.

Andragogy evolved as educators sought to meet the challenges of teaching adults who approach their education based on experience that is very different from that of young learners. Adult learners are more engaged in their learning. They have high expectations, independent learning goals, and a knowledge base that is more varied. They bring agency to their education, have advanced skills for finding information, and prefer application of learning rather than simply recalling or understanding knowledge (Knowles, 1970).

Heutagogy refers to teaching that promotes both learning and appreciation of each individual's agency in their own learning process. It is a student-centered, self-determined teaching strategy that emphasizes the development of autonomy, capacity, and capability. This approach emphasizes goodness-of-fit between the learning experience and outcomes with expectations relevant to the work environment (PowerSchool, 2022).

Pedagogy emphasizes content, suggests interaction with the learner as one who lacks knowledge, and recognizes the educator as significantly responsible for guiding learning. Andragogy emphasizes process and engagement, suggests interaction with the learner to build on existing knowledge and experience, and positions the educator as a facilitator who shares the responsibility of learning with the learner. Heutagogy emphasizes the student's role as director of learning who is accountable for the outcomes. The student and educator increasingly move the emphasis of learning to outcomes and impact.

Social Learning Theory

Social learning theory (SLT) builds on the concepts of classical and operant conditioning established by behavioral theorists. This theory posits that learning behavior is the product of internal, as well as external, factors and motivations. Learning begins with a *stimulus* that is *mediated* and concludes with learning that is evidenced by behavior change (Bandura & Walters, 1977). Instruction is the mediating process and learning outcomes result in behavioral changes. However, SLT suggests that education is an observational experience controlled by the educator and absorbed by the learner.

Metacognition: Thinking About Thinking

In approaching education, it is useful to pause and consider "how we think" in order to enhance the learning process (Pintrich, 2002). "Thinking about thinking," referred to as metacognition, was originally the focus of studies in children (Baker & Brown, 1984; Flavell, 1985). Later, researchers explored application as a means to increase learning (Hatano & Inagaki, 1986; Bransford et al., 2000). Simply put, if one understands the way one thinks and learns, they can do so more effectively. By extension of this logic, a preceptor who understands metacognition can help a learner develop strategies to optimize their learning. This principle was reflective of Socratic thinking. The idea was to give careful thought to how one thinks, to discipline one's reasoning and logic, and to reflect on one's own performance.

Socratic Inquiry

Socratic inquiry calls for the educator to pose challenges, which invites reflection, self-analysis, clarification, and integration of knowledge and experience. Central to law school and medical school pedagogy, the approach seems to have a goal of finding flaws in logic (Meckstroth, 2015). The approach invites integration and application of evidence to specific patients in their particular context.

In its purest application, Socratic inquiry proceeds in five steps: 1) stimulating wonder, 2) generating a hypothesis, 3) posing the elenchus or challenge, 4) acceptance or rejection of the hypothesis, and 5) taking action (Boghossian, 2012). Commonly practiced with small groups led by an educator, students explore antecedents and consequences, blind spots, motivations, affective responses, decisions, context, and outcomes.

In the Socratic method, the learner is challenged to consider not simply the content to be mastered, but also the approach one takes to achieving mastery. In this paradigm, we want to give careful thought to what works and what does not work for a particular learner, what has been learned, and what knowledge gaps remain. The learner focuses on a particular learning need, prepares thoroughly for a learning experience, utilizes an effective learning approach, and participates in debriefing. Socratic learning is particularly effective when the preceptor and learner interact regularly and consistently and individualize learning needs and goals.

This may all sound a bit esoteric for a clinician who is focused on application and results, rather than abstract learning theory. Thus, it is important to understand how this theoretical background applies to real-world situations.

Application of Socratic Method to Clinical Teaching

The Socratic method has been particularly useful as a means to promote deep learning. Its application to instruction of nurses and APRNs in the clinical setting has been found to contribute to development of clinical judgment. Development of clinical judgment includes purposeful, self-regulatory judgment resulting in evidence-based explanations. Skills such as interpretation, analysis, evaluation, and inference are part of the process (Facione, 2011; Makhene, 2019).

Application of the Socratic method requires a safe learning environment, focus on baseline knowledge (strengths), understanding of the learner's goals, and intention of the educator. Commonly practiced with small groups under safe and respectful conditions, the approach enables everyone to learn and strengthen reasoning skills. The process to consider a clinical problem flows accordingly (Boghossian, 2012):

1. Wonder: Instructor poses a question that targets important learning with the goal of provoking thought. (*What is the pain experience for this person and what do you recommend we do about it?*)
2. Hypothesis: Learner provides an answer to the question that becomes the hypothesis and foundation for further discussion. (*Since pain is whatever the patient says it is and their headache is described as constant, burning, and throbbing, I recommend offering acetaminophen.*)
3. Elenchus: The instructor challenges the hypothesis, and the learner "defends" their position. The challenge encourages the learner to provide a coherent, evidence-based rationale. (*What do you consider to be the cause of the pain? What have you ruled out? What else might be going on? Is there a downside to the action you propose? What does the evidence suggest?*)
4. Acceptance or rejection of the hypothesis: Assessment data and evidence are reviewed, and learners test the goodness of fit between their hypothesis, the examined facts, and the evidence. (*How does that evidence fit this patient in this situation?*)
5. Action: Plan is implemented based on deeper understanding. (*What is necessary to implement this plan? How will we determine if the intervention is effective? What negative outcomes might you anticipate and what would be the next step?*)

Bloom's Taxonomy

In the 1950s, a team of educators developed Bloom's taxonomy for documenting learning goals, which is still relevant today. The taxonomy helps educators to articulate the desired outcome and helps learners to understand what is expected of them and what they can expect from their teachers. Language shifts from a focus on content to a focus on application and integration. It distinguishes between development and demonstration of knowledge. Further, learners build knowledge and skills through comprehension, application, analysis, synthesis, and evaluation (Anderson & Krathwohl, 2001).

According to the taxonomy, one might plan knowledge acquisition and describe it using terms like *select, label, list, identify, define, recite, describe, state, memorize* or *recognize*. These behaviors can be attained, demonstrated, and verified with a focus on knowledge development. Higher-level learning terms include *judge, consider, relate, critique, weigh, recommend, criticize, summarize, support, appraise, evaluate*, and *compare*. To demonstrate these behaviors, knowledge must be applied in combination with clinical judgment and more complex behaviors. That is the beauty and utility of the taxonomy. It helps achieve focus and precision, helps reach agreement on what is to be learned and how learning will be evident, increases student agency in their own success, and helps the preceptor be successful in their efforts.

The taxonomy can be used to help the learner develop specific goals for their experience and help the preceptor tailor experiences and feedback related to learner goals and progress (Figure 5.1).

UNDERSTANDING THE LEARNER

Two frameworks are particularly useful to the clinician seeking to understand the learner and promote their success. These are the Novice to Expert Model (Benner, 1982) and the Synergy Model (American Association of Critical Care Nurses, 1992).

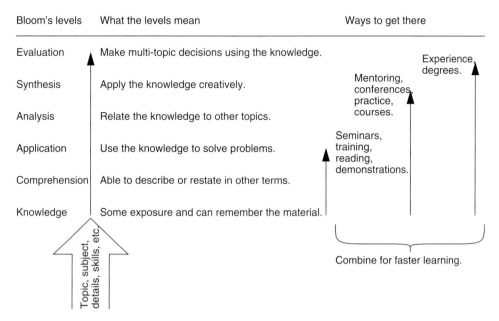

Fig. 5.1 Bloom's taxonomy of learning. (From Jack, H. (2022). People and teams. In Jack, H. (Ed.), *Engineering Design, Planning, and Management* (pp. 149–209). Elsevier Inc.)

Novice to Expert Model

Benner's *Novice to Expert Model* has made a tremendous impact since its introduction (Benner, 1982). The model is broadly adopted and remains relevant today. It describes, explains, and predicts progression of the learner across their career as they develop knowledge, clinical judgment, and capacity for decision-making and informed action. Because of its practicality and clarity, Benner's model is a favorite among clinicians.

The model identifies five levels of development, which move from strict adherence to rules to holistic understanding of phenomena and complex situations. The five levels (Benner, 1982) are described as follows:

- The *novice* nurse possesses basic knowledge but lacks context. Their focus is on specific and measurable aspects of the patient's condition. Because they lack experience, the novice cannot comprehend or process the fullness of patient situations without support and guidance and is unable to anticipate needs and risks.
- The *advanced beginner* nurse slowly develops a fuller understanding of patient conditions, but still cannot fully process the big picture.
- The *competent* nurse, who has been in practice a few years, develops an understanding and appreciation of

their contribution and connection to achievement of patient outcomes and long-term goals. This nurse is aware of plans and able to adapt.
- The *proficient* nurse draws on experience and maxims. They see and comprehend the whole, rely less on rules and more on judgment, and are working to discern components of situations and how those contribute to the big picture and the outcome.
- The *expert* nurse has developed a complex cognitive map that frees them from rules and enables them to reach reliable conclusions and take effective action. They intuitively apply knowledge gained through contextualization, experience, and synthesis. They see the big picture and may even have difficulty deconstructing it into the contributing parts.

Benner's model provides a structure for understanding learner needs, guides the clinician seeking to support learning, and points to helpful educational resources and strategies.

The Synergy Model: Matching Nursing Competency to Patient Needs

The American Association of Critical Care Nurses created a certification process that aligned core

Patient and Family Needs	Competencies of the Nurse	Outcomes
• Resilience • Vulnerability • Stability • Complexity • Predictability • Availability of resources • Participation in care • Participation in decision-making	• Clinical judgment • Clinical inquiry • Collaboration • Systems thinking • Moral agency • Advocacy • Caring practices • Responsiveness to diversity • Facilitation of learning	• Comfort • Healing • Satisfaction • Freedom from complications • Change in function • Change in quality of life • Decreased recidivism • Balanced cost/resource utilization

Fig. 5.2 **Synergy Model components.** (Adapted from Curley, M. (1998). Patient-nurse synergy: Optimizing patients' outcomes. *American Journal of Critical Care, 7*(1), 64–72.)

competencies of nurses with the central needs of patients (Hardin & Kaplow, 2017). The Synergy Model identifies a set of eight patient and family needs and relates those to the competencies of the nurse. It asserts that intentional alignment of patient and family needs generates favorable outcomes. All needs, competencies, and outcomes are presented in Figure 5.2.

Designed to provide a framework to promote ethical practice in challenging critical care settings, this model can help preceptors to understand the goal of their educational efforts. The focus is to develop the nurses' knowledge, abilities, and competencies in alignment with the needs of select patients and families to achieve the best possible outcomes.

THE LEARNING ENVIRONMENT

The learning environment can be understood as having three dimensions: physical, pedagogical, and psychosocial (Closs et al., 2021). The classroom or clinical setting is the *physical dimension* in which learning takes place. Lighting, sound, furniture, tools, and technologies are all considered elements of the physical dimension. Preceptors are the gatekeepers who guide the learner to master the physical space and the learning objectives simultaneously. The *pedagogical dimension* includes the activities, methods, strategies,

and experiences provided while facilitating learning. Preceptors facilitate learner access to assessments, procedures, interventions, and many other kinds of clinical activities. The *psychosocial dimension* comprises the relational and interpersonal role mastery aspects of the learning environment. For this dimension, the preceptor provides the learner with access to caregiving interactions and collaborative activities with other nurses and healthcare professionals (Closs et al., 2021).

The clinical environment presents challenges, which can create feelings of stress and anxiety in the novice. Prebriefing and debriefing, as described here, can help the learner reduce stress, improve learning, and increase the quality of patient care (Brennan, 2021).

Outcomes of instruction can be enhanced by providing challenging yet supportive conditions in the learning environment. Features of a supportive environment include demonstration of respect for the learner, establishment of trust, and recognition of the learners' abilities and experiences. Learners are more likely to take risks and share their vulnerabilities when they perceive the environment as safe and supportive.

The same interpersonal skills that serve nurses well in their interactions with colleagues and patients will be effective in interactions with students and orientees. These skills include maintaining perspective, sharing a good sense of humor, and practicing mindfulness.

BEST PRACTICES OF PRECEPTORS ACROSS CLINICAL SETTINGS

The best learning happens when it is planned, individualized, and supported. Several practices are particularly effective, including prebriefing and debriefing, which are introduced as components of simulation instruction and well worth adapting to clinical instruction. *Prebriefing* occurs in advance of a simulation or clinical experience and helps the learner prepare for and perform effectively in a target situation (Loice et al., 2020). Preceptors may provide focused readings, review patient cases, prepare plans of care, and discuss possible complications and procedures. The goal is to ensure the learner is well prepared for a challenge. Prebriefing enables the learner to consider:

- types of information needed,
- what to assess,
- what to ask,
- findings of a developing problem,
- potential adverse outcomes,
- signs of patient decompensation,
- data reflecting health promotion and disease prevention, and
- additional resources needed.

Debriefing refers to a reflective conversation following a caregiving interaction or collaborative activity. The goal is to take time to reflect on previous patient encounters in a safe environment, to be responsible for caregiving interactions, and to learn from every experience. Several questions can be posed to learners:

- How did you understand the situation?
- Did you see what you needed to see?
- Did you prioritize and act effectively?
- What went well?
- What could have gone better?
- What could you do to be better prepared next time?

Prebriefing and debriefing help learners develop self-awareness and become accountable professionals. Researchers have observed that people do not always know themselves well and may not see themselves as others do. Lack of awareness may be equated with having "blind spots" (Luft & Ingham, 1955). The Johari window model (Figure 5.3) reflects various stages of self-awareness. The four quadrants in the model reflect aspects of an individual's personal and public self-awareness. Acknowledgment of these aspects can be considered

to individualize experiences in support of growth and progress toward learning goals.

The four quadrants of the Johari window provide perspective on how aspects of the learner's awareness interact and influence their strengths and weaknesses. Some aspects present overtly, while others are covert. Some aspects maybe beneficial for preceptors to know to support the learner, while others simply need to be recognized by the learner for self-monitoring. The *open area or arena* reflects interaction of awareness known to self and known to others, and can be useful in goal-setting between the learner and preceptor. The *blind spot* represents that which is known to others but not known to self. In this case, the preceptor may need to overtly call the learner's attention to areas of weaknesses so that the learner can take initiative in strengthening their skills and abilities. The *unknown* quadrant reflects what is not known to others but known to self. In this case, it is up to the leaner to share their needs with the preceptor to set realistic goals. The preceptor can help the student disclose weaknesses by asking the student, "Is there anything I need to know about you to help you learn best and meet your goals?" The *hidden area* or *façade* reflects information that is not known to others and not known to self. Both the learner and preceptor may become aware of the learner's weaknesses during the clinical experience. It is up to the learner or the preceptor, whomever becomes aware first, to identify and name the areas of weakness and discuss goals toward resolution.

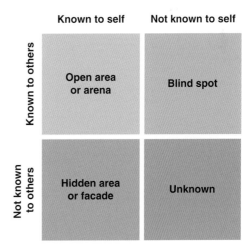

Fig. 5.3 The Johari window model. (From Luft, J. & Ingham, H. (1955). *The Johari window: A graphic model for interpersonal relations.* University of California, Western Training Lab.)

CONCLUSION

Throughout this chapter, multiple learning theories have been presented with the goal of providing an easy and practical foundation for precepting. Preceptors can apply a diverse set of theories and strategies to support learners in their practice setting. The respective strategies will stimulate learning and promote deep understanding and lasting impact on the learner, the care they provide, and the progression of their career. Table 5.1 presents key concepts from many of these theories, along with best practices that can be adopted by preceptors.

REFERENCES

Anderson, L.W., & Krathwohl, D. (Eds.). (2001). *A taxonomy for learning, teaching, and assessing: A revision of Bloom's Taxonomy of Educational Objectives: Abridged* (1st ed). Longman.

Bandura, A., & Walters, R. H. (1977). *Social Learning Theory* (Volume 1). Prentice Hall.

Benner, P. (1982). From novice to expert. *American Journal of Nursing, 82*(3), 402–407. https://doi.org/10.2307/3462928

Boghossian, P. (2012). Socratic pedagogy: Perplexity, humiliation, shame and a broken egg. *Educational Philosophy and Theory, 44*(7), 710–720. https://doi.org/10.1111/j.1469-5812.2011.00773.x

Bransford, J. D., Brown, A. L., & Cocking, R. R. (2000). *How people learn: Brain, mind, experience, and school* (Expanded edition). National Academies Press.

Closs, L., Mahat, M., & Imms, W. (2021). Learning environments' influence on students' learning experience in an Australian faculty of business and economics. *Learning Environment Research, 25*(1), 271–285. https://doi.org/10.1007/s10984-021-09361-2

Facione, P. A. (2011). Critical thinking: What it is and why it counts. *Insight Assessment, 2007*(1), 1–23.

Hardin, S.R., & Kaplow, R. (2017). Synergy for clinical excellence: The AACN Synergy Model for patient care (2nd ed.). Jones & Bartlett Learning.

John, E., & Rice, T. (1994). The Circle of Life [Song]: *On The Lion King: Original Motion Picture Soundtrack.* Walt Disney Entertainment.

Knowles, M. (1970). Andragogy: Adult learning theory in perspective. *Community College Review, 5*(3), 9–20. https://doi.org/10.1177/009155217800500302

Luft, J., & Ingham, H. (1955). *The Johari window: A graphic model for interpersonal relations.* Western Training Lab: University of California.

Makhene, A. (2019). The use of the Socratic inquiry to facilitate critical thinking in nursing education. *Health SA Gesondheid, 24.* https://doi.org/10.4102/hsag.v24i0.1224

Meckstroth, C. (2015). The Socratic Elenchus. *The Struggle for Democracy,* 61–79. https://doi.org/10.1093/acprof:oso/9780190213923.003.0004

PowerSchool. (2022). Heutagogy explained: Self-determined learning in education. Retrieved from: https://www.powerschool.com/blog/heutagogy-explained-self-determined-learning-in-education/

6

Fostering Effective Preceptor-Learner Communication

Cynthia A. Danford

CHAPTER OBJECTIVES

- Describe how social and communication styles can influence preceptor-learner interaction
- Differentiate between four learning styles and related communication techniques

- Describe versatility and its connection with social styles and learning
- Identify generational differences in communication

Effective communication is foundational not only for therapeutic nurse-patient interaction but also for productive preceptor-learner interaction. Diversity in the healthcare workforce adds to the importance of attention to communication style and approach. Data reported from the National Nursing Workforce Study revealed the average age of registered nurses was 52 years in 2020, with 19% of registered nurses age 65 and older (Smiley et al., 2021). This means that preceptors may be verbally communicating with individuals, whether patients or learners, from up to six or seven different generations (the Greatest Generation through Gen Alpha) on any given day. Diverse representation by race, ethnicity, gender, and educational degree further adds to the complexity of communication. Coupled with verbal communication, attention to preceptor-learner social styles is also needed. During the learning relationship, communication and social style blend together to ultimately achieve effective interactions. Flexibility in both communication and social style is required depending on the situation and the individuals involved.

SOCIAL STYLE AS IT INFLUENCES INTERACTIONS

"Social style" refers to observable behaviors through words and actions that present during interactions

and communication with other individuals (Merrill & Reid, 1981). Social style may also be referred to as an "approach." Effective interactions and communication are dependent on how behavioral patterns present, how behaviors are described and perceived, and how behaviors are accommodated. There is no right or wrong way to interact and there is no single style or approach that an individual uses all the time. However, being aware of one's own social style and the social style of others in any given situation can facilitate effective interactions.

Behaviors may be perceived internally by an individual in one way and at the same time interpreted externally by another individual in a completely different way, leading to miscommunication (Hamstra & Blakeslee, 2020). Pausing to reflect on this conundrum can lead the individual to awareness that a change in social style or communication approach may be needed. As an example, a preceptor may perceive their own approach with new nursing students as kind and nurturing, using questioning to guide and facilitate student learning. Some students may observe similar qualities and be comfortable in approaching the preceptor, whereas other students may perceive the questioning as intimidating and fear approaching the preceptor. Such understanding can help the preceptor use different approaches with different students, as the behavior they internally intended may not be the behavior externally perceived.

"Social style" is a theoretical model created by Merrill & Reid (1981), two psychologists who posited that everyone has natural behaviors and preferred styles of communication. This influential model has been used for over 40 years in many organizations to facilitate healthy and effective interactions and relationships. Social style is based on the perception of an individual's behavior by others (Merrill & Reid, 1981; Wilson, 2004). The purpose of the model is to provide a framework to help preceptors understand themselves and others in order to improve communication and avoid misunderstandings (Figure 6.1).

Two behavioral tendencies, assertiveness and responsiveness, intersect to result in four social styles: analytical, driver, expressive, and amiable. Social styles further influence communication techniques or approaches. *Social skill* and *communication* are not discrete, but are used fluidly based on the situation. Individuals may have a tendency to use one style more strongly than another, but most individuals modify their approaches based on circumstances and responses from others.

Four social styles result from the intersection of two behavioral tendencies or continuums: assertiveness and

responsiveness (Merrill & Reid, 1981; Wilson, 2004). How individuals influence the thoughts and actions of others is referred to as "assertiveness." The degree of assertiveness used by individuals can range from an "ask" to a "tell" perspective. Individuals using *ask-directed assertiveness* employ a calm, questioning, process-oriented approach. They are deliberate and methodical in their actions, incorporating a soft tone and slower pace, pausing often to allow for thoughtful interaction without interrupting. Ask-directive assertiveness is useful when preceptors are engaging learners in clinical judgment, often in a controlled situation. Verbal and nonverbal cues may be subtle or indirect as the preceptor guides the learner through a process, especially when collaborating to complete nursing actions while simultaneously addressing rationale. Learners benefit from an ask-directed approach when applying new didactic concepts within the clinical setting. The undergraduate student learning to administer medications or prepare for a procedure, such as urinary catheterization, or the graduate student working to enhance their ability to elicit a focused history and physical examination, are able to embrace new skills when involved actively and

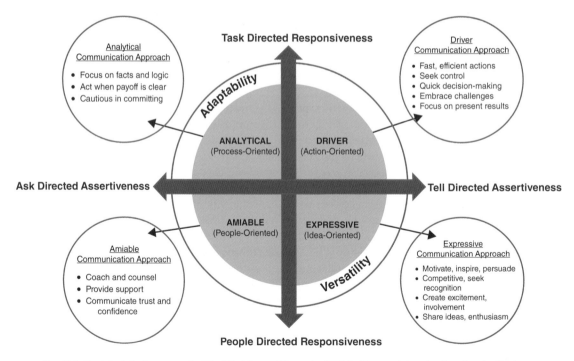

Fig. 6.1 Social style framework. (Modified from Wilson, L. (2004). *The social styles handbook: Find your comfort zone and make people feel comfortable with you.* Nova Vista Publishing.)

constructively. Individuals using *tell-directed assertiveness* employ statements and are focused on results. They are quick to initiate and respond, are emphatic, and often interrupt. Verbal and nonverbal cues are direct, forthright, and move the plan forward. Tell-directed assertiveness is useful when preceptors need to act and make decisions quickly in a less-controlled situation, yet want learners to absorb and embrace the process and relevant concepts. The preceptor managing a rapidly changing patient condition, such as deterioration in respiratory status, will be telling the learner what to do to help versus asking what needs to be done.

Responsiveness refers to the degree to which feelings are expressed during communication and is independent of assertiveness (Merrill & Reid, 1981; Wilson, 2004). Responsiveness ranges from task-directed to people-directed. *Task-directed responsiveness* occurs when the individual is focused on the task or relevant facts without consideration of the people involved. Personal feelings are concealed and the approach may be perceived as reserved or aloof. The individual embracing *people-directed responsiveness* tends to be relationship-focused and may be overtly expressive and empathetic. The belief is that engaging and understanding relationships can contribute to effective completion of tasks. People-directed responsiveness fits well in nursing, as understanding the patient and developing a therapeutic relationship leads to effective completion of tasks as simple as helping a patient with morning care. When precepting, attention to the learner's state of mind can facilitate effective outcomes. The preceptor who recognizes that a learner is fearful of completing a task or engaging with a patient can help the learner modify their approach. In other cases, the preceptor may need to direct the learner to completing a concrete task, such as charting in a timely manner.

The intersection of assertiveness and responsiveness results in four quadrants, reflecting the four learning styles: analytical, driver, expressive, and amiable (Merrill & Reid, 1981; Wilson, 2004). As with assertiveness and responsiveness, social styles are not exclusive. All individuals can exhibit various social styles dependent on changes in situations and their state of mind. Recognizing one's own social style and modifying it based on other's social style and the situational context is a productive approach leading to effective interaction and outcomes. Reflecting on two questions helps to determine one's tendency toward their own social style and that of others: *Does the individual focus more on*

tasks or people? Does the individual ask more questions or tell others what to do? (Wilson, 2004; Woodford, 2023).

Individuals using an *analytical* social style tend to be serious, systematic, and exact in their actions, with an emphasis on facts and logic. Accuracy and attention to how a problem is solved are key foci. With a *driver* social style, individuals tend to be strong-willed, controlling, efficient, and focused on results. Making quick decisions and emphasis on the solution to the problem are of central interest for the driver. Those with *expressive* social styles tend to be outgoing, motivational, and are focused on inspiring and involving others. They are energizing and interested in others who have found solutions to problems. Individuals with *amiable* social styles tend to be confident, supportive, cooperative, and easy-going. They prefer coaching and counseling and often question why a solution is best (Merrill & Reid, 1981; Wilson, 2004).

As a reminder, social styles are not exclusive. One style is not better than another, right or wrong, more or less successful, or better suited for a certain position, such as leadership or preceptorship. Social style qualities vary and can contribute to the type of approach used by the preceptor with the learner (Table 6.1). Additionally, there is no correlation between social style and personality (Wilson, 2004). Assigning one social style to an individual or expecting an individual to behave in one particular manner is not productive. The ability to modify social style depending on the individuals involved and the situation is what contributes to best practice and performance.

When considering social style, it is most beneficial to:
1. Attempt to understand other individual's social style and alter *your own behavior;*
2. Try to adjust your assertiveness and responsiveness behaviors; and
3. Evaluate whether adjustments in your modified behavior or approach have the intended effect. If not, readjust and modify your behavior further.

VERSATILITY

Versatility or adaptability is foundational to the type of social skill used. The ability to modify or adapt social style is learned over time, dependent on previous experiences, and integral to effective interaction and communication (Merrill & Reid, 1981; Wilson, 2004). When precepting, the nurse is exposed to many types of learners, some of whom present unique challenges (see Chapter 17). The learner may be perceived by the

TABLE 6.1 **Social Style Qualities**				
	Analytical	**Driver**	**Expressive**	**Amiable**
Primary attributes	Systematic	Controlling	Energizing	Supporting
Personal approach	Respecting	Controlling	Recognizing	Approving
Preceptor teaching approach	Describing	Responding	Collaborating	Processing
Problem-solving perspective	*How* the problem is solved	*What* the solution will do	*Who* else has used the solution	*Why* the solution is best
Preferred rationale for decisions	Evidence and service	Options and probabilities	Testimony and incentives	Assurances and guarantees
Protective mechanisms	Avoiding	Autocratic	Attacking	Acquiescing

Modified from Wilson, L. (2004). *The social styles handbook: Find your comfort zone and make people feel comfortable with you.* Nova Vista Publishing; and Woodford, C. (2023). *Understanding social style: What they are and why they matter.* http://www. chasewoodford.com/blog/understanding-social-styles/

preceptor as overconfident, shy or reserved, or a know-it-all. Such perceptions can affect relationships, interactions, and communication adversely and may be due to differences between the preceptor's and learner's social style. Recognizing differences and embracing versatility by adapting one's own social style is a useful way to decrease tension or stress resulting from the adversity. Conversely, the preceptor and learner who easily develop a strong relationship resulting in effective and productive interactions may have a similar social style. Essentially, understanding differences in social style and being open to adapting social style to the learner and various situations increases comfort and receptivity in preceptor-learner interactions and facilitates reaching learner objectives. Creating an effective, interactive preceptor-learner relationship contributes to the quality of the learning environment and is foundational to learning (Tuomikoski et al., 2020). In addition to productive interactions, versatility also contributes to effective communication. Versatility is easy to comprehend but it is not easy to apply in actual situations. It takes conscious awareness of variations in social style and communication between oneself and others, as well as time and practice to actively incorporate needed modifications into interactions.

COMMUNICATION INFLUENCED BY SOCIAL STYLE

Social style influences our interactions, which are inclusive of communication. As a component of

preceptor-learner interaction, communication before, during, and after patient and family encounters contributes to successful outcomes. In the case of a disconnect, the preceptor-learner dyad will benefit from determining if social style and communication need to be addressed and how to bridge any identified gaps (Venter, 2017). Direct communication can help novices reflect on their performance, vent frustrations, and consider alternative actions (Shellenbarger & Robb, 2016). For preceptors, reflecting on their own social and communication style is a good beginning point for resolving conflict.

Clear communication can bridge gaps between the preceptor and learner. Communication is described as a balance between content and connection (Hamstra & Blakeslee, 2020). The content needs to be delivered in a clear and concise manner, balanced with a helpful connection, relationship, or social style between the contributor and recipient. Related to content, the preceptor can clarify what skills the learner possesses through discussion and observation and the learner can share what skills they hope to develop and learn in a particular setting. Ongoing bidirectional feedback sets the stage for effective future experiences (Tuomikoski et al., 2020). This includes review of the learner's positive experiences and areas needing further growth, as well as optimal ways the preceptor can support and coach the learner. Ways to direct communication with learners involves encouraging intellectual curiosity through questioning, discussing how to integrate evidence into practice, and analyzing treatment and management decisions (Box 6.1).

BOX 6.1 Communication That Facilitates Learning

- Let's discuss this more...
- Help me to understand...
- Tell me more about *why* you think that?
- Can you expand on that thought?
- Did you consider or rule out anything else?
- Specifically, you did a good job of _____ and this is why it is important...
- You did well based on your knowledge of _____, now how can you include _____?
- I disagree with _____. A more efficient way is _____.
- A different way to look at _____ may be _____.
- The key point that I want you to remember is _____.
- What did we learn from this?

Communication comes in three main forms: verbal, nonverbal, and written. During face-to-face interactions, a balance between nonverbal and verbal communication is needed to offset inconsistent or contradictory interpretations. During in-person communication, the verbal message can be clarified or misconstrued if the nonverbal is misinterpreted. Through their pioneering research, Mehrabian and Ferris (1967) explained that the listener gains 7% of meaning from words spoken verbally, 38% of meaning by how the words are spoken, and 55% of meaning nonverbally, such as through facial expressions. Since the most influential communication is nonverbal, attention to style is essential. With extensive cell phone use and texting, generations are moving into the workforce with expertise in brief, written

---

Exemplar: Avoiding Communication Misunderstandings

Rosie Zeno

Early in my experience as a preceptor, I worked with a student who challenged me to improve my communication skills. I was practicing in a primary care clinic in an urban area with a high patient volume. Before the student's first clinical day, we met to discuss our expectations and educational objectives for the semester. I was impressed with her enthusiasm and learned that she completed one previous clinical rotation in a rural setting that operated at a slower pace with a lower patient volume. We agreed that she would shadow me for the first 2–3 days to orient and acclimate to the flow of the clinical practice. Unfortunately, I became increasingly irritated throughout our first clinical day because the student asked *so* many questions. She would talk to me when I needed to focus, ask me questions while I entered orders, and interject comments while I spoke with families. I appreciated her engagement and enthusiasm in the learning process, but, nonetheless, it felt intrusive. I tried, unsuccessfully, to deter conversation during these times with indirect statements that I assumed would be readily understood by the student. For example, when she continued talking to me and asking questions while I entered orders, I finished what I was working on and said, "I'm sorry. I was trying to concentrate on the order entries. What was your question?"

I took time to reflect before our next shift together and realized I had made assumptions contributing to my frustration. At the start of our second clinical day, I discussed with the student that a fast-paced clinic creates a challenging learning environment. I wanted to encourage her to continue asking great questions, yet I reminded her

that the situation does not always allow for questioning in the moment. I explained, for example, that I sometimes need to focus on what I am doing to avoid making an error. I told her that when I am entering patient orders or in the middle of explaining key issues with a patient and family, it will help if she saves her questions for when I finish. She responded by saying, "This makes complete sense," and said lightheartedly, "Kind of like a no-distraction zone!" I reassured her that I would set aside time for discussion and follow up on her questions each day. From that day forward, the student took the initiative to write down all her questions in a small notebook for discussion when the time was appropriate. Instead of simply telling her what not to do or what I wanted her to stop doing, I was able to better clarify my expectations without diminishing her enthusiasm for learning. My key takeaways from this experience were:

- Do not assume that students will understand the social norms you have come to expect in the professional clinical setting. People interpret social behavior and communication differently, so it is essential to be explicit about your expectations.
- Pause to objectively reflect on how you might have contributed to the concerning dynamic, then attempt to view it from the student's perspective.
- Be willing to adjust your communication approach to achieve the desired results. Preceptors can model meaningful professional attributes by demonstrating a willingness to be vulnerable and engage in open and direct communication.

communication, yet have discomfort with face-to-face communication (McCoy, n.d.). Preceptors need to be attentive to communication approaches used by learners and include effective communication as a learning objective when necessary. Nuances such as eye contact when speaking, posture, head nods, and tone of voice can have a significant influence on patient–nurse/provider relationships and may need to be practiced by the learner (Vogel et al., 2018). Although inconclusive, the use of computers and interference with eye contact has been related to decreased attention to patient concerns, less information sharing, and less awareness of patient emotional responses (Crampton et al., 2016; Meltzer et al., 2022). With digital technology, artificial intelligence, and machine learning on the rise as the preferred mechanism to communicate more than face-to-face encounters, nursing preceptors are on the forefront of helping learners maintain effective communication and interactions with patients and families (Box 6.2).

While being attentive to nurse-patient communication, preceptors and learners also need to be "present" to one another without distraction to facilitate good and effective listening. Listening has been identified as key for interpersonal and business success and is an essential component of effective communication (Altman, 2023). Awareness of social style and communication, being open to adapting to various situations, and *being present* will contribute to an effective precepting experience. In other words, "where you are, be there" (Ramsey, n.d.).

While reflecting on communication and social style, generational differences also need to be given consideration (Table 6.2). Bi-directional in nature, the effect of generational variations can lead to gaps in communication and misunderstandings. Generational differences may be part of why interactions are successful or not successful, and awareness may inform approaches to modify communication (Venter, 2017). Differences can be overcome with understanding and practice. Preceptors are encouraged to respond thoughtfully to learners and clarify any questions or concerns regardless of age.

FUTURE ADVANCES IN COMMUNICATION THAT INTEGRATE TECHNOLOGY

Technology is evolving quickly and may require attention from preceptors to facilitate interactions with learners. Growing advances in healthcare technology

---

BOX 6.2 Etiquette When Using Technology During Healthcare Interactions

Patients or healthcare provider or peer engagement
- Remember that the patient, provider, peer, or colleague is *physically in your presence*.
- Acknowledge those present at the beginning of an interaction and throughout by using eye contact when speaking.
- Avoid "hiding" behind the computer screen or keeping your head down in a smart phone or tablet.
- Talk to the patient or individual when searching the web or engaging with digital technology; inform the patient or individual on what is being searched, found, or documented to help them feel respected.
- Avoid texting or talking on the phone when physically interacting with others.

Documented messages
- Stay focused on the topic and main point.
- Avoid using all capital or all lower case letters. For emphasis, use bullet points or highlight.
- Add an appropriate subject in the subject line of emails.
- Use caution when using abbreviations or acronyms to minimize confusion.

Technology logistics
- Set up and test video conferencing ahead of the time; test internet connection, webcam, chat software, and volume.
- Check the environment to verify the area visible is professional in appearance.

Data from Kumar, M. S., Krishnamurthy, S., Dhruve, N., Somashekar, B., & Gowda, M. R. (2020). Telepsychiatry netiquette: Connect, communicate and consult. *Indian Journal of Psychological Medicine, 42*(5 Suppl), 22S–26 S; McCoy, W. (n.d.). Cell phones and social skills. *CHRON.* https://smallbusiness.chron.com/cellphones-social-skills-28929.html.

---

include: brain–computer interfaces facilitating communication without keyboards, mice, or touchscreens; apps for screening disease in various populations; and artificial intelligence for processing orders and evaluating patterns in symptoms, laboratory data, and clinical decision (Bresnick, 2018). Technological advances, including in-depth digital information and patient care algorithms, will require preceptors to modify their approach to clinical education.

In the future, preceptors may be expected to teach learners about the nuances of how technology is utilized within various clinical settings. The greater challenge

TABLE 6.2	**Generational Variations in Workplace Communication**			
	Baby Boomers	**Generation X**	**Millennials**	**Generation Z**
Age	55–73 years (1946–1964)	39–54 years (1965–1979)	23–38 years (1980–2000)	≤22 years (Born after 2000)
Technology	• Digital immigrants • Embracing digital technology: smart phones and social media • Adjusting to working remotely but want to maintain face-to-face communication	• Digital immigrants • Comfortable using technology in the workplace • Want technology that supports professional development	• Digital natives • Technology influences where they decide to work • Want mobile technology to facilitate collaboration and teamwork • Leaders in embracing cloud-based technology	• Digital natives • Have never known a world without technology • Prefer use of their own devices and expect seamless use of apps in the workplace
Values	• Respect • Tradition	• Shared responsibility • Partners to provide, help and support • Often provide emotional and financial support to others	• Self-expression • Having their opinion represented	• Direct and fun communication • Prefer brief, succinct, exact communication (sound bites)
Tips for communication	• Respect is key • Respect life experiences • Respect opinions	• First, offer help versus asking for help • Remove pressures, if possible	• Include their opinion • Value their ideas • Include in problem-solving and brainstorming	• Get to the point • Use preferred communication method • Short, "bite-size," interesting information • Avoid lectures
Work expectations	• Strict, stable, and centralized hierarchies • Loyalty, respect, and obedience	• Leadership, management roles important • Likely to stay at their company longer and take on heavier workloads • Prefer coaching from outside consultant	• Frequently shifting jobs and careers • Expectations often tentative and flexible • Loyalty and obedience contingent on continued support • Emphasis on mental health more than previous generations	• Expect communication to be instantaneous and tech-enabled • View flexibility and frequent career shifts as the norm

Data from Sevitz, E. (2022, February 12). How to improve communication across generations at work. Office by Eptura. https://www.iofficecorp.com/blog/improve-communication-workplace; Van Edwards, V. (n.d.). *Social skills: How to communicate with people from different generations.* Science of People. https://www.scienceofpeople.com/communication-generations/

may be verifying clinical judgment and decision-making. Although technology will provide many answers, it does not replace the ability to understand and apply concepts in real-world situations with patients and families. Digital technology may provide easy access to information; however, the application of the knowledge must be individualized to meet the specific needs of the patient and family. Challenging learners to think beyond the guidelines and algorithms and embrace a holistic perspective on patient and family needs will lead to consistent and safe care with effective outcomes. Thinking outside of algorithms or "outside of the box" involves intellectual curiosity. Not only does it enhance learning and facilitate communication (Hole, 2020), but it brings an individualized human element to care, which is innate to nursing and beyond the rote qualities of technology. Intellectual curiosity is the driver to deep understanding (Hole, 2020). Without intellectual curiosity, knowledge becomes superficial, articulation of rationale and justification of actions and interactions is minimized, communication becomes clouded, individual nuances may be missed, and patient care may become unsafe. New and innovative solutions in healthcare will continue as technological advances become increasingly sophisticated. Preceptors, learners, and all nurses are responsible for maintaining a deep human connection with patients and families through clear verbal, nonverbal, and written communication.

REFERENCES

Altman, L. (2023). *Being fully present to others*. Intentional Communication Consultants. https://intentionalcommunication.com/giving-our-presence/

Bresnick, J. (2018, April 30). *Top 12 ways artificial intelligence will impact healthcare*. Xtelligent Healthcare Media. https://healthitanalytics.com/news/top-12-ways-artificial-intelligence-will-impact-healthcare

Crampton, N. H., Reis, S., & Shachak, A. (2016). Computers in the clinical encounter: A scoping review and thematic analysis. *Journal of the American Medical Informatics Association*, 23(3), 654–665. https://doi.org/10.1093/jamia/ocv178

Hamstra, C., & Blakeslee, J. (2020). Communicating effectively: Balancing content and connection In A. J. Viera & R. Kramer (Eds.), *Management and Leadership Skills for Medical Faculty and Healthcare Executives* (pp. 13–21). Springer. https://doi.org/10.1007/978-3-030-45425-8_2

Hole, G.A. (2020, August 15). *Intellectual curiosity is the key for successful development and lifelong learning*. https://www.linkedin.com/pulse/intellectual-curiosity-key-successful-development-hole-ph-d-mba

Kumar, M. S., Krishnamurthy, S., Dhruve, N., Somashekar, B., & Gowda, M. R. (2020). Telepsychiatry netiquette: Connect, communicate and consult. *Indian Journal of Psychological Medicine*, 42(5 Suppl), 22S–26S. https://doi.org/10.1177/0253717620958170

McCoy, W. (n.d.). Cell phones and social skills. *CHRON*. https://smallbusiness.chron.com/cellphones-social-skills-28929.html

Mehrabian, A., & Ferris, S. R. (1967). Inference of attitudes from nonverbal communication in two channels. *Journal of Consulting Psychology*, 31(3), 248. https://doi.org/10.1037/h0024648

Meltzer, E. C., Vorseth, K. S., Croghan, I. T., Chang, Y. H. H., Mead-Harvey, C., Johnston, L. A., Strader, R. D., Yost, K. J., Marks, L. A., & Poole, K. G. (2022). Use of the electronic health record during clinical encounters: An experience survey. *The Annals of Family Medicine*, 20(4), 312–318. https://doi.org/10.1370/afm.2826

Merrill, D. W., & Reid, R. H. (1981). *Personal styles & effective performance*. CRC Press.

Ramsey, B. (n.d.). *Seize the moment with key people*. Bob Ramsey. https://bobramseyseminars.com/2011/01/14/seize-the-moment-with-key-people/

Sevitz, E. (2022, February 12). How to improve communication across generations at work. Office by Eptura. https://www.iofficecorp.com/blog/improve-communication-workplace

Shellenbarger, T., & Robb, M. (2016). Effective mentoring in the clinical setting. *AJN The American Journal of Nursing*, 116(4), 64–68. https://doi.org/10.1097/01.NAJ.0000482149.37081.61

Smiley, R. A., Ruttinger, C., Oliveira, C. M., Hudson, L. R., Allgeyer, R., Reneau, K. A., Silvestre, J. H., & Alexander, M. (2021). The 2020 national nursing workforce survey. *Journal of Nursing Regulation*, 12(1), S1–S96. https://doi.org/10.1016/S2155-8256(21)00027-2

Tuomikoski, A. M., Ruotsalainen, H., Mikkonen, K., & Kääriäinen, M. (2020). Nurses' experiences of their competence at mentoring nursing students during clinical practice: A systematic review of qualitative studies. *Nurse Education Today*, 85, 104258. https://doi.org/10.1016/j.nedt.2019.104258

Van Edwards, V. (n.d.). *Social skills: How to communicate with people from different generations*. Science of People. https://www.scienceofpeople.com/communication-generations/

Venter, E. (2017). Bridging the communication gap between Generation Y and the Baby Boomer generation. *International Journal of Adolescence and Youth*, 22(4), 497–507. https://doi.org/10.1080/02673843.2016.1267022

Vogel, D., Meyer, M., & Harendza, S. (2018). Verbal and non-verbal communication skills including empathy during history taking of undergraduate medical students. *BMC Medical Education*, 18(1), 1–7. https://doi.org/10.1186/s12909-018-1260-9

Wilson, L. (2004). *The social styles handbook: Find your comfort zone and make people feel comfortable with you*. Nova Vista Publishing.

Woodford, C. (2023). Understanding social style: What they are and why they matter. http://www.chasewoodford.com/blog/understanding-social-styles/

7

The Learning Curve: A Parallel Venture for Preceptors and Learners

Cynthia A. Danford

CHAPTER OBJECTIVES

- Describe clinical reasoning as it relates to nursing practice
- Discuss the simultaneous effect the learning curve can have on the preceptor and learner
- Identify stages of skill acquisition as they relate to preceptor and learner progress
- Incorporate principles of experiential learning when precepting learners

LEARNING IN NURSING

Learning is a lifelong endeavor for professional nurses that ensures safe patient care and effective outcomes. Learning needs are influenced by changes in technology and advances in science incorporating evidence-based practices. Learning in nursing involves more than memorizing principles from the biopsychosocial sciences (e.g., anatomy, physiology, psychology, sociology) and their relevance to patient care. Application of principles is emphasized in educational programs and is an early step in developing nursing skill, yet there is more to the process of nurses advancing in their respective roles. A nurse who excels in their role learns the art of effective clinical reasoning. Additionally, the intricacies of learning needs change with variations in patient populations, settings, and acuities, as well as during transitions. A learning continuum is ongoing and may present as a vacillating experiential curve faced by both the preceptor and learner.

CLINICAL REASONING

When caring for patients, nurses incorporate reason while assessing and understanding changes in patient conditions (Benner, 2004). With experience, nurses develop clinical reasoning by incorporating intellect and perception to determine what science is relevant to apply to each patient situation. Knowledge, judgment, and intuition blend, resulting in a holistic approach to patient care. This has been referred to as the *logic of reasoning in translation* (Benner, 1994). Nurses assess for changes in patient status ranging from improvement to deterioration. Assessment may occur in acute care settings where changes are subtle or dramatic or in primary care settings, where more nuanced changes require preventive measures or radical changes require referral to acute care settings. The key is identifying trends in symptoms or patient conditions (Benner, 2004). Trends need to be considered in context, where the patient's personal and family life, as well as their general environment, are considered.

Understanding the depth of learning can be articulated to some extent and varies depending on experience. The knowledge and evidence that each individual nurse, whether an experienced practitioner or novice student, acquires is often driven by the role they are in or the role they are pursuing. The depth of learning subsequently advances with incorporation of clinical reasoning.

INTRODUCING THE LEARNING CURVE

Clinical reasoning as an abstract component of learning is different than the concrete acquisition of skills and competencies. Clinical reasoning involves a fusion of skill, judgment, and wisdom—or, in some cases, intuition—which is cultivated with experience (Benner, 2004). The challenge presents in determining how clinical reasoning can be taught and how this type of learning is leveled based on the learner's present knowledge and experience. This can be especially difficult when a novice preceptor is assigned to precept a novice nurse. The novice preceptor may be threatened by the inquiring questions of the novice nurse. While navigating learning and skill acquisition, the novice nurse may rely heavily on their previous experiences and exhibit rigidity to change. The novice nurse tends to be dependent on rules and guidelines and has difficulty integrating individual variations or synthesizing exceptions to the norm. The novice preceptor needs to understand that the novice nurse is not challenging or evaluating, but trying to learn and maintain a degree of comfort or confidence in an unfamiliar setting. Both nurses, as novice preceptor and novice nurse, are simultaneously experiencing a learning curve. When the curve is steep, the individual is challenged, leaving them vulnerable, insecure, and sometimes questioning their abilities. With time and experience, the curve plateaus and the individual becomes more comfortable with their abilities and contributions. Identifying where the learner *thinks* they are on the learning curve in parallel with the preceptor's learning will help provide more effective precepting experiences.

SKILL ACQUISITION AND THE LEARNING CURVE

The Dreyfus skills acquisition model (Benner, 2004; Dreyfus & Dreyfus, 1980) gives perspective on the role-transition path that all nurses and preceptors have experienced and sometimes still experience. The model does not represent professional career development, but focuses on specific skill and competency development that occurs within a profession. Specifically, the path does not culminate with a final endpoint or career achievement. Even for the expert, the path continues as the nurse encounters new challenges and experiences. The model depicts developmental levels of acquiring

skills and competencies and can be applied in many situations and across many disciplines inside and outside of healthcare. Five developmental stages are included: novice, advanced beginner, competent, proficient, and expert. The *novice* is learning basic, fundamental skills and specific rules. They tend to adhere to the rules with little deviation and tend to be inflexible in making judgments. The *advanced beginner* is learning to make connections between rules and factual knowledge in an environmental context. Although growing in knowledge, they have not developed the ability to prioritize effectively and tend to treat all situations with equal importance. The *competent* individual selectively applies rules and principles dependent on the situation through active reasoning and takes responsibility for the approach and outcomes. With further experience, the individual described as *proficient* recognizes problems and effortlessly implements problem-solving, blending concrete reasoning and abstract intuition. Although usually effective, their approach is not always effective and intermittent errors may result. The *expert* easily identifies needs and intuitively takes action by tailoring their approach. The problem-solving abilities of the expert almost always lead to effective resolution with few, if any, inaccuracies (CABEM Technologies, 2021). In the end, mastery is a product of commitment and experience, combined with embodiment of skills and knowledge (Brykczynski, 2009).

Recognition of the level of skill development is helpful in maintaining a realistic perspective of one's progress and the progress of others, increasing awareness of limitations or *what one knows and does not know* and minimizing imposter syndrome (see Chapter 18). Through self-reflection, the learner can have opposing thoughts about their skills and abilities, often in the same day. In one instance, they may think, "I am doing well and really excelling." Later, they may have an experience that leads to them to reflect, "I thought I was doing well, but I still have so much more to learn." Skill acquisition, learning, and development of clinical expertise does not occur on a straight or smooth trajectory. For new learners and new nurses, the learning curve generally proceeds on an upward path with checks, pauses, and regrouping along the way. Nurses transitioning to a new clinical setting or advancing their education may experience great vacillations in learning when they move from a state of being proficient or an expert back to a novice state. The vacillations in learning continue as they gradually build new expertise. All nurses, as learners and preceptors, can find themselves somewhere on the skill acquisition trajectory (Figure 7.1). Even as they practice in their area of expertise, nurses learning the role of preceptor may find themselves at a novice or advanced beginner level.

The path to proficiency or becoming an expert is not cleanly linear, but involves accelerations and decelerations, as well as peaks and valleys (Benner, 1984; Benner et al., 2009; Dreyfus & Dreyfus, 1986). During any role transition, acknowledgment of individual learning needs of both the learner and the preceptor will facilitate optimal planning. A visualization of the learning trajectory is provided by Brykczynski (2009) in the application of the Dreyfus skills acquisition model to the development of advanced practice registered nurses (APRNs) (Figure 7.2).

In Figure 7.2, advanced practice nursing (APN) students begin graduate school as proficient or expert nurses (1a) or as competent RNs with limited practice experience (1b). Depending on previous experience, the new APN student returns to a novice or advanced

beginner level (2). Direct-entry APN students with no experience begin role transition as novices. Upon graduation, the APN student may reach the competent level, but has no experience practicing as a licensed APN (3). Progress plateaus as the graduate searches for a position and attains certification (4). Once employed, the new APN returns to an advanced beginner level (5) while learning a new system and perspective. As the new APN acclimates to the new site, they rebuild to a level of competence (6), where they may plateau or experience an erratic, unpredictable path to the proficient level (7). The expert level is achieved with time and experience (8) (Brykczynski, 2009).

EXPERIENTIAL LEARNING

Preceptors guide experiential learning in the clinical site, where the learner becomes integrally involved in specific experiences. Experiential learning involves integrating theoretical concepts into actual practice with the learner actively engaged at all stages (Murray, 2018). Learning can

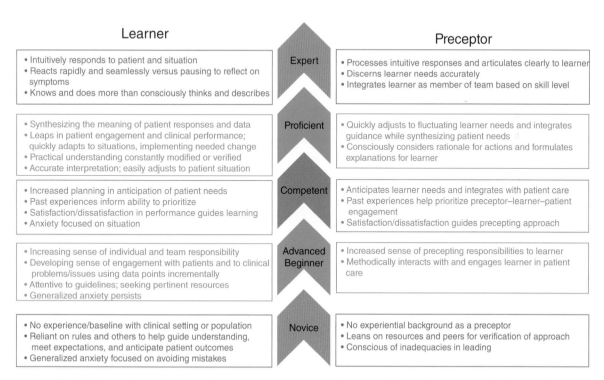

Fig. 7.1 The novice to expert trajectory for preceptors and learners. (Created from content by: Benner, P. (2004). Using the Dreyfus model of skill acquisition to describe and interpret skill acquisition and clinical judgment in nursing practice and education. *Bulletin of Science, Technology & Society, 24*(3), 188–199.)

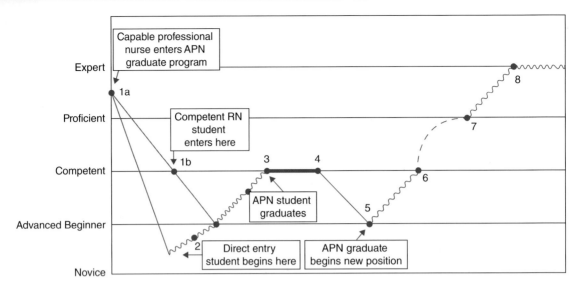

Fig. 7.2 Dreyfus skills acquisition model applied to advanced practice registered nurses. APN, advanced practice nurse; RN, registered nurse. (From Hamric AB, Spross JA, Hanson CM. *Advanced nursing practice: An integrative approach.* 6th edition. 2018. Elsevier.)

be described as a cyclic process where knowledge develops through the transformation of experience. Knowledge and skills are developed and strengthened when applied through practical, hands-on experiences, thereby creating a foundation for problem-solving. Kolb identified four stages of experiential learning: two stages reflect "grasping" experiences (concrete experience and abstract conceptualization); and two stages reflect "transforming" experiences (active experimentation and reflective observation) (Cherry, 2022) (Figure 7.3). Concrete experience involves learning through active involvement. The learner must be open to new experiences and perspectives and learn in part through feelings or awareness of emotions. During phases of reflective observation, learning occurs by observing, listening, and reflecting on the experience. Reflection allows for evaluation and consideration of different perspectives on the experiential outcomes (Murray, 2018). Abstract conceptualization occurs when the learner uses reason to systematically combine new ideas and concepts to apply in future encounters. Active experimentation occurs when learners test new knowledge and ideas further in clinical practice, which are further influenced by other extraneous factors (Kolb, 1984). Throughout the learning process, new information is actively gathered with each experience and transformed or processed to inform the next experience. The cyclic nature of experiential learning results in added

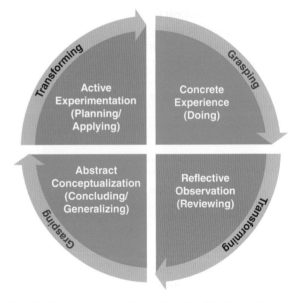

Fig. 7.3 Kolb experiential learning. (Modified from McLeod, S. (2017). *Kolb's learning styles and experiential learning cycle.* SimplyPsychology. https://www.simplypsychology.org/learning-kolb.html; Informed by Cherry, K. (2022). *The experiential learning theory of David Kolb.* https://www.verywellmind.com/experiential-learning-2795154; and Konak, A., Clark, T. K., & Nasereddin, M. (2014). Using Kolb's experiential learning cycle to improve student learning in virtual computer laboratories. *Computers & Education, 72*, 11–22.)

depth as similar or new experiences with variations in the situation present for the learner. Appropriate for nursing, Kolb describes how learning is holistically influenced by environmental or situational factors, as well as emotion and cognition, all blended within an experience (Cherry, 2022).

Awareness of the stages of experiential learning provides a modifiable framework for preceptors as they guide learners on the novice-to-expert continuum. Some learners may require repetition of similar experiences, whereas other learners may require added time for reflection and synthesis of content before advancing in ability. The learning process will vary with each learner and situation. Experiential learning coupled with conscious engagement leads to a productive and valuable learning experience for both the learner and preceptor.

EXPERIENTIAL LEARNING APPLIED WITH THE APRN STUDENT

An APRN student with expertise as a school nurse begins her first clinical experience in a primary care pediatric clinic. The APRN student identifies that she is most confident working with school-age children. On the third clinical day, the preceptor informs the APRN student that they will conduct a patient encounter together with a toddler and accompanying parent.

The concrete experience includes the APRN student gathering the patient history, and observing the preceptor augment the history and conduct a physical examination. Reflective observation occurs when the preceptor and student reflect on the process and the student expresses feelings about her interactions with the toddler. Abstract conceptualization results when the APRN student identifies better ways to approach toddlers based on her observations and knowledge of developmental expectations. Active experimentation occurs when the APRN student applies a modified approach with the next toddler and parent encounter. The preceptor can guide active experimentation by asking the APRN student to discuss their modified approach before the actual patient encounter.

EXPERIENTIAL LEARNING WITH THE UNDERGRADUATE NURSING STUDENT

An undergraduate student in their final year of nursing school began their first clinical rotation in a transition course. The nursing student identified that he is confident in caring for one or two patients at one time but has never managed more.

A concrete experience occurred when the nursing student shadowed the preceptor, observing how the preceptor balanced care for six patients. At the end of the day, the preceptor engaged the student in reflective observation by asking the student what he learned and how he felt about caring for several patients during a shift. Abstract observation resulted when the student identified ways he could balance a heavier patient load. Active experimentation occurred when the nursing student applied his modified approach in managing three patients. The process continued under the guidance of the preceptor, with the student building his skills to efficiently care for four or five patients by the end of the clinical experience.

LEARNING TO LEAD

Although the learning curve is filled with peaks, valleys, and plateaus for all who are seeking a new role, learning to lead has added layers that need consideration. To strengthen the workforce, a leader needs to be available and visible to pave the way. Principles of leadership may be taught in a classroom setting; however, knowledge of such principles alone do not make a leader. Nursing leaders often learn essential components of leadership while working daily in the healthcare environment. Learning to precept is no exception. Social interaction combined with engagement in the practice setting are key to actualizing leadership potential (Nilsson & Furåker, 2012; Van Dam & Ford, 2019).

Similar to Kolb's theory of experiential learning, leadership learning involves reflection. In their work with nursing leaders, Van Dam and Ford (2019) determined that learning to lead involves social interaction within the context of the healthcare setting. Self-awareness was identified as a thread increasing throughout the leadership learning process. Their model includes four steps: 1) reflecting, 2) discovering, 3) deciding, and 4) choosing (Figure 7.4). The tipping point is the crossroad where the leader decides whether or not to make changes in their behavior that would strengthen their leadership abilities. For example, the decision to be more vocal or conversational contributes to building an assertive approach. Thinking of the preceptor as a leader, these steps can be applied to the nurse building their proficiency as an effective preceptor.

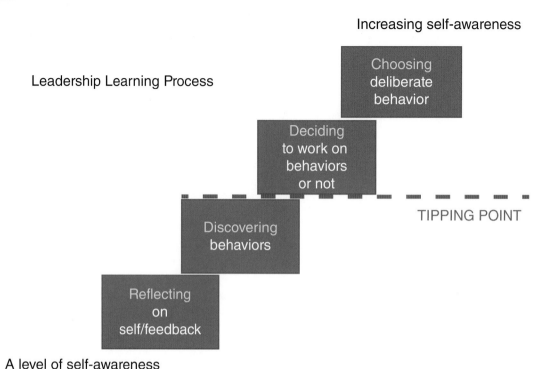

Increasing self-awareness

Leadership Learning Process

Choosing deliberate behavior

Deciding to work on behaviors or not

TIPPING POINT

Discovering behaviors

Reflecting on self/feedback

A level of self-awareness

Fig. 7.4 **Leadership learning process.** (From Van Dam P. J., & Ford K. M. (2019). Nursing leadership learning in practice: A four-stage learning process. *International Archives of Nursing and Health Care 5*:132.)

In consideration of the interactive relationship between the learner and preceptor, especially a novice preceptor, the zone of proximal development provides valuable insight (Smith & Sweet, 2019). The zone of proximal development (Vygotsky, 1978) allows for differentiation of what can be self-learned, for instance, by the novice; and what is learned with the help of someone experienced, such as the preceptor. The model can be applied to the novice preceptor who seeks help from experienced preceptors or even the student learner's faculty. Seeking help from those with experience is especially relevant given that age and degree of experience have been identified as contributing factors influencing preceptors' confidence, ability, and comfort in guiding the novice nurse (Chang et al., 2013).

Nurse preceptors can expect to experience a learning curve when precepting students, novice nurses, or nurses transitioning to a new setting. The degree of the learning curve will be dependent on the individual level of healthcare experience. Preceptors are not expected to navigate their learning curve in isolation, but are encouraged to reach out to others for support and assistance at any time throughout the precepting experience. Social interaction and reflection between the learner and preceptor will create a strong, effective precepting experience.

REFERENCES

Benner, P. (1984). *From novice to expert: Excellence and power in clinical nursing practice.* Menlo Park, CA: Addison-Wesley.

Benner, P. (1994). The role of articulation in understanding practice and experience as sources of knowledge in clinical nursing In J. Tully (Ed.), *Philosophy in an age of pluralism: The philosophy of Charles Taylor in question* (pp. 136–155). Cambridge University Press.

Benner, P. (2004). Using the Dreyfus model of skill acquisition to describe and interpret skill acquisition and clinical judgment in nursing practice and education. *Bulletin of Science, Technology & Society, 24*(3), 188–199. https://doi.org/10.1177/0270467604265061

Benner, P., Tanner, C., & Chesla, C. (2009). *Expertise in nursing practice: Caring, clinical judgment, and ethics.* Springer.

Brykczynski, K. A. (2009). Role development of the advanced practice nurse In A. B. Hamric, J. A. Spross, & C. M. Hanson (Eds.), *Advanced practice nursing: An integrative approach* (pp. 95–120). Saunders Elsevier.

CABEM Technologies. (2021). *Dreyfus model of skill acquisition*. CABEM Technologies, LLC. https://www.cabem.com/dreyfus-model-of-skill-acquisition/

Chang, A., Douglas, M., Breen-Reid, K., Gueorguieva, V., & Fleming-Carroll, B. (2013). Preceptors' perceptions of their role in a pediatric acute care setting. *Journal of Continuing Education in Nursing*, 44, 211–217. https://doi.org/10.3928/00220124-20130315-81

Cherry, K. (2022). *The experiential learning theory of David Kolb*. https://www.verywellmind.com/experiential-learning-2795154

Kolb, D. A. (1984). *Experiential learning: Experience as the source of learning and development*. Prentice-Hall.

Konak, A., Clark, T. K., & Nasereddin, M. (2014). Using Kolb's experiential learning cycle to improve student learning in virtual computer laboratories. *Computers & Education*, 72, 11–22. https://doi.org/10.1016/j.compedu.2013.10.013

McLeod, S. (2017). *Kolb's learning styles and experiential learning cycle*. SimplyPsychology. https://www.simplypsychology.org/learning-kolb.html

Murray, R. (2018). An overview of experiential learning in nursing education. *Advances in Social Sciences Research Journal*, 5(1). https://doi.org/10.14738/assrj.51.4102

Nilsson, K., & Furåker, C. (2012). Learning leadership through practice–healthcare managers' experience. *Leadership in Health Services*, 25(2), 106–122. https://doi.org/10.1108/17511871211221037

Smith, J. H., & Sweet, L. (2019). Becoming a nurse preceptor: The challenges and rewards of novice registered nurses in high acuity hospital environments. *Nurse Education in Practice*, 36, 101–107. https://doi.org/10.1016/j.nepr.2019.03.001

Van Dam, P. J., & Ford, K. M. (2019). Nursing leadership learning in practice: A four stage learning process. *International Archives of Nursing and Health Care*, 5(3), 1–8. https://doi.org/10.23937/2469-5823/1510132

Vygotsky, L. (1978). Interaction between learning and development: *Mind and Society* (pp. 79–91). Harvard University Press.

8

Special Precepting Tools for Clinical Judgment

Heather L. Bartlett and Anne Marie Michon

CHAPTER OBJECTIVES

- Enhance the clinical nurse preceptor's ability to develop clinical judgment skills in the advanced practice registered nurse (APRN) student or learner
- Utilize reflective journaling as a tool to deconstruct a particular clinical situation and aid in evaluation of the clinical judgment process the student uses during a patient encounter

- Apply the One-Minute Preceptor (OMP) tool to probe and guide student reasoning skills
- Implement the SNAPPS model to guide students/learners in efficiently presenting clinical cases

Nurses develop clinical judgment skills in their undergraduate educational programs and utilize them throughout their clinical practice. Registered nurses (RNs) and advanced practice registered nurses (APRNs) who are preceptors take these skills to a new level. One of the most challenging aspects of precepting all learners is encouraging clinical judgment and developing a process for assessment and treatment planning for each patient and family. This chapter will focus on tools utilized in the clinical environment by both the preceptor and the learner to guide clinical judgment skills.

Clinical judgment is one of the most essential skills utilized by both RNs and their APRN counterparts. Development of these skills is necessary for all learners, including pre-licensure nursing students or orientees new to a specific clinical setting. Clinical teaching integrates three key learning domains that involve clinical judgment skills: 1) clinical knowledge and skills, 2) professionalism, and 3) communication (Burgess et al., 2020). Consequently, the preceptor's role includes nurturing and developing the learner's ability to think critically and exercise good clinical judgment (Seibert, 2020).

clinical judgment in nursing is a purposeful self-regulatory judgment associated with clinical decision-making, diagnostic reasoning, the nursing process, clinical judgment, and problem-solving. The result is safe, competent clinical practice (Turner, 2005). Clinical judgment in education and clinical practice involves analysis, explanation, inference, interpretation, knowledge, open-mindedness, reflection, and synthesis (Turner, 2005), all of which must be taught, reinforced, and role-modeled.

On one of my assigned days to precept, my clinic schedule included a 12-year-old female who, due to the COVID-19 pandemic, missed her wellness exam the previous year. The nurse practitioner (NP) student with whom I was working was in their first clinical rotation. Prior to the visit, we discussed what immunizations were to be given. After completing the visit, the NP student returned to discuss the case with me. She was clearly upset and stated the parent became angry that she discussed the human papillomavirus (HPV) vaccine in front of her child. The parent stated there was "no way that my daughter will receive that shot today." The student tried to explain to the mother what the rationale was for the immunization at this age. However, the patient's mother stopped the student from further discussion. The NP student complied and completed the physical exam before reporting to me.

When we sat down to discuss this case, I explained to the student that she encountered a mother who was vaccine hesitant. As a NP student, it can feel intimidating when encountering a caregiver hesitant to immunize their child. Before finishing the visit with the student, I gathered HPV vaccine information sheets. The student and I planned to ask the mother if she would be open to discussing this information in a room separate from her daughter.

The mother agreed to discuss the vaccine and followed us into a consultation room. I asked the mother if she was willing to share her reasoning for not wanting her daughter to have information about HPV nor receive the vaccine. She simply stated it was because it was a "sex virus," and her daughter did not need this right now. We discussed the benefits and risks of the HPV vaccine in more detail. I then asked her to review the written materials and reconsider the vaccine in the future. I also suggested that we include her daughter in a future discussion so that an informed and shared decision could be made.

Later, I explained to the student that when encountering vaccine hesitant caregivers, it is best to listen with empathy. Caregivers deserve the chance to express their reasoning for declining immunizations. As a preceptor, it is important to model shared decision-making when discussing whether or not to immunize. My best advice is to give information in an unbiased manner and respect the parent's decision regarding their child. As an experienced advanced practice nurse, I have learned to sometimes employ the concept of agreeing to disagree.

Educators and preceptors are challenged to adapt teaching strategies to promote clinical judgment and foster perseverance (Seibert, 2020). The need for flexibility in clinical judgment intensifies depending on local, national, and international clinical situations. For example, the recent COVID-19 pandemic presented as a global challenge where rapidly changing patient conditions and evolving evidence-based treatments created a dynamic environment that demanded clinical judgment. The clinical preceptor has an integral role in encouraging the learner to persist when confronted with difficulties or even perceived failure. Nurses who develop perseverance will have an ongoing motivation to learn throughout their careers (Seibert, 2020).

TOOLS AND STRATEGIES FOR DEVELOPING CLINICAL JUDGMENT

There are quick, easy-to-use tools for the development of clinical judgment that can be utilized by the learner in many different learning environments. These tools can be adapted for many types of learners, such as undergraduate nursing students, graduate students, and those who are transitioning to a new clinical area.

Reflective Journaling

Reflective journaling is a structured way for the learner to reflect on a patient situation and debrief. Using a written tool to "deconstruct" a patient care moment facilitates evaluation of the thinking process used at the time. Reflective thinking and journaling help learners to review clinical situations and infer what was learned (Raterink, 2016). The learner writes a one-page journal entry about a specific clinical experience. They review how they applied clinical judgment skills or habits to the clinical situation. The learner reflects on their initial actions and thoughts, and then focuses on enhancing their clinical judgment skills to improve clinical decision-making. The expectation is that the learner will reflect on what they have journaled and learn from their own experience as well as from feedback by the preceptor or faculty.

Reflective journaling may be used as an adjunct or alternative to writing subjective, objective, assessment, planning (SOAP) notes. When learners are unable to document in the electronic health record (EHR) because of program or institutional barriers, journaling about the patient encounter can be a meaningful assignment (Box 8.1). Feedback can be objectively provided using

---

BOX 8.1   Steps to Writing a One-Page Reflective Journal Entry

1. **Identify** clinical scenario/patient problem/interaction for reflection as it relates to the nurse's or advanced practice nurse's role
2. **Analyze** the actions of the clinical scenario, how it relates to the relevant nurse's role, and its significance to the role
3. **Reflect** on actions for similar situations in order to demonstrate clinical judgment habits

---

a journal rubric. Reflective journaling also allows for ongoing self-evaluation and critique of clinical performance (Wedgeworth et al., 2017).

For additional information, see Appendix H: Examples of Reflective Journaling, and Appendix I: Example of Journaling Rubric.

THE SNAPPS MODEL

The SNAPPS model is a learning tool that fosters collaborative learning between the APRN student and clinical preceptor (Wolpaw et al., 2003). This mnemonic describes an efficient way for the student to present patient cases and discuss clinical reasoning. The SNAPPS model condenses the reporting of facts while encouraging clinical reasoning. Presenting a case using the steps of SNAPPS enables the process of deductive reasoning and self-directed learning (Jain, 2019). The SNAPPS model is learner-led and ultimately can create a bi-directional interactive clinical learning environment. This method can encourage continued interest in self-directed learning.

Step 1: **S**ummarize the history and physical exam findings briefly

Step 2: **N**arrow the differential diagnoses

Step 3: **A**nalyze the differential diagnoses

Step 4: **P**robe the clinical instructor with questions and express case uncertainties (The learner is responsible to lead this discussion)

Step 5: **P**lan management for patient case (The learner initiates the plan)

Step 6: **S**elect a case-related issue for self-directed learning

THE ONE-MINUTE PRECEPTOR

The One-Minute Preceptor (OMP) is an evidence-based, time-efficient, learner-centered teaching approach

(Gatewood & De Gagne, 2019). The OMP is composed of two phases. The "inquiry phase" allows the preceptor to probe the learner's understanding of the case using open-ended questions. The "discussion phase" gives the preceptor the opportunity to make a targeted teaching point and provide positive, corrective feedback. The OMP consists of five micro-skills for probing and guiding student reasoning. See Appendix J for One-Minute Preceptor Exemplars. The five micro-skills are as follows:

- **Prompt** the learner to verbalize and commit to a diagnosis. *(What do you think is going on? What do you do next?)* This encourages the learner to process the experiences and problem solve.
- **Probe** for underlying reasoning and supporting evidence for the learner's assessment. *(What are major findings that lead you to that conclusion? Why would you choose that treatment?)*
- **Teach** general rules at the level of the learner's understanding. Discuss common findings and general rules associated with the patient's issue. *(When this happens, do this…)*
- **Provide** positive feedback. *(You did an excellent job of _____.)*
- **Correct** errors. Provide the learner an opportunity to critique their performance. *(Do you feel you addressed the patient/family's questions?)* Provide constructive feedback. *(Next time this happens, try ___.)*

ENHANCING CLINICAL KNOWLEDGE AND SKILLS

Decision-making increases in complexity as the nurse transitions into a new setting or an advanced practice role. To be effective, the preceptor needs to guide clinical judgment parallel to the learner's current level of experience. Asking the learner stimulating questions promotes in-depth learning, sound decision-making, and effective provision of evidence-based care (Box 8.2).

CONCLUSION

Clinical faculty rely on the preceptor's ability to teach clinical judgment skills in real time with real patients. Often, the preceptor has progressed to the point that these skills become innate and automatic. Clinical teaching requires that preceptors think consciously about their decision-making and articulate their thought process to the learner.

BOX 8.2 Questions to Stimulate Clinical Judgment in APRN Students

Formulating the diagnosis and treatment plan:
- What are the presenting symptoms?
- What do you need to know *now* in order to know what to do next?
- What assessment strategies must you use?
- What do you know from the patient's history? What is missing?
- What do the physical exam findings mean? What is abnormal? What is normal?
- What are the differential diagnoses?
- What further diagnostic information is needed?
- Can you make a diagnosis now?
- What is the most appropriate treatment?
- How will you evaluate treatment?

Medications:
- What is the evidence for the best choice in medication?
- What are the dosing parameters?

- What do you need to know about medication dosing and side effects?
- What do you need to teach the patient about medication dosing and side effects?

Procedures (either diagnostic or treatment):
- What has already been done? What were the results?
- What is the evidence for suggesting this as the most appropriate procedure?
- What do you need to teach the patient regarding the procedure?
- Do you have the necessary skills and equipment to perform this procedure now?
- To whom should you refer the patient?
- Who is the best consultant to involve in this patient's plan of care and treatment?
- What information does the patient need to schedule an outside procedure?

REFERENCES

Burgess, A., van Diggele, C., Roberts, C., & Mellis, C. (2020). Key tips for teaching in the clinical setting. *BMC Medical Education, 20*(S2), 463. https://doi.org/10.1186/s12909-020-02283-2

Gatewood, E., & De Gagne, J. C. (2019). The One-Minute Preceptor model. *Journal of the American Association of Nurse Practitioners, 31*(1), 46–57. https://doi.org/10.1097/jxx.0000000000000099

Jain, V., Rao, S., & Jinadani, M. (2019). Effectiveness of SNAPPS for improving clinical reasoning in postgraduates: Randomized controlled trial. *BMC Medical Education, 19*(1). https://doi.org/10.1186/s12909-019-1670-3

Raterink, G. (2016). Reflective journaling for critical thinking development in advanced practice registered nurse students. *Journal of Nursing Education, 55*(2), 101–104. https://doi.org/10.3928/01484834-20160114-08

Seibert, S. A. (2020). Problem-based learning: A strategy to foster generation Z's critical thinking and perseverance. *Teaching and Learning in Nursing, 16*(1), 85–88. https://doi.org/10.1016/j.teln.2020.09.002

Turner, P. (2005). Critical thinking in nursing education and practice as defined in the literature. *Nursing Education Perspectives, 5*(26), 272–277.

Wedgeworth, M. L., Carter, S. C., & Ford, C. D. (2017). Clinical faculty preceptors and mental health reflections: Learning through journaling. *The Journal for Nurse Practitioners, 13*(6), 411–417. https://doi.org/10.1016/j.nurpra.2017.01.011

Wolpaw, T., Wolpaw, D., & Papp, K. (2003). SNAPPS: A learner centered model for outpatient education. *Academic Medicine, 78*(9), 893–898.

9

Expectations: Preceptors, Faculty, and Academic Programs

Amy Bieda and Jessica L. Spruit

CHAPTER OBJECTIVES

- Identify the responsibilities of the academic institution and healthcare system for both undergraduate and graduate nursing students

- Describe the role and responsibilities of both undergraduate and graduate nursing students during a precepted experience

PART 1: PRECEPTING AN UNDERGRADUATE SENIOR NURSING STUDENT

Ideally, during a baccalaureate nursing program, a fourth year (senior) nursing student enters their last semester with the skills and knowledge necessary to participate in a precepted experience with a qualified registered nurse who has an unencumbered license. The purpose of this one-on-one precepted experience is to give the experienced (senior) undergraduate nursing student the opportunity to function successfully as a new graduate in the work force. A preceptorship helps the student identify their strengths, as well as areas for development and improvement.

A precepted experience gives the undergraduate student the opportunity to take responsibility for a full patient care assignment under the guidance of an experienced clinician. The intent is to help the student develop time management skills, demonstrate accountability and ethical behavior in the practice of nursing, cultivate interprofessional communication, advocate for patients

and their families, develop leadership skills, and integrate best current evidence to deliver safe, high-quality nursing care. The precepted experience also gives the student time to learn the culture of the unit and begin socialization into the profession.

Healthcare systems are becoming increasingly complex due to rapid changes in technology and advances in clinical knowledge. Electronic health records (EHR), medication dispensing systems, and point of care diagnostic devices have all evolved rapidly. Beyond technological advances, patient outcomes and quality of care remain the primary focus of healthcare teams (Kavanagh & Sharpnack, 2021). Appropriately, healthcare institutions have long recognized and reported concerns to nursing programs regarding new graduates' inability to think critically, reason clinically, and apply clinical judgment soundly. The difficulty linking theoretical knowledge to practical application has been well-documented. The student or early career nurse may not recognize when a patient's condition is deteriorating, which is one of the four key elements of failure to rescue (Burke et al., 2022).

The fourth-year transitional rotation pairs a senior nursing student in the clinical setting with a capable and experienced nurse and establishes the structure and support necessary to both prepare the student and ensure quality of care for patients. It is the best evidence-based approach to support entry to practice at all levels and in all types of practice environments (American Association of Colleges of Nursing [AACN], 2021).

Reciprocal Benefits of Precepting for Universities and Healthcare Systems

Academic institutions and healthcare systems both benefit from collaborating to provide fourth year/senior undergraduate preceptorships. The university cannot provide a high-quality, transformative, and integrative clinical experience without the assistance of clinical partners. Additionally, healthcare providers need new graduates to be as well prepared as possible to enter the nursing workforce. A good working relationship between partners helps to accomplish these complementary goals (Markaki et al., 2021).

Often, a capable student will decide to join the nursing staff in a hospital system where they feel welcomed, supported, included, and respected. Students are able to experience the practice culture and see the opportunities available to them, and may select or de-select sites accordingly. Likewise, staff may recognize the potential of a student to become a valued and trusted colleague and nursing employee or may shy away from bringing a student onto staff if they observe poor ethics, unprofessional behavior, or lack of accountability.

Role of the Hospital Administration and Leadership

Nursing leadership (managers, directors, educators, and clinical nurse specialists) all play vital roles in the success of preceptors and the students. They are sensitive to the nursing unit culture, acuity, and conditions. Nursing leaders are generally aware of nurses who are high performers, effective role models, and good candidates to serve as preceptors.

Hospital administration must intentionally support nurse preceptors by adjusting schedules and responsibilities to allow for success in the role, providing preparation for preceptor responsibilities, as well as developing and documenting clear expectations for preceptors. Creating a balance in responsibilities helps prevent the preceptor from becoming overloaded (e.g., preceptors should not serve simultaneously in the role of charge nurse or resource nurse). Preceptors may be asked to take on leadership responsibilities, such as leading the code response team, which can facilitate student learning.

Staff shortages, call-offs, and heavy workloads can create challenges during the clinical day. It is not uncommon for a student to be assigned a second preceptor as a backup. However, this may not work well when the backup preceptor is not as familiar with the student's learning needs. Consequently, accepting students for preceptorships requires meaningful leadership support and the support of the entire team on the unit.

Faculty, Preceptor, and Clinical Nurse Educator Collaboration

The best clinical experiences are grounded in a strong collaboration between a university or school of nursing faculty member, the preceptor, and a clinical educator who is employed by the healthcare facility. They work together to ensure the best clinical experience, patient care, and professional cooperation. Clear understanding of roles and responsibilities is a key to the success of this partnership, as is respectful commitment to the mission and values of each partner.

The faculty member is responsible for the structure, process, and outcomes of the course. Faculty collaborate to establish learning outcomes, develop course content and assignments, create assessment tools, and provide guidance for the practicum experience. The faculty member assigns the course grade and retains accountability for the outcome of the course. They are responsible for ensuring that students have the knowledge and skills necessary to be successful in the practice setting.

The preceptor follows the education plan as developed by the faculty. They provide real-time support and coaching. The preceptor provides ongoing, individualized feedback that helps the student progress toward goals. They identify when student performance does not meet expectations, and work with the faculty and clinical educator to plan experiences that promote student success and ensure patient safety.

The clinical educator provides training, experiences, and resources to support the preceptor in their role and promote student success, while ensuring patient safety and quality care. The educator may provide coaching for preceptors and design resources to promote their success. The educator also engages with the faculty to ensure quality student experiences.

Open lines of communication between the healthcare system, administration, faculty of the academic institution, unit directors, and nurse educators are vital for this undertaking to be successful, particularly when a student is not performing up to expectations. Providing clear and constructive feedback in this situation can be challenging for the preceptor. Support from the educator and faculty will prove useful in improving student outcomes and maintaining positive relationships between the clinical setting and the university program.

Roles and Responsibilities of the Academic Institution, Faculty, Preceptor, and Undergraduate Student

Academic Institution Responsibilities

A responsibility of the academic institution is to verify that students are compliant with all regulations and have up-to-date health records prior to the start of the clinical rotation. Each student is required to complete onboarding expectations according to individual healthcare system mandates. The academic institution should provide useful, easily accessible resources for preceptors. These resources may include: nursing program policies, student handbook, course syllabus, student course objectives, nursing program goals, specific policies related to emergencies and attendance, as well as contact information for course faculty and other helpful individuals or teams.

The Faculty Nurse Educator Role

Faculty need to remain current on healthcare systems policies and procedures. The nurse educator is typically the liaison between the student, preceptor, and academic institution, and needs to be available to the preceptor and the student throughout the semester. It is their responsibility to make site visits during the clinical rotation (e.g., midterm and final) (Table 9.1). Meetings with the preceptor and student should occur regularly to ensure the student is meeting clinical objectives. The faculty liaison can also support the preceptor's teaching and learning needs as well as assist the preceptor when difficult student issues arise.

Preceptor Role

Preceptors usually have a minimum of two years' experience working in a specific area. The most effective preceptors have demonstrated clinical competence,

TABLE 9.1 Expectations of Preceptors During Faculty Site Visits for Undergraduate Nursing Students	
Faculty questions for preceptor	• Does the student arrive on time, dressed appropriately? • Does the student have any knowledge deficits that the faculty and preceptor need to address? • Does the student conduct themself in a professional, ethical manner with patients and staff? • Is the student meeting the competencies of the clinical experience? • Is the student seeking new learning opportunities (e.g., patient teaching, procedures with other patients)? • Does the student advocate for their patients?
Faculty observations at the site	• Is the student assigned a safe number of patients to provide quality nursing care? • Is the student accepting of positive reinforcement and constructive criticism? • Is the student utilizing current resources (e.g., journals, textbooks, and online reference materials)? • Is the student building on foundational clinical skills and displaying professional, ethical behavior? • Is the student using any "downtime" effectively for learning and collaboration?

Courtesy Amy Bieda, PhD, RN.

problem-solving skills, and excellent communication skills. They have also been observed teaching and mentoring nurses, recognized as role models, seen to consistently promote nursing as a profession, and have demonstrated cultural sensitivity (Loughran & Koharchik, 2019).

The preceptor role is multifaceted with undergraduate nursing students and requires advanced planning. The knowledge, experience, and values of the preceptor are paramount to establishing a good working preceptor–student relationship. The preceptor needs to communicate with the student prior to beginning the clinical experience to discuss orientation and unit logistics, including expectations for communication during and between clinical days, when the shift starts and ends, and where they are to meet the first day.

Orientation sets the tone for a good experience for both student and preceptor. The preceptor introduces the student to the unit culture to foster understanding of the diverse care needs for the patient population. A directive conversation between preceptor and student can reveal the student's preferred learning style and pace, as well as perceived strengths and weaknesses. The preceptor may consider reaching out to the faculty for further clarification. Ultimately, individual healthcare systems decide what nursing students can and cannot do.

The preceptor directly supervises student performance of tasks and procedures, preparation and administration of medications, patient care, and evaluation. The student must also be oriented to the EHR system and often will have their own access in order to document. Preceptors ensure that documentation is done in real time and need to provide feedback to the student regarding accuracy. Additionally, the preceptor monitors student progress with regard to: number of assigned patients and acuity; time management skills; prioritizing patient care and needs; communicating with staff and families; attending physician rounds to advocate for the patient; obtaining report at the beginning of the shift; asking pertinent questions; updating care plans; and learning to give an accurate report at the end of the shift. Preceptors also monitor development of clinical judgment skills, which can be facilitated by asking questions such as: "What would you do?" and "What do you think?" (Loughran & Koharchik, 2019).

The preceptor provides formative and summative evaluations as required by academic institutions at mid-term and the end of the clinical experience (See Chapter 21). Positive reinforcement provides validation to the student and helps strengthen the learning process. Constructive feedback throughout the day is much more effective than providing a litany of information at the end of a shift. However, an overall synopsis of the day can provide vital information for the student. The preceptor has the freedom to assign exercises to enhance learning, especially when knowledge deficits are identified.

Part of the preceptor role is to identify when a student is not integrating and applying evidence-based knowledge and clinical skills to establish competence during the clinical experience (Figure 9.1). Additionally, the student's attitude may influence their learning, often reflected in the confidence and commitment the student displays. If the preceptor has concerns about the students' abilities, it is their responsibility to notify the faculty member and discuss the issues so a meeting can be held with the student and a remediation plan formulated. Suggesting remediation may be difficult for preceptors because this is a high-stakes decision that can influence the student's progression in the academic program (Oermann, 2021). Safe practice is always a priority and must be established during the student's formalized learning process. Often, a nursing program will extend a clinical rotation for a student that needs to meet the competencies.

One question that often arises from preceptors relates to liability. Healthcare systems carry malpractice insurance for nurses and often nurses additionally carry their own. Students are provided liability insurance through the academic institution where they are enrolled and have the ability to purchase additional insurance. The student nurse is responsible for their own negligent acts. Communication between the preceptor and student, as

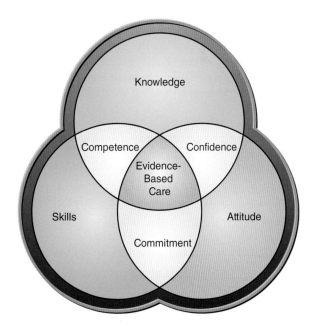

Fig. 9.1. Competencies for evidence-based nursing care.

well as documentation in real time, is instrumental in preventing litigation.

Undergraduate Student Role

This is an exciting time for senior undergraduate nursing students as they finish their rigorous nursing program, prepare to graduate, take the NCLEX, and seek employment as a registered nurse (RN). The primary goal is for the student to gain experience and continue to develop as a pre-licensure nurse that practices in a safe and competent manner.

Students need to understand the purpose of the precepted experience. It is the academic institution's responsibility to review clinical judgment and clinical reasoning to aid students in developing clinical judgment. Students are accountable and responsible for their own learning. They need to be open with the preceptor about learning opportunities in which they would like to observe or participate (e.g., setting up a sterile procedure at the bedside, accompanying a patient to a diagnostic procedure).

Not every clinical day is going to be exciting and some days may be overwhelming for the student. Students can be reassured that the successes and challenges they experience are all part of the learning process. Interpersonal conflicts that present between the student and others in the healthcare setting should be addressed with the preceptor. If a student has an issue with the preceptor, they need to discuss it with faculty. Miscommunication is often the issue, and a meeting between all parties can resolve the problem. However, if a poor working relationship is the issue, the faculty member should consider finding another preceptor for the student.

PART 2: PRECEPTING AN ADVANCED PRACTICE REGISTERED NURSE STUDENT

The need for advanced practice registered nurses (APRNs), most notably nurse practitioners (NPs), has increased for multiple reasons, including an aging population, lack of access to primary healthcare, increased mental health issues, and a continuous decline in and maldistribution of primary care physicians and non-primary care specialty physicians (American Association of Medical Colleges [AAMC], 2021; Li & Jones, 2021). As a result, the need for well-prepared preceptors has grown exponentially.

Graduate nursing students are professional RNs aspiring to develop their careers through further education. Differing in many ways from pre-licensure students, graduate nursing students have overcome many of the initial challenges that pre-licensure students encounter. They typically have an increased maturity level and may have different motivations for learning. Additionally, they have participated in various clinical experiences and have developed some expertise in nursing. Advanced communication skills and time management skills are often well-established. Therefore, the preceptor's role is to assist the APRN student in developing advanced practice skills, and higher-level clinical reasoning.

ROLES AND RESPONSIBILITIES OF THE ACADEMIC INSTITUTION, FACULTY, PRECEPTOR, AND GRADUATE STUDENT

Responsibilities of the Academic Institution

A contract or memorandum of understanding (MOU) between the academic institution and clinical site must be in place before the start of a clinical rotation. Academic institutions must retain documentation regarding fulfillment of all requirements to enter the clinical setting, including drug screening, fingerprinting, immunizations, health clearance, background check, and an unencumbered nursing license. Academic nursing programs and the clinical sites may have additional requirements for graduate nursing students.

Academic institutions are also required to maintain certain documentation on preceptors including: a resume or curriculum vitae (CV), documentation of an unencumbered license, and national certification through a specialty organization (National Task Force, 2022). Both academic institutions and clinical sites may have their own requirements for preceptors.

Academic programs support preceptors by providing orientation materials. The academic program should provide faculty contact information and links to resources (Pitts et al., 2019), skills checklists, and communication that is goal-directed and student-specific (Burt et al., 2022). Preceptors will benefit from a preceptor manual, a copy of the course syllabus with course objectives, and a schedule of didactic lectures. Due to the shortage of APRN preceptors, it is the responsibility of the academic institution to incentivize preceptors appropriately (See Chapter 1).

Academic Faculty Role

The faculty is responsible for the student and review of the student's clinical experience, including their learning progression (Pitts et al., 2019). In conjunction with the preceptor, faculty evaluates the student's knowledge, attitudes, and competencies.

Faculty schedule site visits with the preceptor and student during their clinical rotation to discuss the student's progression, attainment of competencies, and any areas of concern. This is an opportunity to observe the student in the clinical site. Faculty make themselves available to both the preceptor and student for questions, issues, or concerns in person or via phone, text, or virtual platform.

Faculty review both the preceptor evaluation of the student *and* the student's evaluation of the preceptor and the site. Meeting with the preceptor and student to review the student evaluation allows discussion of the students' strengths and areas for improvement. A remediation plan may need to be implemented (Pitts et al., 2019).

Preceptor Role

Preceptors should consider the dynamics on their team and within their clinical environments prior to agreeing to precept a student. Several factors can compromise the clinical experience for the student. Clinical teams that are short-staffed, precepting their own newly hired colleagues, or undergoing significant change may not be optimally positioned to precept a student during that semester (Renda et al., 2022). While it is important for students to observe adversity and the inevitable challenges experienced in healthcare today, it is equally important that they are provided clinical opportunities in environments that can support their training and need for additional attention and oversight. Even when the clinical environment is not ideal, preceptors model professional behavior, respectful interactions, and embrace constructive criticism from colleagues.

As previously discussed, preceptors should engage the APRN student in conversations about their learning styles and strive to offer educational opportunities that align with their preferences and program course objectives. The preceptor role with APRN students is more focused on a specific area than a preceptor role for a pre-licensure nursing student. Preceptors and program faculty should encourage students to develop site-specific

---

Exemplar: Family-Focused Specialty Care in an Interdisciplinary Clinical Setting

Donna J. Marvicsin

Nurse practitioner (NP) students often experience unnecessary anxiety in their clinical rotations despite their eagerness to learn and experience as much as possible. They may have high and unrealistic expectations of their abilities and clinical skills. The pressure they self-impose can contribute to an inability to absorb detailed clinical information. Their anxiety can be compounded by the need to incorporate clinical decision-making within a limited time frame, especially in focused specialty clinics. As preceptors, we know that it can take a year or more to fully grasp the nuances of clinical practice.

As an NP in a pediatric endocrinology clinic, I was precepting an NP student who was anxious because she had no clinical experience in this specialty. One of her learning objectives was to educate and support children and families living with a chronic illness. The first patient we cared for was a child newly diagnosed with diabetes, and the student's priority was focused on insulin management. My first action was to help the student focus instead on the *impact* of the condition on the child and family, *not* to immediately teach them to become experts in adjusting insulin. Expanding the assessment process to include the family's adjustment to living with the patient's chronic disease state is a priority. Using the "see one, do one, teach one" approach, I introduced the student to a simple assessment tool that emphasizes family strengths and areas of concern.

I later framed the clinical encounter as a learning opportunity for the student to practice therapeutic communication. We discussed motivational interviewing and role-play simulation to facilitate the NP student's interactions with children and families. Since many specialty clinics include multidisciplinary team members to provide high-quality care for those with chronic conditions, I structured the student's experience in our clinic to spend time with the dietician, social worker, and endocrinologists. This provided the student with the opportunity to observe team-based interdisciplinary care and build collaborative skills as an advanced practice provider.

The NP student continued to develop foundational assessment and therapeutic communication skills with each patient encounter. By providing structured opportunities in this specialty setting, the student's anxiety decreased and she was able to be proactive in her learning experience instead of being a passive observer.

objectives for their clinical experience (Appendix N: Examples of NP Student Learning Needs and Clinical Objectives).

The preceptor in a hospitalist role might expect the student to engage in learning activities that include inpatient rounds, radiology rounds, patient care conferences, grand rounds, consultations, and specific patient procedures. Students should be encouraged to prepare for the clinical experience by reviewing relevant content and site-specific policies and protocols.

Teaching specialized skills and procedures. Students in acute care NP tracks need to learn specific skills and procedures. Prior to performing procedures in the clinical setting, most academic programs incorporate procedural skills labs and simulation for hands-on practice. This is an opportunity for the student to receive feedback and refine their skills before attempting a procedure in the actual clinical environment.

Preceptors need to be adept at teaching hands-on procedures when translating from simulation to bedside. The process should be interactive and follow a "see one, do one, teach one" methodology (Box 9.1).

Evaluation. It is *never* the responsibility of the preceptor to fail a student or determine whether they can progress within a program. It *is* the responsibility of

---

BOX 9.1   Steps to Teaching Hands-On Procedures

Preceptor role
- Provide rationale for required procedure
- Verbally explain procedural steps
- Demonstrate procedure while providing verbal narrative
Note: Student may need more than one demonstration before performing

Student role
- Review written procedure
- Demonstrate equipment setup
- Verbally explain the process to the preceptor
- Perform procedure with preceptor guidance

Preceptor and student role
- Debrief
  – Preceptor providing constructive feedback
  – Student self-evaluates

---

the preceptor to provide objective information and alert the course faculty to any concerns regarding the student or faculty member assigned to the student. Concerns may be presented to faculty verbally or in writing, and should be reflected in formative and summative evaluations (See Chapter 21). The preceptor is a critical and highly valued extension of the academic program faculty and should feel empowered to reach out to the responsible faculty with any concerns. Thorough documentation of issues supports the faculty ability to address problems and take appropriate action, such as development of a remediation plan (Pitts et al., 2019).

Graduate Nursing Student Role

The graduate student must be responsible and accountable for a significant portion of their own adult learning. Graduate nursing education provides many opportunities for learning and professional growth, but the student must demonstrate a desire to identify and take advantage of these opportunities. Students are encouraged to pursue patient interactions with complex disease processes that they are not familiar with as a means to learn new knowledge and skills. These new opportunities facilitate students' ability to formulate differential diagnoses and expand their critical reasoning skills. As part of being accountable, students maintain a record of completed procedures, which may also required by the academic institution to track competencies.

If a graduate nursing student has interpersonal issues with their preceptor, they need to contact the faculty assigned to them. Students should not be expected to resolve conflicts with preceptors on their own. The faculty should always be available to mediate issues whether presented by the student or the preceptor. Directly addressing concerns that arise through mediation often helps to clarify and resolve difficult situations.

CONCLUSION

The creation of an excellent precepted clinical experience goes beyond "just" the preceptor–student interaction. Collaboration must occur between students, preceptors, faculty, and academic institutions. Truly great experiences occur when all parties meet their responsibilities and work together to maintain clear expectations, open communication, and respect for each other's time and effort.

REFERENCES

American Association of Colleges of Nursing. (2021). *The Essentials: Core competencies for professional nursing education.* https://www.aacnnursing.org/AACNEssentials

American Association of Medical Colleges. (2021). Aging patients and doctors drive nation's physician shortage. https://www.aamc.org/news-insights/aging-patients-and-doctors-drive-nation-s-physician-shortage#:~:text=That%20shortage%20includes%20shortfalls%20of%2017%2C800%20to%2048%2C000

Burke, J. R., Downey, C., & Almoudaris, A. M. (2022). Failure to rescue deteriorating patients: A systematic review of root causes and improvement strategies. *Journal of Patient Safety, 18*(1), e140–e155. https://doi.org/10.1097/pts.0000000000000720

Burt, L., Sparbel, K., & Corbridge, S. (2022). Nurse practitioner preceptor resource needs and perceptions of institutional support. *Journal of the American Association of Nurse Practitioners, 34*(2), 348–356. https://doi.org/10.1097/jxx.0000000000000629

Kavanagh, J. M., & Sharpnack, P. A. (2021). Crisis in competency: A defining moment in nursing education. *Online Journal of Issues in Nursing, 26*(1). https://doi.org/10.3912/ojin.vol26no01man02

Li, Y., & Jones, C. B. (2021). Care received by patients from nurse practitioners and physicians in U.S. primary care settings. *Nursing Outlook, 69*(5). https://doi.org/10.1016/j.outlook.2021.02.007

Loughran, M. C., & Koharchik, L. (2019). Ensuring a successful preceptorship. *AJN, American Journal of Nursing, 119*(5), 61–65. https://doi.org/10.1097/01.naj.0000557917.73516.00

Markaki, A., Prajankett, O. O., Shorten, A., Shirey, M. R., & Harper, D. C. (2021). Academic service-learning nursing partnerships in the Americas: A scoping review. *BMC nursing, 20*(1), 1–15. https://doi.org/10.1186/s12912-021-00698-w

National Task Force on Quality Nurse Practitioner Education. (2022). *Standards for quality nurse practitioner education: A report of the national task force on quality nurse practitioner education.* (6th ed.) https://cdn.ymaws.com/www.nonpf.org/resource/resmgr/2022/ntfs_/ntfs_final.pdf

Oermann, M. (2021). Some principles to guide the assessment of competency. *Nurse Educator, 47*(1). https://doi.org/10.1097/nne.0000000000001143. 1–1

Pitts, C., Padden, D., Knestrick, J., & Bigley, M. B. (2019). A checklist for faculty and preceptor to enhance the nurse practitioner student clinical experience. *Journal of the American Association of Nurse Practitioners, 31*(10), 591–597. https://doi.org/10.1097/JXX.0000000000000310

Renda, S., Fingerhood, M., Kverno, K., Slater, T., Gleason, K., & Goodwin, M. (2022). What motivates our practice colleagues to precept the next generation? The *Journal for Nurse Practitioners, 18*(1), 76–80. https://doi.org/10.1016/j.nurpra.2021.09.008

10

Providing a Well-Rounded Clinical Experience

Annette Peacock-Johnson, Sue Anderson, and Daniela Edson

CHAPTER OBJECTIVES

- Appraise various models and guidelines for clinical site selection as an essential first step for providing a well-rounded clinical experience
- Design diverse learning opportunities for graduate and undergraduate students that promote the integration of quality and safety competencies in clinical practice
- Develop graduate patient care experiences within the four spheres of care that include commonly seen clinical situations by body system or service type
- Incorporate planned and unplanned teachable moments to facilitate learning
- Describe the complementary role of simulation in facilitating clinical judgment and the acquisition of skills

Well-rounded clinical experiences involve careful preparation and collaboration between preceptors and faculty to meet required quality and safety competencies for graduate and undergraduate students. This chapter presents preceptors with concepts related to developing effective clinical experiences.

Pre-planning for clinical experiences is essential in laying the groundwork for a well-rounded clinical experience. The selection of an appropriate clinical site is a necessary first step in creating an environment that fosters the application of theoretical concepts to the practice setting. Site selection should be made based on the ability of the setting to provide learning opportunities to meet the course and clinical learning objectives.

> Appropriate clinical sites that meet learning objectives are essential in providing a well-rounded educational experience.

UNDERGRADUATE CLINICAL SITES

A variety of clinical placement models have been identified and utilized in the clinical education of undergraduate nursing students (Nyoni et al., 2021) (see Table 10.1). The model used is often determined by the type of clinical experience, the level of the student in the academic program, and the size of the student group(s).

Block Clinical Placement Model

A traditional model used in undergraduate nursing programs is the block clinical placement model. Block clinical models are frequently used in healthcare agencies, such as hospitals or long-term care institutions, that care for larger populations of patients or residents. In this model, the faculty member *is* the preceptor who directly supervises a group of undergraduate students over a specified number of weeks or block of time using the same clinical setting. The faculty develops relationships with students and provides guidance of nursing care. Further, faculty are responsible for assessing student clinical performance, including the completion of formative and summative student evaluations (see Chapter 21). A strength of the block clinical placement model is consistency in the faculty–student relationship and clinical environment, which can facilitate confidence and growth in clinical knowledge and skills. Additionally, block placements allow for a larger group of

TABLE 10.1	Comparison of Undergraduate Clinical Teaching Models		
	Block Clinical Placement (BCP) (Traditional)	**Dedicated Education Unit (DEU)**	**Collaboration Clinical Placement (CCP)**
Preceptor	Faculty from school of nursing oriented to the patient unit to provide clinical oversight	All staff registered nurses specifically trained to precept	Multiple nurses or nursing leaders selected to precept
Setting	Multiple units throughout one facility for student experiences	One unit in facility dedicated to student learning	Multiple special experiences throughout facility
Predominant relationship	Faculty–student	Staff–student	Faculty–student and/or Staff–student
Grouping	Group of students from multiple programs	Group of students from one program	~1–3 students
Level of student	Beginning	Beginning–advanced	Advanced–fourth year

Data from Hunt, D. A., Milani, M. F., & Wilson, S. (2015). Dedicated education units: An innovative model for clinical education. *American Nurse Today, 10*(5), 46–49; Nyoni, C. N., Hugo-Van Dyk, L., & Botma, Y. (2021). Clinical placement models for undergraduate health professions students: A scoping review. *BMC Medical Education, 21*(598).

students in one setting, enhancing the ability of students to develop team relationships with peers and members of the healthcare team.

Dedicated Education Unit Model

An innovative model for undergraduate clinical instruction is the Dedicated Education Unit (DEU). The DEU is created by a contractual agreement between the healthcare agency and the specific nursing program. Students work consistently with the same nurses on the same unit over the course of the clinical rotation. This approach facilitates understanding of the educational outcomes by nursing staff on the unit (Walker et al., 2012; Hunt et al., 2015). The staff nurse functions as preceptor and mentor, providing clinical supervision and guidance for assigned nursing students, and is primarily responsible for assessing student clinical performance. Unlike the block model, the nursing faculty does not provide direct patient care and supervision of the nursing student. Instead, faculty engages in routine collaboration with the DEU preceptor to receive feedback and input regarding the student's progress. Further, faculty coach the preceptor and provide guidance when a student is not meeting clinical learning objectives or is demonstrating unprofessional behaviors, which may necessitate intervention. Frequent and clear communication is needed between the preceptor, faculty, and student to determine a plan for clinical improvement and progression when unsatisfactory performance is identified. Strengths of

this model include consistency in the preceptor–student relationship and clinical environment, thus building student knowledge acquisition and confidence.

Collaboration Clinical Placement Model

The collaboration clinical placement model relies on the assignment of one to three students to a preceptor who may or may not be the same preceptor throughout the clinical rotation (Nyoni et al., 2021). This model is often used for advanced undergraduate nursing students who may be working with a nurse preceptor during a transitional clinical rotation. Collaboration clinical placement models are also seen in community or outpatient settings such as clinics, schools, or other community healthcare settings that meet the course and clinical learning objectives. Students develop collaborative relationships with assigned preceptors who guide them in providing direct patient care. Similar to the DEU clinical placement model, the nurse faculty member collaborates continuously with assigned preceptors to assess the nursing student's performance. Formative and summative clinical evaluations are completed by faculty. Strengths of this model include the ability to assign students to a wide variety of clinical sites that may not accommodate large groups of students. Other clinical placement models for undergraduate healthcare students have been identified, but are less commonly used in nursing (Nyoni et al., 2021). All models provide clinical placements that best meet the clinical learning objectives.

GRADUATE CLINICAL SITES

The 2022 National Task Force (NTF) on Quality Nurse Practitioner Education Standards provides clarity on the appropriateness of advanced practice registered nurse (APRN) clinical placements. There must be an alignment of clinical placement sites to provide the student with opportunities to meet course and program objectives within the population focus of the program (NTF, 2022). Students in primary care–focused programs must engage in clinical experiences in primary care settings. Likewise, students in acute care–focused programs must engage in clinical experiences in acute care settings. To meet the latest NTF criteria, students must participate in interprofessional educational (IPE) experiences within their didactic learning and clinical rotations.

According to the *Essentials: Core Competencies for Professional Nursing Education* (American Association of Colleges of Nursing [AACN], 2021), nursing programs must ensure that clinical placements are "safe, supportive, and conducive to learning" (p. 20). While students may be involved in securing clinical placements, ultimately, the nursing programs are required to ensure that clinical placements are *available* and *appropriate* for the clinical learning experience. Students may be in the best position to find a preceptor and clinical site that can meet their personal learning needs (Gigli & Gonzalez, 2022). While course faculty have the ultimate responsibility for providing APRN student evaluations, preceptors are generally invited to provide formative and summative feedback on student clinical performance.

FACILITATING CLINICAL COMPETENCIES

Balanced clinical experiences for undergraduate and APRN students should incorporate patient care assignments, which provide diverse opportunities to apply theoretical concepts and psychomotor skills in the clinical setting. Historically, frameworks for clinical experiences were centered on the performance of technical skills and the application of knowledge related to physiologic systems (Preheim et al., 2009). Such an approach lacked a systems perspective that was needed to develop competency in quality and safety for professional nursing practice. A ground-breaking report by the Institute of Medicine (IOM) in the late 1990s documented preventable medical errors stemming from deficiencies in the delivery of safe, quality patient care (Kohn et al., 2000).

As a result, the national Quality and Safety Education for Nurses (QSEN) initiative was implemented in 2006 to meet the needs of contemporary healthcare systems and transform nursing education (Cengiz & Yoder, 2020). An outgrowth of the initiative was the establishment of the QSEN Institute, whose mission is to meet the challenge of preparing future nurses to improve quality and safety within healthcare systems (QSEN.org).

A panel of nursing leaders developed six quality and safety competencies for nursing education, known as the QSEN competencies. The six competencies are: 1) safety, 2) patient-centered care, 3) teamwork and collaboration, 4) evidence-based practice, 5) quality improvement, and 6) informatics. Beginning in 2022, the QSEN competencies were aligned with the new *Essentials: Core Competencies for Professional Nursing Education* (QSEN.org, 2022; AACN, 2021) to create domains and concepts that integrate quality and safety into baccalaureate and graduate education and practice.

Nursing programs are working to align students' knowledge, skills, and attitudes with the QSEN competencies. Patient-centered care, in particular, is cited by nursing students as the most widely implemented competency in clinical experiences (Cengiz & Yoder, 2020).

> Well-rounded clinical experiences foster the development of knowledge, skills, and attitudes essential for providing safe, quality care. The use of planned experiences, as well as unpredictable clinical events, can create teachable moments that enhance learning.

While quality and safety competencies are often introduced through didactic content, the *application* of competencies is a vital component of the clinical experience and should be incorporated by the clinical preceptor. Students are responsible for tracking their clinical and academic experiences to justify the competencies they have met. Documentation of competencies can be organized in ePortfolios as a reflection of student growth (Box 10.1).

DIVERSE LEARNING OPPORTUNITIES

Graduate Students

There are six population foci within the realm of APRN education: 1) adult-gerontology (primary and acute care), 2) pediatrics (primary and acute care), 3)

BOX 10.1 The Nursing Student e-Portfolio

Electronic portfolios (e-portfolios) are an innovative way for academic institutions to assist students in organizing their accomplishments *and* providing preceptors with an overview of the student's achievements. E-portfolios provide a digital record that combines information about students' knowledge, skills, and previous achievements. Links are provided so that there is a clear record of teaching assessments and clinical evaluations. By reviewing a digital record of the student's activities, clinical instructors (faculty) and clinical preceptors can better design student learning experiences. The portfolio provides a clear record of student progress toward the achievement of required competencies.

Examples of e-Portfolio Content:
- Record of clinical experiences and hours
- Assignments that meet the AACN *Essentials* requirements
- Graduate or undergraduate thesis, or Doctorate of Nursing Practice (DNP) project
- Academic papers reflecting nursing theory, health policy, ethical issues, etc.
- Curriculum vitae or resume
- Clinical evaluations
- Copies of reference letters
- Awards and grants

family/individual across the lifespan, 4) neonatal, 5) women's health/gender-related, and 6) psychiatric/mental health across the lifespan. At the advanced practice education level, students engage in direct patient care in their chosen clinical specialty, including face-to-face care of individuals and families and patient care via telehealth. Rather than observing, the clinical preceptor facilitates student–patient interactions, guiding students' performance of comprehensive patient assessments in which they obtain demographic, subjective, and objective data. Students must then interpret and use advanced clinical judgment to synthesize these data to derive diagnoses and develop a patient-centered plan of care that is evidence-based (NTF, 2022) (See Appendix E: **Site Specific APRN Clinical Experiences**).

The Essentials (AACN, 2021) requires that students engage in person-centered care, which means that the nurse respects diversity, recognizing that a patient is a person who is a full partner and the source of control in team-based interaction. Person-centered care requires the nurse to be intentionally present to understand the person's lived experiences and life connections. Person-centered care emphasizes diversity, equity, and inclusion. Well-rounded clinical experiences include opportunities for nursing students to engage in a vast array of patient circumstances. For more information on championing diversity, see Chapter 1.

To provide a well-rounded clinical experience, primary care nurse practitioner preceptors should incorporate clinical experiences within the four spheres of care, as defined by the AACN: 1) wellness and disease prevention, 2) chronic disease management, 3) regenerative and restorative care, and 4) hospice and palliative care (AACN, 2019). Preceptors should consider the previous experiences of APRN students when selecting and delegating learning opportunities. Priority is placed on experiences that provide opportunities to integrate the latest evidence-based practices with previous knowledge, skills, and attitudes.

Wellness and Disease Prevention

Wellness and disease prevention care focuses on the diagnosis and treatment of acute illness in otherwise healthy individuals. The preceptor prompts the primary care APRN student on the completion of head-to-toe wellness physical assessments, including evidence-based screening guidelines for vision, hearing, cardiovascular disease, cancer, mental health, and gender/reproductive health.

APRN students are coached in the delivery of preventive services, including immunizations and education on evidence-based risk reduction strategies for smoking cessation, nutritional deficiencies, physical inactivity, substance abuse, domestic violence, obesity, and falls. Commonly seen clinical conditions vary by the patient population and clinical site (acute versus primary setting). The preceptor strives to assign or delegate patients representing a broad range of health conditions to achieve a well-rounded graduate clinical experience. A range of more commonly seen clinical situations by body system or service type for wellness and disease prevention are listed in Table 10.2 for the primary care setting and Table 10.3 for the acute care setting.

Regenerative and Restorative Care

Regenerative and restorative care incorporates critical or trauma care, complex acute care, and exacerbations of chronic conditions. Integral to the provision of regenerative and restorative care is the need for interprofessional

TABLE 10.2	**Common Medical Conditions Seen in Primary Care**	
System	**Acute or Episodic**	**Chronic**
Head, Eyes, Ears, Nose, Throat (HEENT)	Hearing loss (conductive and sensorineural), visual disturbance/blurry vision, foreign body (eyes, ears, nose), acute angle glaucoma, otitis media/externa, acute sinusitis, viral upper respiratory infection, viral/bacterial/allergic conjunctivitis, oral candidiasis, rhinitis (non-allergic, vasomotor, allergic), dentition, tonsils/throat (pharyngitis, tonsillitis, tonsilloliths, peritonsillar abscess), snoring, temporomandibular joint symptoms, mastoiditis, mononucleosis, vertigo, epistaxis, sialadenitis	Hearing loss, visual disturbance, glaucoma, chronic sinusitis, head and neck neoplasms
Cardiovascular	Heart tones, heart rhythm, valve placement in correlation with anatomy, murmurs, rhythm, dysrhythmias along with rates, rubs, cardiomegaly, congenital heart diseases, hypertension, chest pain, syncope, edema	Hypertension, peripheral arterial disease, varicose veins, congestive heart failure, congenital heart disease
Pulmonary	Asthma, bronchitis, pneumonia, rhonchi, rales, crackles, pulmonary edema, respiratory distress, sleep apnea, spontaneous pneumothorax, chronic obstructive pulmonary disease (COPD)	Chronic obstructive pulmonary disease, emphysema, asthma, chronic cough
Gastrointestinal	Nausea, vomiting, heartburn/gastroesophageal reflux disease (GERD), diarrhea, constipation, appendicitis, cholecystitis, acute abdominal pain, acute gastroenteritis, diverticulitis, hemorrhoids, acute pancreatitis, viral hepatitis, hernias, intussusception, ulcers, irritable bowel syndrome, hematochezia	Crohn's disease, fatty liver disease, viral hepatitis, Hirschsprung's disease, diverticular disease
Integumentary	Acne, eczema, dermatitis (contact, atopic, diaper, seborrheic), skin cancer, spider bites, impetigo, insect stings, skin cancer, tinea, viral rash (fifth disease; hand, foot, and mouth disease; herpes zoster; herpangina; rubella; rubeola; varicella), tinea, scarlet fever, pediculosis, warts, pityriasis rosacea, rosacea, scabies, bacterial skin infections, cellulitis	Actinic keratosis, burns, Lyme disease, psoriasis, skin cancer
Neurological	Bell's palsy, carpal tunnel syndrome, headaches (tension, migraine, cluster), concussion, febrile seizures, meningitis, syncope, vertigo, neuropathy	Seizures, epilepsy, Alzheimer's disease, dementia, multiple sclerosis, Parkinson's disease, restless leg syndrome, cerebrovascular accident (CVA), transient ischemic attack (TIA), post-cerebrovascular accident sequelae
Musculoskeletal	Congenital hip dysplasia, sprains, strains, scoliosis, Osgood-Schlatter, slipped capital femoral epiphysis (SCFE), bursitis, tendonitis, soft tissue syndromes, osteoarthritis, fractures, gout, sciatica, polymyalgia rheumatica, fibromyalgia	Rheumatoid arthritis, osteoporosis, disk herniation, sciatica, gait disturbance, fall risk
Hematology	Neonatal hyperbilirubinemia, anemia (iron deficiency, folic acid deficiency, thalassemia, sickle cell, chronic disease, vitamin B-12 deficiency, glucose-6-phosphate dehydrogenase deficiency [G6PD]), lead toxicity, leukemias, lymphoma, thrombocytopenia purpura	Anemia (iron deficiency, folic acid deficiency, thalassemia, sickle cell, chronic disease, vitamin B-12 deficiency, glucose-6-phosphate dehydrogenase deficiency [G6PD]), lead toxicity, leukemias, lymphoma

Continued

TABLE 10.2	Common Medical Conditions Seen in Primary Care—cont'd	
System	Acute or Episodic	Chronic
Reproductive	*All*: Sexual identity, preferences; satisfaction with sexual experiences; sexually transmitted infection (STI) testing *Women*: fertility, menstrual cycles (history, symptoms, dysmenorrhea, abnormal uterine bleeding, amenorrhea), urinary incontinence, breast disorders (fibroadenoma, fibrocystic breast disease, intraductal papilloma, breast cancer, mastitis), cervical cancer, contraception, premenstrual syndrome, premenstrual dysphoric disorder, vaginal foreign body, Bartholin's gland cyst/abscess *Men*: fertility, erectile dysfunction, nocturia, dysuria	Menopause history and symptoms, polycystic ovarian syndrome, cervical cancer, ovarian cancer, vulvar cancer, prostate cancer, genitourinary syndrome of menopause
Endocrine	Thyroid nodule, diabetes mellitus type 1, diabetes mellitus type 2, obesity	Diabetes mellitus type 1, diabetes mellitus type 2, hypoglycemia, hypothyroidism, hyperthyroidism, precocious puberty, Addison's disease, Cushing's disease, chronic kidney disease, gynecomastia
Mental health	Depression, suicide, anxiety, panic disorder, alcohol and substance abuse disorder, overdose, sleep quality/insomnia, smoking cessation, sexual assault	Attention deficit hyperactivity disorder (ADHD), anorexia nervosa, bulimia, post-traumatic stress disorder, bipolar disorder, schizophrenia, obstructive sleep apnea
Urology	Acute pyelonephritis, asymptomatic bacteriuria, enuresis, hematuria, post-streptococcal glomerulonephritis, urethritis, incontinence, urinary tract infection (UTI), urolithiasis, vesicoureteral reflux, acute cystitis, acute prostatitis	Chronic kidney disease, Wilms' tumor, interstitial cystitis

collaboration to promote coordinated safe, quality care. The preceptor guides the graduate student in the identification of patients with acute or chronic conditions requiring multidisciplinary services. Well-rounded learning experiences include opportunities for the student to initiate referrals to physical or occupational therapy, speech and language pathology, or social work, among others; or in ordering durable medical equipment to meet identified patient needs.

Hospice and Palliative Care

Well-rounded clinical experiences incorporate opportunities for graduate students to manage the care for persons with complex, chronic disease, or end-of-life concerns. Students should be encouraged to engage in conversations with patients and families that focus on values and preferences for care and the completion of advanced directives. The preceptor mentors the student on management

options and resources, including referrals for hospice or long-term care placement when appropriate.

Undergraduate Students

A well-rounded clinical experience for undergraduate nursing students includes a range of learning opportunities. Using a block clinical model, preceptors focus on patient assignments that provide opportunities to cultivate knowledge, skills, and attitudes for safe and optimal patient care. Preceptors should consider the complexity of the patient assignment reflecting the level of the learner and previous clinical experience.

Student Assignments

Student assignments for the block clinical placement model are made most often by nursing faculty who screen patients and assign students accordingly. In addition to reviewing the electronic health record (EHR) for

System	Acute	Chronic
Head, Eyes, Ears, Nose, Throat (HEENT)	Pupillary changes and their correlation, ruptured ear drums, head injuries, tracheostomy and reconstructions, airway obstruction (upper), tracheal stricture, cranial nerves and their correlating function, ocular hypertension, recognize cerebrospinal fluid leak from ear/nose, Battle's sign, ocular trauma, orbital cellulitis, corneal abrasions, barotrauma to the head/neck, vertigo (traumatic), epiglottitis, Mallampati classifications	
Cardiovascular	Types of heart failure, hypertension (emergency, urgency), malignant hypertension, classification of hypertension, coronary artery disease, angina, myocardial infarction (MI), acute coronary syndrome, venous thrombosis, peripheral vascular disease, chronic venous insufficiency, pericarditis, endocarditis, cardiac transplant, cardiogenic shock, cardiogenic syncope, cardiomyopathies (stress, hypertrophic, restrictive), valvular diseases (stenosis, regurgitation), aortic stenosis, aortic aneurysm, cardiac arrhythmias, cardiac complications with pregnancy, shock	Congestive heart failure (CHF), hypertension
Pulmonary	Status asthmaticus, chronic obstructive pulmonary disease (COPD), tuberculosis, pneumonia (Hospital-acquired pneumonia (HAP), Community-acquired pneumonia (CAP), adult respiratory distress syndrome (ARDS), respiratory failure, pulmonary embolism, pulmonary function studies, pleural effusion, pneumothorax, hemothorax, cystic fibrosis (CF), interstitial lung disease, pulmonary hypertension, alveolar hemorrhage, pneumonitis	Asthma, chronic obstructive pulmonary disease (COPD)
Gastrointestinal	Peptic ulcer disease, *Helicobacter pylori*, hepatitis (A, B, C, D), gastroesophageal reflux disease (GERD), diverticulitis, ileus, bowel obstruction (small and large), cholecystitis, acute pancreatitis, ulcerative colitis, mesenteric infarct, appendicitis, *Clostridioides difficile*, gastrointestinal bleeding, peritonitis, refeeding syndrome, acute liver failure, hepatorenal syndrome, cirrhosis, portal hypertension	Cirrhosis, portal hypertension, esophageal varices, diverticulitis, Crohn's disease
Integumentary	Burns, cellulitis, dog/cat bites, dermatitis, fungal infections of the skin, herpes complex 1, angioedema, Stevens-Johnson syndrome, papules, Kaposi's sarcoma, skin ulceration, allergic vasculitis	
Neurological	Transient ischemic attack (TIA), cerebrovascular accident (CVA) both hemorrhage and infarct, seizures, status epilepticus, myasthenia gravis, multiple sclerosis, Guillain-Barre syndrome, head trauma, Monro-Kellie doctrine, spinal cord trauma, Brown-Sequard syndrome, cauda equina syndrome, Parkinson's disease, delirium, dementia, Alzheimer's disease, suicidal ideations, brain death	Seizures, epilepsy, Parkinson's disease, cerebrovascular accident, multiple sclerosis, myasthenia gravis, Alzheimer's disease, suicidal ideations
Musculoskeletal	Traumatic fractures, spinal surgeries	

TABLE 10.3 **Common Medical Conditions Seen in Acute Care**

Continued

TABLE 10.3	Common Medical Conditions Seen in Acute Care—cont'd	
System	**Acute**	**Chronic**
Hematology	Anemia (iron deficiency, thalassemia, folic acid deficiency, pernicious anemia, chronic disease, sickle cell), Von Willebrand's disease, acute nonlymphocytic leukemia, acute lymphocytic leukemia, chronic lymphocytic leukemia, chronic myelogenous leukemia, lymphomas (non-Hodgkin's, Hodgkin's), idiopathic thrombocytopenic purpura (ITP), disseminated intravascular coagulation (DIC), neutropenia, thrombocytopenia, leukopenia, amyloidosis, blood compatibility	Anemia (iron deficiency, thalassemia, folic acid deficiency, pernicious anemia, chronic disease, sickle cell), Von Willebrand's disease, acute nonlymphocytic leukemia, acute lymphocytic leukemia, chronic lymphocytic leukemia, chronic myelogenous leukemia, lymphomas (non-Hodgkin's, Hodgkin's), idiopathic thrombocytopenic purpura (ITP)
Reproductive	Gonorrhea, syphilis, chlamydia, vulvovaginitis, chancroid, herpes, embryologic embolization, pre-eclampsia	
Endocrine	Cushing's disease, Grave's disease, thyroid storm, thyroidectomy, diabetes mellitus (including Somogyi effect, dawn phenomenon, diabetic ketoacidosis, hyperosmolar hyperglycemic non-ketosis), hyperthyroidism, hypothyroidism, Addison's disease, syndrome of inappropriate antidiuretic hormone (SIADH), diabetes insipidus (DI), pheochromocytoma, myxedema	Cushing's disease, Grave's disease, diabetes mellitus type 1, diabetes mellitus type 2, Addison's disease.
Mental health	Suicidal ideations, schizophrenia, post-traumatic stress disorder, bipolar disorder, depression disorder, substance abuse disorder, overdose	
Urology	Urinary tract infections (UTI), acute pyelonephritis, renal insufficiency, acute renal failure, renal calculi, benign prostatic hypertrophy, prerenal, intrarenal, postrenal disease, acute epididymitis, acute cystitis, acute prostatitis	Chronic kidney disease, benign prostatic hypertrophy

appropriate patient assignments, staff nurses or managers who are familiar with the patients can provide valuable information about student learning opportunities. Additionally, they can identify patients who may not be suitable for student assignments. Knowledge of important psychosocial or family circumstances or patients who prefer not to have a student nurse facilitates the ability of the faculty to make optimal student assignments that promote learning.

Faculty may encourage students to self-select their patient assignment based on their own learning needs. This encourages student initiative and ownership for learning. Faculty should provide students with clear guidelines for selecting suitable patient assignments that

address learning outcomes. On occasion, faculty may identify patient circumstances that may prevent them from directly supervising all patient care by students. Faculty cannot supervise students caring for patients with neutropenic precautions when overseeing students caring for patients in contact isolation. In this instance, faculty should collaborate with the staff nurse who is responsible for direct oversight of the care provided by the nursing student.

Patient assignments by faculty or students should reflect a wide representation of medical conditions over the clinical rotation. Diverse medical conditions can provide students with opportunities to apply knowledge of specific body systems. Faculty guide students in

---

Exemplar: Enhancing Family-Centered Communication

Lorraine M. Novosel

I worked as a clinical instructor on an inpatient medical unit, supervising a group of fourth-year undergraduate nursing students. Each student was assigned to a registered nurse (RN) preceptor. One student assisted an RN in conducting an intake assessment of an 88-year-old gentleman. He was admitted to the unit after a tiring 14-hour stay in the emergency department. His wife of 62 years and his daughter accompanied him.

I watched as the RN welcomed the patient and his family and helped him settle into the bed. I listened carefully as the RN talked to the patient, and listened just as carefully as she directed the intake questions toward his daughter: "How old is your father?"; "What did he do for a living?"; "How many children does he have?"; "How many people does he need to help him get out of bed and walk?" I stood still and remained quiet. As a faculty member, I was there to observe and guide the student.

The precepting RN then suggested the student complete the intake interview and the student eagerly agreed. Again, I listened carefully as the student directed the patient history questions to the patient's wife: "How active is your husband at home?"; "How many hours of sleep does [he] get each night?" His wife responded, and I, as faculty, redirected the discussion to the patient. I said, "Five or six hours each night? I don't think there is any way I could function if I only got five or six hours of sleep at night!" The patient responded, "Well, that's the way it's been all my life and it works for me. I feel good, except for this little bump on my leg that I got while I was out mowing the lawn. Now that you got me in here, I'm afraid I'm not going to be able to get the job done before the rains come. And next week I've got to paint the outside of the garage."

In our brief exchange, I learned much about the patient. He was a vibrant, 88-year-old gentleman who had an accident outside while he was doing yardwork. His hearing was intact, he could speak clearly, and he understood my words and responded appropriately. He knew quite well how old *he* was, what *he* did for a living, and how many children *he* had. And he didn't need anyone to help him get out of bed and walk.

I stayed with the nursing student, and we completed the intake assessment together. Later, I sat down with the student and asked her what she learned during the encounter. She said she found the gentleman charming, and that she initially "assumed" he couldn't speak for himself. When asked why, the student stated, "Well, I followed what my preceptor did, and she was talking with the daughter." We talked at length about the experience, including making assumptions, as well as the importance of speaking directly to *the patient*. This is particularly important when caring for an older adult. By engaging the patient directly in conversation, we laid a foundation for better patient–nurse communication. It is vitally important for preceptors to remember they are always role-modeling in their words and actions. My hope is that the student will remember the lessons learned from this encounter the next time she observes someone acting on assumptions rather than directly engaging the patient in conversation.

---

knowledge acquisition of pathophysiology and clinical manifestations, as well as understanding pharmacologic and other medical treatments. Additionally, faculty guide students in the implementation of assessment skills, including health history and physical assessment skills.

> The preceptor is instrumental in delegating and designing learning opportunities that incorporate diverse populations.

In addition to a range of medical conditions, well-rounded clinical experiences should incorporate assignments of diverse patients, thereby cultivating knowledge and attitudes that foster patient-centered care. Faculty should consider patient factors that may be specific to

the clinical site or patient population. For example, students in pediatric rotations should have opportunities to care for children across the age spectrum, from infancy through adolescence. Caring for children of differing ages allows students to incorporate developmentally appropriate care. Assignment of students to children across the age spectrum will also expose students to a wider range of medical conditions that are age-specific, acute, or chronic.

Faculty assigning patients should consider diverse patient assignments that expose students to patients with differing values and preferences. Student attitudes are cultivated through the care of patients with various spiritual beliefs, cultural practices, sexual orientation, gender preferences, and economic status. Faculty should guide students in assessing holistic factors that affect patient care and coach students on approaches that support patient preferences. Guidance may include helping students contact appropriate interdisciplinary professionals. For example, providing care for individuals who are homeless challenges students to consider psychosocial needs, including economic resources to access care and essential resources. Since nutrition is influenced by religious practices or cultural preferences, students can collaborate with dieticians or nutritionists to meet patient dietary needs. Mentoring students in assessing and providing gender-sensitive care includes respecting the patient's preferred name and preferences for care. Assigning patients with differing gender preferences or sexual orientation facilitates student knowledge and the formation of positive professional attitudes.

Clinical Skills

A well-rounded clinical experience also incorporates the opportunity for students to implement a range of technical skills, ranging from simple to complex. The preceptor should consider opportunities to apply new skills, as well as the repetition of skills to increase accuracy and efficiency. Medication administration provides a range of skill levels, from the delivery of oral and topical to enteral, injectable, and intravenous medications. Medication administration also provides an excellent opportunity for the preceptor to assess student skill proficiency, as well as the ability to provide safe care.

Undergraduate students implement psychomotor skills as part of routine care for the assigned patient. However, the preceptor should encourage students to seek additional learning opportunities that are available on the clinical unit. Opportunities may arise for students to perform skills, such as performing injections, inserting nasogastric tubes, or managing urinary catheterizations on patients who are not directly assigned to students. Faculty maintain collaborative relationships with staff, encouraging nurses to include students in these additional learning opportunities. Additionally, preceptors can further facilitate learning and a well-rounded experience through shared student experiences. Not all students have an equal opportunity to perform the same type or number of skills during a clinical rotation. Tracheostomy care, urinary catheterizations, administration of a bolus tube feeding, or ostomy care are several examples of skills that may occur on an infrequent basis depending on the clinical unit. By asking a student to assist another peer in completing a skilled procedure, the preceptor can increase the number of students exposed to these learning opportunities.

Faculty will maintain an anecdotal record of the types of patients and specific skills completed by each student for every clinical experience. Anecdotal information is necessary to ensure making subsequent patient assignments that provide for ongoing well-rounded clinical experiences.

TEACHABLE MOMENTS

Teachable moments are valuable in facilitating learning in all nursing students. Teachable moments are circumstances or events that provide the opportunity for students to receive and integrate new knowledge. Such moments may be introduced by the clinical preceptor, or result from an unintended or unanticipated event. Patient falls and medication errors are examples of unintended or unanticipated events that can cause an emotional response from the student. Such circumstances require guidance and support from the clinical preceptor to help the student analyze and reflect on the occurrence. Integration of new learning enhances student growth and prevents future clinical mistakes. When addressing errors in patient care, the clinical preceptor provides feedback in a safe, confidential environment. Reflection by the student is necessary to identify contributing factors for the incident and propose alternative approaches for providing safe care. The clinical preceptor avoids shaming but rather, frames the error as an opportunity for learning and growth.

Teachable moments can be created by the preceptor. Of importance is the use of guided questions to facilitate clinical judgment (Wagner & Ash, 1998). Guided questions go beyond the use of questions that simply ask for recall information. Medication administration is one example where recall still fulfills a vital role by asking the student to identify a drug dosage or classification, describe a mechanism of action, or list important adverse effects. Guided questions, however, go beyond recall, enhancing the development of clinical judgment. A guided question on medication evaluation might ask the student to describe what assessment is needed to determine if the medication is effective, including specific lab or diagnostic results, as well as the follow-up assessment findings that are needed to determine a therapeutic response.

Teachable moments may also arise from students who encounter unique patient circumstances. Novice learners may demonstrate uncertainty in a new or unfamiliar situation, lacking the knowledge or experience for responding in a timely or effective way. Examples might include a patient who demonstrates aggressive or inappropriate behaviors. The student's perception of inadequacy may undermine the student's confidence and hence their ability to integrate new learning. Student behaviors demonstrating anxiety or emotional responses to clinical events should be recognized and addressed by the clinical preceptor as soon as possible after an event. Listening is essential for the preceptor to understand the student's perspective. The clinical preceptor should invite the student to reflect in private or during a postconference to promote reflection and insights that contribute to attitude formation and clinical decision-making (Wagner & Ash, 1998).

Unplanned Clinical Experiences

A well-rounded clinical experience can be enhanced through student participation in unplanned learning opportunities. Spontaneous situations frequently arise on the nursing unit, where patients may be involved in various procedures or diagnostic tests. These activities can occur at the bedside or in a specific hospital department during the clinical day. Students are encouraged by the preceptor to identify and participate in these learning activities when appropriate. As an example, the insertion of a peripherally inserted central catheter (PICC) is a procedure that may be done at the bedside or in the interventional radiology department, depending on the clinical agency. Observation of a PICC line insertion can enhance students' knowledge of the procedure, sterile technique, and indications for insertion, along with necessary nursing assessments needed preinsertion and postinsertion. Knowledge gained from direct observations strengthens a student's understanding and subsequent ability to provide future patient teaching.

Clinical emergencies during the clinical day also contribute to student learning. A cardiac arrest is an infrequent but critical patient event. Such emergencies can generate anxiety in the inexperienced student or novice nurse. The preceptor encourages observation or participation in the resuscitation response based on the level of the learner and the institutional protocol. Additionally, the preceptor provides opportunities individually or

---

Exemplar: Clinical Experience Debriefing With Undergraduate Students

Jennifer M. Brown

I was a new clinical faculty assigned eight undergraduate students on a medical-surgical floor. Each student was assigned a patient and worked with the registered nurse (RN) to complete the physical assessment, administer medications, and provide other patient care needs for an 8-hour shift. One student was assigned a female patient who was admitted with a diagnosis of cardiac murmur. The patient's husband brought her to the hospital the night before and was still at the bedside. I accompanied the student to the patient's room and stayed as the student introduced herself, established rapport with the patient and her husband, and began the patient's assessment. I then left to assist another student. Later, I was urgently called back to the patient's room. The student expressed that while documenting the assessment, she noticed a change in the patient's husband's appearance. He suddenly seemed "out of it," less responsive than earlier, and she sensed something was amiss beyond the stress of his wife's admission. After quickly observing the patient's husband, I, as faculty, immediately called for a code and alerted the RN assigned to the patient. When the code team arrived, I allowed the student and a classmate to observe the code from a safe distance. After the patient's husband was transported from the unit, I quickly pulled the two students to a quiet room for debriefing.

I knew the student's observation, quick thinking, and clinical decision-making led to her swift actions. My goal, however, was to get the student and her classmate to a place where we could debrief the events without interruption. Once there, I asked both students to share their recollections and reactions to the events as they occurred. I allowed them as much time as needed to share their thoughts about what may have caused the events. After reflecting on the chain of events, they agreed the code went well. Still, the student noted how easily she could have missed the signs had she only paid attention to the patient and not engaged with the patient's husband. I reassured her that her keen observation skills, along with the fact that she took time to engage with the caregiver and not just the patient, were the reasons he quickly received emergency care. I shared the value of the teamwork they had witnessed and its importance to nursing. While I knew that I would need to debrief with the entire clinical group, my approach was to ensure that the two students had time to process what they had seen before they were exposed to all the questions that would follow from their classmates.

during postclinical debriefings for students to share their experiences. Reflection is a valuable tool that allows students to process their emotional responses and assimilate new knowledge.

Planned Experiences

Student learning can be augmented through the use of planned special experiences. The type, duration, and degree of student participation in planned learning activities is contingent on the clinical objectives. A formal agreement with the hospital department or clinical agency is generally required to assign students to specialty experiences. Clear learning objectives should be individualized for the specialty experience and understood by both students and department or agency staff. As an example, the preceptor may arrange for a student or limited number of students to participate in a perioperative learning experience during one clinical day as a part of medical-surgical clinical rotation.

Planned specialty experiences can have multiple benefits. A perioperative experience can facilitate the acquisition of knowledge, skills, and attitudes. Perioperative experiences can reinforce classroom concepts, such as surgical asepsis or factors that create a culture of safety, including the surgical time-out. Supervised participation in the immediate preoperative or postoperative assessment can strengthen the student's skills. For example, students gain experience by assessing vital signs, auscultating the heart and lungs, determining outputs from postoperative surgical drains or tubes, or reinforcing postoperative surgical dressings. Observing interprofessional collaboration during the surgical time-out can reinforce the critical role of teamwork and facilitate professional attitude formation.

Other benefits of planned special experiences include the exposure of students to unique clinical settings and nursing roles, and introduce students to future career paths or opportunities. The use of special experiences can facilitate the ability of the preceptor to accommodate additional students while maintaining an appropriate clinical ratio of faculty to students on the clinical unit.

Planned special experiences may be agency- or community-based, and can include:

- An emergency department or cardiac catheterization lab experience for an advanced medical-surgical course
- An experience observing a clinical nurse leader or nursing unit manager for a nursing leadership course

- A hospice home care experience for an adult chronic care nursing course
- An observational experience at a community-based Alcoholics Anonymous meeting for a psychiatric-mental health nursing course
- A prenatal community-based clinic experience for a maternal-child nursing course
- A hospital or community-based pediatric clinic for children with disabilities or cancer for a pediatric nursing course

INTERDISCIPLINARY EXPERIENCES

A knowledge of teamwork and collaboration can be facilitated by planned clinical experiences that incorporate interdisciplinary experiences. Participation by students in unit-based interdisciplinary rounding can facilitate students' understanding of the role of various team members in delivering coordinated, quality patient care. Additionally, the preceptor should encourage students to interact with providers who are involved in the patient's care to foster interprofessional collaboration and coordination of care. Examples of multidisciplinary professionals include:

- Respiratory therapists who administer breathing treatments or care for persons on mechanical ventilation
- Physical therapists who work with orthopedic populations or persons with gait or mobility disorders
- Speech therapists who work with children or adults who experience speech or swallowing impairment from congenital conditions or stroke
- Occupational therapists who work with individuals across the lifespan to learn or regain independence in fine motor skills
- Dieticians who complete nutritional assessments on vulnerable individuals of all ages
- Medical specialists to whom referrals are often made
- Medical imaging or interventional radiology specialists
- Social workers who engage discharge planning or in-home care
- Certified medical interpreters

SIMULATION

A well-rounded clinical experience can be enhanced by the use of simulation. The International Nursing Association for Clinical Simulation and Learning

(INACSL) has defined simulation as "an array of structured activities that represent actual or potential situations in education and practice. These activities allow learners to develop or enhance their knowledge, skills, and attitudes, or to analyze and respond to realistic situations in a simulated environment" (INACSL Standards Committee, 2021) (p. 40.) Substantial existing and emerging evidence supports the use of simulation to promote clinical decision-making and clinical judgment in undergraduate and graduate nursing students (Hayden et al., 2014; Jeffries et al., 2019). Simulation has been shown to improve technical skills, improve student preparation for clinical, and build self-confidence in a safe, controlled environment that allows students to learn from their mistakes (Bridge et al., 2022; Jeffries et al., 2019). Additionally, simulations can provide critical scenarios for learning that may not be encountered during clinical experiences (Perez et al., 2022).

Various simulation modalities have been described in the literature. Low fidelity simulations that use role-play, anatomical models, static manikins, standardized patients, unfolding case studies, or video recordings have long been used in nursing education (Olson et al., 2018; Jeffries et al., 2019). Static manikins can facilitate technical skill development in undergraduate and APRN nursing students. Examples include the insertion of intravenous or urinary catheters by undergraduate students, or the performance of defibrillation, intubation, or chest tube insertion by APRN students. A combination of modalities uses two or more types of simulations to create realistic scenarios. One example is the use of standardized patients and video recordings for undergraduate nursing student physical assessments or standardized patients with free video conferencing to depict telehealth conferences for APRN nursing students. The development of high-fidelity manikins with haptic technology has contributed to a significant growth in the use of simulation in nursing education (Olson et al., 2018). Haptic technology creates the experience of touch for the user by providing vibration or motion.

A scarcity of clinical placements and shortage of qualified faculty have led to changes in regulations by individual state boards of nursing regarding undergraduate nursing programs. These changes permit the substitution of instructional simulation hours for a percentage of clinical patient care hours for undergraduate nursing programs. Instructional simulation hours must meet specific criteria or standards to meet the requirement for substitution. While simulation education enhances clinical judgment and decision-making for APRN students, the NTF on Quality Nurse Practitioner Education states that simulation hours cannot be used to replace the required direct patient care hours (Jeffries et al., 2019).

High-quality simulation experiences are facilitated by qualified nursing faculty and staff development nurses within a hospital system. Clear communication between the preceptor and course faculty facilitates a shared understanding of complementary learning experiences. Preceptors can play a key role in identifying and referring undergraduate and APRN students who would benefit from additional skills practice and simulation experiences to build clinical competence.

▮ CONCLUSION

The ability to provide safe, patient-centered quality nursing care is facilitated by well-rounded clinical experiences for undergraduate and APRN students. Appropriate clinical sites that meet learning objectives are essential in providing well-rounded educational experiences. Attention to planned and unplanned clinical experiences can create teachable moments that enhance learning. The preceptor, in collaboration with faculty, is instrumental in delegating and designing learning opportunities for students to develop the knowledge, skills, and attitudes necessary for competent nursing practice.

REFERENCES

American Association of Colleges of Nursing. (2021). *The Essentials: Core competencies for professional nursing education.* https://www.aacnnursing.org/Portals/42/AcademicNursing/pdf/Essentials-2021.pdf

American Association of Colleges of Nursing Task Force on AACN's Vision for Nursing Education. (2019). *AACN's Vision for Academic Nursing: Executive Summary*. Retrieved from: https://www.aacnnursing.org/Portals/42/News/White-Papers/Vision-Academic-Nursing.pdf

Bridge, P., Adeoye, J., Edge, C. N., Garner, V. L., Humphreys, A.-L., Ketterer, S.-J., Linforth, J. G., Manning-Stanley, A. S., Newsham, D., Prescott, D., Pullan, S. J., & Sharp, J. (2022). Simulated placements as partial replacement of clinical training time: A Delphi consensus study. *Clinical Simulation in Nursing*, 68, 42–48. https://doi.org/10.1016/j.ecns.2022.04.009

Cengiz, A. C., & Yoder, L. H. (2020). Assessing nursing students' perceptions of the QSEN competencies:

A systematic review of the literature with implications for academic programs. *Worldviews on Evidence-Based Nursing, 17*(4), 275–282. https://doi.org/10.1111/wvn.12458

Gigli, K. H., & Gonzalez, J. D. (2022). Meeting the need for nurse practitioner clinicals: A survey of practitioners. *Journal of the American Association of Nurse Practitioners*, Publish Ahead of Print. https://doi.org/10.1097/jxx.0000000000000749

Hayden, J. K., Smiley, R. A., Alexander, M. A., Kardongedgren, S., & Jeffries, P. R. (2014). The NCSBN national simulation study: A longitudinal, randomized, controlled study replacing clinical hours with simulation in prelicensure nursing education. *Journal of Nursing Regulation*(suppl), S3–S40. https://doi.org/10.1016/s2155-8256(15)30062-4

Hunt, D. A., Milani, M. F., & Wilson, S. (2015). Dedicated education units: An innovative model for clinical education. *American Nurse Today, 10*(5), 46–49.

INACSL Standards Committee, & Miller, C., Deckers, C., Jones, M., Wells-Beede, E., & McGee, E.. (2021). Healthcare simulation standards of best practiceTM outcomes and objectives. Clinical Simulation in Nursing, 58, 40–44. https://doi.org/10.1016/j.ecns.2021.08.013

Jeffries, P. R., Bigley, M. B., McNelis, A. M., Cartier, J. M., Pintz, C., Slaven-Lee, P. W., & Zychowicz, M. E. (2019). A call to action: Building evidence for use of simulation in nurse practitioner education. *Journal of the American Association of Nurse Practitioners, 31*(11), 627–632. https://doi.org/10.1097/jxx.0000000000000335

Kohn, L. T., Corrigan, J., & Donaldson, M. S. (2000). *To err is human: Building a safer health system.* National Academy Press.

National Task Force on Quality Nurse Practitioner Education. (2022). *Standards for quality nurse practitioner education* (6th ed.). American Association of Colleges of Nursing; National Organization of Nurse Practitioner Faculties.

Nyoni, C. N., Hugo-Van Dyk, L., & Botma, Y. (2021). Clinical placement models for undergraduate health professions students: A scoping review. *BMC Medical Education, 21*(598). https://doi.org/10.11186/s12909-021-030323-w

Olson, J. K., Paul, P., Lasiuk, G., Davison, S., Wilson-Keates, B., Ellis, R., Marks, N., Nesari, M., & Savard, W. (2018). The state of knowledge regarding the use of simulation in pre-licensure nursing education: A mixed methods systematic review. *International Journal of Nursing Education Scholarship, 15*(1), 1–12. https://doi.org/10.1515/ijnes-2017-0050

Perez, A., Gaehle, K., Sobczak, B., & Stein, K. (2022). Virtual simulation as a learning tool for teaching graduate nursing students to manage difficult conversations. *Clinical Simulation in Nursing, 62*, 66–72. https://doi.org/10.1016/J.ECNS.2021.10.003

Preheim, G. J., Armstrong, G. E., & Barton, A. (2009). The new fundamentals in nursing: Introducing beginning quality and safety education for nurses' competencies. *Journal of Nursing Education, 48*(12), 694–697. https://doi.org/10.3928/01484834-20091113-10

Quality and Safety Education in Nursing. (2022). QSEN.org. https://qsen.org/about-qsen

Wagner, W., & Ash, K. L. (1998). Creating the teachable moment. *Journal of Nursing Education, 37*(6), 278–280. https://doi.org/10.3928/0148-4834-19980901-14

Walker, E., Springer, P. J., Lazare, P., Jensen, N., Clavelle, J. T., Johnson, P. L., & Lind, B. K. (2012). The ABCs of DEUs. *Nursing Management, 43*(12), 38–44. https://doi.org/10.1097/01.NUMA.0000419446.58986.f8

11

Special Considerations When Precepting Nurse Practitioner Students

Celeste M. Schultz, Cynthia A. Danford, and Beth Heuer

CHAPTER OBJECTIVES

- Describe components of faculty site visits
- Review key elements of coding and billing related to student experiences
- Describe progression of skills utilizing RIME framework
- Provide an overview of effective patient care reporting
- Discuss legal implications of precepting, including student and preceptor liability

When preparing a nurse practitioner (NP) student for clinical experiences, a great deal of planning occurs "behind the scenes" between faculty, the clinical site, and the academic institution. There are issues related to site visits, insurance, referrals, coding and billing, telehealth encounters, and legal responsibilities that are often not priorities of the preceptor but require special consideration.

FACULTY SITE VISITS

The faculty site visit is meant to focus on the NP student's overall progress. During the site visit, faculty verify that the types of patients seen in the clinic setting are suitable for meeting course requirements, that course and individual student clinical objectives are being met, and the student is making progress and performing competently with increasing autonomy. In addition, faculty can determine if the student and preceptor are interacting effectively. Site visits should be scheduled early and at a convenient time for the preceptor. However, allowing time for the student and preceptor to establish a working relationship prior to the first visit is recommended. Extra site visits may be scheduled for new preceptors or when students are having trouble. Preceptors may also request that faculty schedule a site visit at any time to help problem-solve concerns. The primary objective of the site visit is to evaluate student progress and preceptor–student interaction, *not* evaluate preceptor performance. During site visits, preceptors can expect faculty to take time observing the student during patient encounters as well as ask questions about the student's progress (Table 11.1).

Not all academic programs require in-person or virtual site visits from faculty unless mandated by state law or other regulations, especially in the case of distance learning programs. Communication technologies, such as video conferencing, email, phone, and group messaging can be utilized to maintain ongoing contact between faculty and preceptors. Technology can also be used to facilitate observation of a student–patient encounter. Faculty must assess whether students are seeing an appropriate volume and variety of patients. Student clinical documentation should also be reviewed by faculty throughout the rotation to augment assessment of progress towards meeting course and national NP competencies.

TABLE 11.1	What Preceptors of Nurse Practitioner Students Should Expect During Faculty Site Visits
Faculty questions for preceptors	• Does the student arrive on time and remain on site for the full duration of the clinical experience? • Does the student conduct themselves in a professional manner with patients and staff? • Does the student interact with their patients in a caring and professional manner? • Does the student present the H&P, patient complaint, assessment, differential diagnosis and treatment plan to the preceptor after seeing the patient? • Does the student see a variety of patients and is able to see a full complement of patents during a clinical day? • Does the student discuss with the preceptor patient management, protocols, guidelines, treatment options and nurse practitioner documentation? • Does the student have any issues that the faculty and preceptor need to address?
Faculty observations of students	• Does the faculty observe effective communication between staff members, student and preceptor • Is the student receiving positive feedback and constructive criticism from the preceptor? • Is the student integrating exemplary clinical skills and professional ethical behavior? • Is the student utilizing evidence-based practice (EBP) resources and seeking additional information? • Is the student exhibiting the level of autonomy expected for the assigned rotation? Are they learning to work independently? • Does the student see patients within the allotted time given? • Is the student accurately documenting the patient visit?

Courtesy Amy Bieda, PhD, RN.

CLINIC OPERATIONAL PROCESSES

In acclimating the student to the clinical site, the preceptor provides a description of the general patient population served. This description includes the overall socioeconomic status, age range, gender identification, race, ethnicity, and level of health literacy. Insurance coverage and referral processes may be introduced or reviewed with NP students, who may not be familiar with utilizing this information in creating a plan of treatment.

Patient Insurance Coverage

Students benefit from discussions about types of healthcare insurance coverage, (e.g., Medicare, Medicaid, private, fee for service/cash, or free services). They utilize this information differently in the NP role when considering the need for consultations and diagnostic testing, as well as prescribing medications. In this discussion, preceptors review what services are allowed and covered, as well as where information about insurance coverage can be located.

With attention to confidentiality, preceptors can role-model patient communication about insurance coverage for healthcare treatments and medications to enhance student learning.

The Referral Process

In outpatient and inpatient specialty areas, a beneficial experience for the NP student is participating in the process for referrals or consultations. Review of the process includes: 1) assuring the referral/consulation is appropriate and necessary, 2) documentation in the medical record is accurate and reflects the need, and 3) communication with the new provider is complete. The preceptor may also invite the student to observe a peer-to-peer review with the insurer to justify the need for the referral.

CODING AND BILLING FOR THE NURSE PRACTITIONER STUDENT

During clinical experience, preceptors have a prime opportunity to introduce NP students to the intricacies

TABLE 11.2 Coding Terminology for Nurse Practitioner Students

Code Set	Abbreviation	Purpose
Current Procedure Terminology	CPT	Procedures and services
CPT Evaluation/ Management	CPT-E/M	Specific subset of codes for services provided by qualified providers, including NPs. There are four levels of outpatient E/M codes for new patients and five levels for established patients. Coding levels increase as care delivery needs increase
International Classification of Diseases, 10th Revision, Clinical Modification	ICD-10-CM	Diagnosis and health status in the U.S.
Healthcare Common Procedure Coding System	HCPCS	Level 1: Synonymous with CPT codes Level 2: Medications, supplies, equipment

Adapted from Bischof, A. L. (2023). Understanding the 2021 evaluation and management coding guidelines. *The Nurse Practitioner, 48*(2), 6–12.

of practice management. One critical area of practice management is coding and billing and understanding the relevant terminology (Table 11.2). Including the NP student in determination of proper codes with each patient encounter will facilitate understanding related to this complex process. Improper coding can lead to decreased revenue *or* concerns about fraudulent billing practices. Additionally, coding and billing is used to quantify productivity for providers. Preceptors can review the importance of how documentation supports reimbursement. Attention to coding and billing helps NP students think about and build organizational skills as they transition to independent clinical practice.

Coding and billing discussion points for preceptors to review include identification and assignment of appropriate ICD-10 diagnostic codes (e.g., J02.0 streptococcal pharyngitis), CPT-E/M codes based on medical complexity or time spent (Codes 99202-99215), and any codes for procedures (e.g., cerumen removal). In addition, preceptors can discuss the differences in preventive and episodic codes for new and established patients and the amount of time spent in counseling during the office visit (e.g., more than 25 minutes out of 30 minutes spent in counseling). Further, a modifier (e.g., additional 25 minutes) may be used to append a visit for reimbursement due to additional time addressing a significant illness, abnormality, or condition (The Bright Futures/American Academy of Pediatrics, 2022). Preceptors may consider disclosing reimbursement amounts from private and public insurers to distinguish payment differences (Shanahan et al., 2022; Suzewits, 2003). With guidance from preceptors and faculty, NP students should graduate from their programs confident in choosing appropriate billing codes to maximize revenue and accurately reflect provided services (Bischof, 2023).

PRESENTING PATIENT CLINICAL INFORMATION

Development of case presentation skills is a core component in clinical nursing education. Not all nurses have the opportunity to develop concise patient handoff or reporting skills during their baccalaureate education or in their primary clinical work setting. Preceptors can educate NP students on developing effective reporting skills by consistently providing a short, accurate snapshot of the patient's presenting concerns, history, physical examination, and recommendations. Encouraging students to practice repeatedly and providing consistent feedback helps NP students solidify this skill. The OLDCARTS and OPQRST mnemonics are useful in characterizing the patient's chief complaint and may be inclusive of subjective information from the review of systems (ROS). These mnemonics can be utilized to help the student present comprehensive information to the preceptor in an organized manner (Box 11.1). Two additional and frequently used mnemonics for clinical presentation skills are SBAR (situation, background, assessment, recommendation) and SNAPPS (See Chapter 8).

SBAR

The SBAR mnemonic stands for Situation, Background, Assessment, and Recommendation. SBAR provides a consistent and concise framework for the discussion of patient information (Singh et al., 2017). However, when using SBAR, important social information may be missed, such as family dynamics and health literacy.

- **S**ituation: observations and concerns
- **B**ackground: patient diagnosis and current treatment plan
- **A**ssessment: subjective and objective data related to the problem
- **R**ecommendation: changes in treatment plan

PROGRESSION IN CLINICAL PERFORMANCE

The RIME Framework

The RIME framework is utilized in medical education to guide both teaching and evaluation as medical students and residents progress in the clinical setting (Pangaro, 1999; Ogburn & Espey, 2003). This framework can also be utilized to assess NP student readiness for independence (Johnson et al., 2022). The elements of the RIME framework are presented as a logical progression of the student role, with clinical skills building on each prior element.

1. **Reporter:** The NP student gathers comprehensive patient information, communicates effectively to the preceptor, and accurately documents findings in the EHR.
2. **Interpreter:** NP student interprets data, prioritizes information, and analyzes patient problems. At this stage, the student is still learning to identify differential diagnoses and develop plans of care.
3. **Manager:** The NP student autonomously develops differential diagnoses and evidence-based plans of care incorporating patient preferences.
4. **Educator:** The NP student demonstrates consistent knowledge and application of current evidence to patient care, with the ability to effectively teach patients, family, and staff.

   Note: This framework has also been presented as ORIME, with the "O" standing for the observer, who shadows and engages in passive learning.

BOX 11.1 Assessment Mnemonic Tools

Students are directed to use a systematic approach to gaining pertinent information from the patient when assessing chief complaints. The following mnemonic tools are introduced in undergraduate nursing programs, and remain helpful to advanced practice registered nurses:

OLD CARTS
Onset
Location
Duration
Character
Aggravating/alleviating factors
Radiation
Timing
Severity

OPQRST
Onset
Provocative/palliative
Quality/quantity
Region/radiation
Severity/scale
Timing (frequency/duration)

TELEHEALTH CONSIDERATIONS

Precepting Students Using Telehealth

Susan Nickel Van Cleve

Nurse practitioner (NP) students and faculty are struggling to find high-quality clinical sites and preceptorships. One way to broaden NP student experiences is for preceptors to involve NP students in telehealth visits. Since the COVID-19 pandemic, the use of telehealth has skyrocketed, with telehealth visits being conducted throughout different types of health systems. Telehealth has multiple benefits, including increasing access to care, improving health equity, and providing patients and clinicians with real-time interactions conducted easily from home. When using a telehealth format, several elements should be considered:

PREPARATION

When preparing for the telehealth visit with an NP student, the following questions need to be addressed:

- Will the student be present with the preceptor in the office, or will the student be at a remote location during the telehealth visits?
  - If both student and preceptor are in the same office, strategies on how each will interact with the patient need to be determined.
  - If at different locations, can the telehealth format allow for a three-way connection (to include the student) versus a two-way connection with only the patient and provider? If a three-way connection is possible, it is important to practice ahead of time using the technology.

THE PATIENT ENCOUNTER

- What is the best way to obtain permission from the patient for the student to participate in the telehealth visit?
  - Should contact be made ahead of time to obtain permission?
  - Who will make this contact and how will it be documented in the electronic medical record (EMR)?
- How will the student participate in the telehealth visit?
  - Will the NP student lead the history?
  - Will the NP student inquire about the review of systems and address components of the physical examination?
- How will the preceptor and student allow for a private discussion of differential diagnoses and clinical decision-making before presenting the plan of care to the patient and family?

FOLLOW-UP

- Scheduled time outside of telehealth visits to review patients, conditions, documentation, and student performance is needed. These sessions should be frequent and provide the NP student with time for questions, debriefing and feedback.

Exemplar: Precepting Students Using Telehealth

Susan Nickel Van Cleve

During the COVID-19 pandemic, I transitioned my integrated behavioral and pediatric mental health pediatric practice to a remote telehealth model. During this time, I was able to precept several students using telehealth. Before conducting any visits, I met with each student virtually and reviewed the types of patients I see, types of visits I conduct, and conditions I commonly manage. I provided an overview of interventions used to treat the most common disorders. Each student received the most recent evidence-based treatment guidelines, presentations handouts summarizing these conditions, and my most commonly used resources. I also reviewed the behavior rating scales we use and how to score them.

Prior to the visit, the student and I practiced using the telehealth technology. One of the biggest challenges was providing student access to the patient electronic medical record (EMR) when both of us were remote. At times, I had to read pertinent sections of the EMR to the student before the visit.

As we began each telehealth session, I introduced the student to the patient and family. The student would conduct the history, any relevant exam, and provide feedback on behavior rating scales. After the student became more comfortable with the encounter format and patient diagnoses, they were encouraged to share their diagnostic impression and develop the treatment plan. There were times when the student was clearly struggling, so I would jump in and complete the visit.

During the visit, the student documented the visit information in a Word document and securely emailed it to me after the visit. This enabled us to more easily review the information and modify as needed. Due to time constraints, we usually completed these reviews at the end of the day. The students appreciated learning to use telehealth as part of their NP educational experience.

LEGAL IMPLICATIONS WHEN PRECEPTING NURSE PRACTITIONER STUDENTS

Two legal questions related to who is responsible for care when precepting NP students include: 1) Who is ultimately responsible for the care that the NP student provides to the patient? and 2) Who is ultimately responsible for documenting the patient's condition and healthcare? Individually or in combination, the student, the preceptor, the nursing program, or the institution may be responsible.

Faculty clearly provide expectations of the student and preceptor, as well as nursing program course objectives. Student expectations include performing a clinically relevant history and physical assessment, determining appropriate differential diagnoses, developing an appropriate management and follow-up plan, and accurately documenting the patient encounter. Preceptor expectations include being available to the student, incorporating experiences to facilitate student understanding, encouraging clinical judgment, as well as overseeing and critiquing student performance. Objectives may vary by nursing course and level of student.

Preceptors are legally, professionally, and academically accountable for preparing safe, competent healthcare providers (Luhanga et al., 2010). Scope of practice, which has a significant impact on liability, is legislatively defined by each state and is also subject to hospital rules, policies, and bylaws (Szalados, 2021).

Preceptor liability related to students is described as *supervisory* liability. Whether or not the preceptor is directly involved in patient contact, providing patient care, or teaching patients, they are still responsible for the actions of the NP student they are supervising (Szalados, 2021). Students are held to the same professional standards as that of the preceptors. Thus, the student and preceptor can be jointly liable for malpractice arising from patient care.

According to the nurse's code of ethics (Fowler, 2015), preceptors share responsibility and accountability for the care provided by students when they make clinical assignments. The knowledge and skill of the student must be *sufficient* to provide the assigned care under appropriate supervision. Legal responsibilities of the preceptor include:

- Selecting appropriate activities based on learning objectives
- Determining that students have the prerequisite knowledge, skills, and attitude necessary to complete their assignments (Fowler, 2015)
- Providing appropriate guidance and supervision (Cherry & Jacob, 2002; Gaberson & Oermann, 1999)
- Delegating tasks that the student is *properly trained* to perform; the preceptor cannot delegate activities that are prohibited by their state nurse practice acts

Preceptors must acknowledge when student performance is unsatisfactory or unsafe. There is a disturbing trend in nursing education literature called "failure to fail," where reluctance to report unsatisfactory student performance persists despite the need to safeguard the public and ensure adequate standards of practice (Adkins & Adcoin, 2022). Simply stated, "failure to fail" means passing a student who cannot adequately demonstrate safe and competent clinical practice. Some preceptors and faculty are uncomfortable when directly confronting a student who is performing poorly and do not clearly articulate the concern. Reasons for avoiding confrontation vary from worrying about the student's reaction to lacking confidence in how to approach a difficult conversation with a student (Dibble, 2014). Concrete examples of the student's deficiencies will enhance clarity during discussions and/or summative evaluations (See Chapter 21).

An unsafe student compromises patient safety and public trust for the nursing profession (Brown et al., 2019). The long-term consequences for the student who has not received an honest evaluation may end in future failure (e.g., course failure, certification examination failure, future employment failure, disciplinary board action) (Litten, et al., 2023). Preceptors play an integral role in identifying students at-risk for unsafe practice and with the assistance of the faculty, provide effective guidance. The end result is assurance that the preceptor has done everything to safeguard future patients and families and contribute to preparing a competent and safe student, better prepared for providing effective health care for the public. In addition, the risk for legal action against the preceptor and faculty is minimized due to "failing to fail" an unsafe or incompetent student (Chasens et al., 2000; Osinski, 2003; Smith et al., 2001).

REFERENCES

Adkins, D. A., & Aucoin, J. W. (2022). Failure to fail—Factors affecting faculty decisions to pass underperforming nursing students in the clinical setting: A quantitative study. *Nurse Education in Practice*, 58, 103259. https://doi.org/10.1016/j.nepr.2021.103259

Bischof, A. L. (2023). Understanding the 2021 evaluation and management coding guidelines. *The Nurse Practitioner*, 48(2), 6–12. https://doi.org/10.1097/01.npr.0000000000000007

Brown, H., Lisk, L. E., & Scruth, E. A. (2019). Applying an ethical approach to building great preceptorships. *Clinical Nurse Specialist*, 33(6), 250–252. https://doi.org/10.1097/nur.0000000000000479

Chasens, E. R., DePew, D. D., Goudreau, K. A., & Pierce, C. (2000). Legal aspect of grading and student progression. *Journal of Professional Nursing*, 16(5), 267–272.

Cherry, B., & Jacob, S. R. (2002). *Contemporary nursing: Issues, trends & management* (2nd ed.). St. Louis: Mosby.

Dibble, J.L. (2014). Breaking good and bad news: Face-implicating concerns as mediating the relationship between news valence and hesitation to share the news. Communication Studies, 65(3), 223–243. https://doi.org/10.1080/10510974.2013.811431

Fowler, M. (2015). *Guide to the code of ethics for nurses with interpretive statements: Development, interpretation, and application* (2nd ed.). American Nurses Association.

Gaberson, K. B., & Oermann, M. (1999). *Clinical teaching strategies in nursing.* New York: Springer.

Johnson, H. L., Beatty, J. R., Archer, H. R., Best, N. I., Trautmann, J. L., Williams, J. K., Williamson, J. M., Seibert, D. C., & Taylor, L. A. (2022). Applying the RIME framework to level nurse practitioner curriculum competencies. *Nurse Educator*, 48(1), 43–48. https://doi.org/10.1097/nne.0000000000001258

Litten, K.P., McQuade, B.M., Wettergreen, S.A., Nardolillo, J.A, & Stewart, M.P. (2023). Failure to fail—Perspective from junior faculty preceptors on the challenges of evaluating underperforming students in the experiential learning environment. Currents in Pharmacy Teaching and Learning, 15(3), 238–241. https://doi.org/10.1016/j.cptl.2023.03.002

Luhanga, F., Myrick, F., & Yonge, O. (2010). The preceptorship experience: An examination of ethical and accountability issues. *Journal of Professional Nursing, 26*(5), 264–271. https://doi.org/10.1016/j.profnurs.2009.12.008

Ogburn, T., & Espey, E. (2003). The R-I-M-E method for evaluation of medical students on an obstetrics and gynecology clerkship. *American Journal of Obstetrics and Gynecology, 189*(3), 666–669. https://doi.org/10.1067/s0002-9378(03)00885-8

Osinski, K. (2003). Due process rights of students in cases of misconduct. *Journal of Nursing Education, 42*(2), 55–58. https://doi.org/10.3928/0148-4834-20030201-05

Pangaro, L. (1999). A new vocabulary and other innovations for improving descriptive in-training evaluations. *Academic Medicine, 74*(11), 1203–1207. https://doi.org/10.1097/00001888-199911000-00012

Shanahan, T. D., Gurley, L. E., Chatman, S. H., & Cunningham, J. L. (2022). Promoting understanding of medical decision making coding for nurse practitioner students. *Journal of the American Association of Nurse Practitioners, 34*(11), 1235–1241. https://doi.org/10.1097/JXX.0000000000000789

Singh, D., Purva, M., & Gupta, S. (2017). SBAR (Situation, Background, Assessment, Recommendation)—An exploration of transfer of learning to clinical workplace. *Metric Journal, 2*(1), 8–11.

Smith, M., McKoy, Y., & Richardson, J. (2001). Legal issues related to dismissing students for clinical deficiencies. *Nurse Educator, 26*(1), 33–38. https://doi.org/10.1097/00006223200101000-00015

Suzewits, J. (2003). Medical student education in practice management. *Family Medicine, 35*(10), 697–698

Szalados, J. E. (2021). Laws and liability relating to the education and supervision of trainees and allied health professionals In J. Szalados (Ed.), *The medical-legal aspects of acute care medicine: a resource for clinicians, administrators, and risk managers* (pp. 171–190). Springer. https://doi.org/10.1007/978-3-030-68570-6

The Bright Futures/American Academy of Pediatrics (2022). *Coding for Pediatric Care 2022.* https://downloads.aap.org/AAP/PDF/Coding%20Preventive%20Care.pdf

12

Precepting the Undergraduate and Graduate-Entry Nursing Student

Celeste M. Schultz, Beth Heuer, and Cynthia A. Danford

CHAPTER OBJECTIVES

- Identify similarities and differences in precepting prelicensure students from various pathways
- Understand the process and structure around precepting students in various settings
- Recognize teaching strategies to promote clinical judgment
- Recognize strategies to augment learning experiences, as well as preceptor–faculty relationships

There are several educational paths to licensure as a registered nurse (RN). Students graduating from a traditional program may be receiving a bachelor of science in nursing (BSN), associate degree in nursing (ADN), or a diploma. RN to BSN programs provide the option for nurses to advance their education, often while working full time. Graduate entry (GE) programs may be referred to as "accelerated option" or "second degree" nursing programs, and may enroll international students who have completed advanced degrees in other fields. Students from these educational programs present with similar yet distinct challenges for preceptors. Each learner brings knowledge that may differ based on educational preparation and life experiences. This chapter focuses on precepting "traditional" and GE students.

Preceptors may find that traditional students are more amenable to constructive criticism and exploration of alternative learning strategies when applying nursing content in patient care settings. Preceptors may also find that GE students tend to be less flexible in learning and applying nursing content in the clinical setting. The difference in learning style may be a result of GE students bringing prior life experiences and maturity in understanding diverse life situations, as well as confidence in their abilities (Jarden et al., 2021).

Moreover, GE students typically prefer one mode of learning (e.g., active experimentation) compared to traditional students, who prefer and are more comfortable with multiple modes (McKenna et al., 2018). As a result, traditional and GE students have different learning preferences and require different teaching styles during their clinical practicum. A conversation addressing learning style during orientation to the clinical setting can help set the stage for a productive preceptor–learner experience (refer to Chapters 6 and 7). To individualize student experiences, learning objectives need to be clearly delineated.

UNDERGRADUATE NURSING PROGRAM OUTCOMES

Nursing programs determine student learning outcomes based on the American Association of Colleges of Nursing (AACN) *Essentials: Core Competencies for Nursing Education* (AACN, 2021). The Commission on Collegiate Nursing Education (CCNE) evaluates that program learning outcomes reflect the competencies, knowledge, values, or skills attained by students (CCNE, 2018). Awareness of entry-level nursing program outcomes can help guide preceptor–learner interactions. Examples include the following.

Students will:

- Assume accountability for the autonomous provision of generalist nursing practice.
- Engage with clients to improve outcomes through health promotion across the lifespan and the continuum of care.
- Use primary, secondary, and tertiary levels of prevention to maximize quality of life and prevent disease.
- Demonstrate principles of collaboration with interprofessional team members, patients, and families to resolve complex health problems and promote, improve, or optimize health.
- Engage in ethical professional practice.
- Apply evidence-based practice (EBP) and research findings to improve nursing care and the healthcare system.
- Incorporate knowledge of developmental processes in the design of care.
- Exhibit leadership attributes in a variety of settings to improve health outcomes.
- Utilize informatics to recognize, locate, evaluate, store, and classify information to mitigate errors and support clinical decision-making.
- Participate in service learning.
- Demonstrate professionalism by accepting responsibility and accountability for nursing practice, patient outcomes, and a commitment to lifelong learning.
- Foster healthy communities through health promotion and advocacy that is informed by local and global perspectives (Adapted from: Nursing BSN Accreditation, Temple University, n.d.).

LOGISTICS OF PRECEPTING IN DIVERSE CLINICAL SETTINGS

Nursing program faculty typically have ongoing, collaborative relationships with preceptors and unit managers in a variety of clinical sites. Student clinical experiences are scheduled by designated clinical placement coordinators or directly by faculty (Kamolo et al., 2017). Faculty often function in the clinical instructor role, and collaborate with preceptors to facilitate students' clinical learning experience (Shellenbarger & Robb, 2016). Preceptors do not work with students in isolation, but interface regularly with faculty throughout each clinical day.

Traditional and GE clinical practicums typically involve rotating to various sites, including inpatient units, outpatient clinics, and community settings, such as federally qualified health centers, public health departments, immunization clinics, and schools. Students may also be afforded the opportunity to participate in national or international learning experiences in underserved areas. Nursing electives allow students to have precepted experiences in specialty clinical areas, including the emergency department, perioperative, oncology, hospice or palliative care, rehabilitation, and global health (Smith, 2022).

AMBULATORY CARE EXPERIENCES

Preparing nurses for roles beyond acute care inpatient settings is highlighted in the *Essentials: Core Competencies for Professional Nursing Education* (AACN, 2021). With more nurses entering ambulatory care, precepted prelicensure experiences are needed (Wojnar & Whelan, 2017). For successful ambulatory care experiences, clear perimeters need to be defined. Clarifying expectations and boundaries can be accomplished by explicitly defining specific skills that nursing students are permitted to perform in the clinics, as well as verifying clinical objectives. A focused orientation can also set the stage for an effective experience between both preceptor and student. Frequent follow-up with preceptors by faculty helps to diminish anxiety experienced by preceptors (Fritz et al., 2020).

Preceptors can introduce students to issues of population health, equitable healthcare, and social determinants of health (Fritz et al., 2020; Woodward et al., 2022). Experiences with phone triage are unique and often not covered in academic programs. Toward the end of their clinical experience, students benefit from precepted experiences in specialty areas, such as chemotherapy centers and urgent care (Fritz et al., 2020). Blended environments have been suggested, where students participate in more than one setting within one practice (Park et al., 2019).

SERVICE LEARNING EXPERIENCES

Service learning is an educational method that actively engages students in organized reflection and community service to meet needs and diversify learning experiences. As one type of authentic learning environment, it provides students with immersion in real-world settings for application of classroom knowledge and skills. Preceptors working in public health settings may be actively engaged with students in service learning experiences.

Exemplar: Care of Vulnerable Populations: Understanding the Homeless Community

Dr. Judith M. Fouladbakhsh

When I precept undergraduate community health nursing students and meet them for the first time, I typically see concern and hesitation in their faces about the upcoming clinical experience. Vastly different from previous clinical experiences within specific and often confined healthcare environments, we venture into diverse community neighborhoods, homeless shelters, and street-corner encounters. I discuss what to expect at each site and encourage the nursing students to openly express their concerns and expectations. It is critically important that I identify what students envision for this experience, and recognize their biases, beliefs, and values. I ask thought-provoking questions such as, "How do we begin to understand the journey into homelessness?", and "Are these individuals just addicts or criminals who have avoided responsibility in their lives? Or have they fallen on hard times due to job loss, economic downfall, and more?"

As a preceptor, I begin to explore the nursing students' perceptions and beliefs about their field experiences with those who are homeless. Illuminating the diversity of life experience increases their awareness and empathy, thereby highlighting the importance of holistic nursing care. These learning experiences are welcomed by most students. Their interest in learning about diverse cultures, family dynamics, community groups, and availability of resources is evident.

One winter day, a 62-year-old woman with severe cardiac disease arrived at the shelter following her hospital discharge, using her walker to ambulate through the snow. Her medical history revealed she was on a blood thinner and multiple other medications. The nursing students were anxious and fearful for her safety as they questioned how she became homeless and why she was navigating snow-covered streets with her walker. This woman revealed that she had been evicted from her home during her hospital stay. The students listened supportively as this homeless guest shared her story and showed photos of her extended family. In processing the history, the students provided evidence-based care tailored to maximize her safety, assessed and assured proper medication use, safe mobility, nutrition guidance, and transportation for healthcare visits. During the postclinical seminar, the students questioned why, despite her current situation, this guest was seemingly proud of and engaged with her family. They struggled with their perception that she was "abandoned" by her family.

As preceptor, my role was to promote the exploration of student feelings, values, and biases about homelessness. Sharing observations and emotional reactions helps students to understand the patient's situation, reduces bias, and subsequently fosters evidence-based clinical judgments. I modeled interactions with all of the homeless shelter guests to strengthen perceptions of holistic nursing care, maximizing understanding of each individual's decisions and current situation. The students were encouraged to listen with empathy, process the guests' stories, and address health concerns without bias. I promoted learning about communities and families and addressing needs of diverse vulnerable populations from a holistic integrative community model of care. Finally, we highlighted and honored the essence of community health nursing by addressing needs, collaborating with the homeless shelter team, and engaging with the shelter guests.

However, because not all nursing courses are affiliated with authentic learning experiences, it is possible students may not see service learning course content as applicable to their future careers or may not feel comfortable translating didactic course content to a community setting (Horning et al., 2020). The preceptor has the unique opportunity to bridge classroom knowledge with service learning to facilitate public healthcare.

INTERPROFESSIONAL EXPERIENCES

Interprofessional education (IPE) provides an opportunity for collaboration across disciplines and can occur in all settings, whether inpatient or community-based (Institute of Medicine, 2010). Consequently, nurse preceptors may be invited to interact with students from other disciplines. In nursing, collaboration may occur with pharmacy, medicine, dentistry, and social work professionals and students, leading to new and varying perspectives on patient care. The nurse preceptor guides clinical education with the nursing student while facilitating interprofessional experiences between the student and other members of the healthcare team (Woolforde et al., 2022). (Figure 12.1).

Increased understanding of communication, teamwork, and the interconnectedness of professional roles are key outcomes of IPE, in addition to increased readiness and self-confidence in the clinical role (Figure 12.2)

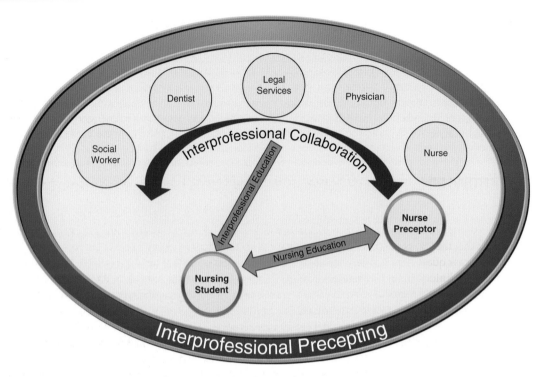

Fig. 12.1 Interprofessional precepting model. (Data from Woolforde, L., Mercado, N. R., Pawelczak, M., Callahan, B., & Block, L. (2022). Interprofessional precepting: A nursing–medicine partnership. *Journal for Nurses in Professional Development*, *38*(5), 302–307.)

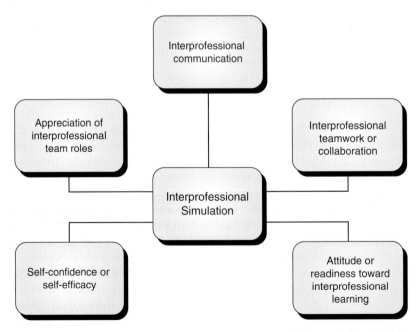

Fig. 12.2 Interprofessional simulation. (Modified from Labrague, L. J., McEnroe–Petitte, D. M., Fronda, D. C., & Obeidat, A. A. (2018). Interprofessional simulation in undergraduate nursing program: An integrative review. *Nurse Education Today, 67*, 46–55.)

(Interprofessional Education Collaborative, 2022; Temple & Mast, 2016). To be effective, barriers need to be minimized and facilitators optimized. The preceptor may be engaging students with a variety of experiences, including novice nursing students and seasoned medical students in residency rotations. Understanding the roles and expectations of students in their respective roles will facilitate a collaborative experience for all (Leubbers et al., 2017).

BUILDING KNOWLEDGE AND EVIDENCE-BASED SKILLS

Faculty and preceptors need to develop a relationship with students such that there is mutual trust and respect. All parties are free to ask questions and provide feedback to students to build clinical judgment, clinical skills, and confidence (Kantar, 2021). Faculty and preceptors need to review the content of health education, as well as its developmental and health-literacy appropriateness prior to presentation to patients and families. Faculty or preceptors should be present during health-related education to support students and clarify any information. Faculty and possibly preceptors may also need to assist students with the use of the electronic health record (EHR) and review the student's documentation for completeness. This review is an opportune time to gain insight into the student's understanding of the patient's condition and to emphasize the importance of accurate documentation.

EVIDENCE-BASED PRACTICE

Evidence-based practice (EBP) must be addressed and integrated into the clinical experience (Melnyk et al., 2018). When reviewing patient charts and preparing for patient care, preceptors and faculty can facilitate students thinking about what evidence will guide their actions and interactions. Preceptors can guide students by directing them to unit or institution policy and guidelines or research relevant to a specific patient population and illness. Preceptors and faculty can remind students to ask themselves "what" and "why" questions related to all nursing activities. "What" refers to an action, activity, or intervention, and "why" refers to the rationale or evidence regarding whether the action is necessary, important, and safe given the patient's condition. If the student cannot clearly discuss

the "what" and "why" questions related to any type of nursing care with the patient or family, then the preceptor and faculty need to facilitate clinical judgment in the student to build their rationale. Once the rationale is developed, students can be redirected to further explore the literature. Similar to administering medications, all interactions with patients must be justified to maintain patient safety, promote patient and family health, and support the profession and science of nursing. Preceptors who role-model the process of applying or connecting didactic knowledge and evidence with actual clinical practice are contributing to a sustainable EBP culture (Melnyk et al., 2021). Regular exposure to EBP will help students systematically incorporate the clinical judgment process in their role as a student and, in the future, as a nurse.

HELPING STUDENTS STRUCTURE NURSING CARE

A concept in helping students organize their nursing care is called *cognitive stacking*, which refers to workflow processes for prioritization and time management. Cognitive stacking involves determining the level, type, and delivery of necessary care given available resources and time. Nurses require mental flexibility as they constantly reorganize tasks when higher priority items arise. Mental flexibility requires practice; the inability to do so results in frustration for both student and preceptor. Being organized involves developing basic routines for each clinical day. Inpatient nurse routines include: 1) obtaining patient assignments, 2) receiving patient handoffs, 3) reviewing EHRs, 4) performing patient assessments, 5) administering scheduled medications, 6) documenting, and, 7) providing patient handoff to the incoming nurse (Kohtz et al., 2017).

Prioritization

Prioritizing patient care is a necessary, albeit overwhelming, skill for students to master. Preceptors guide students as they learn to sort their core responsibilities from other activities. Core responsibilities include: completing patient assessments, administering medications, performing dressing changes and treatments, and admitting and discharging patients. Important yet often less-urgent tasks include: documenting, assisting team members, providing patient and family teaching, organizing and restocking supplies; and taking personal

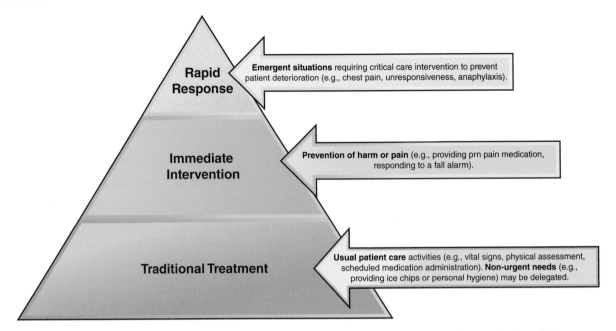

Fig. 12.3 Prioritizing patient care with undergraduate students. Preceptors help students apply theoretical content while prioritizing patient care needs in real time. This hierarchy can be used by preceptors to facilitate prioritization and delegation of patient care needs. Low priority needs may be delegated in the event of a more critical situation.

time for breaks (Kohtz et al., 2017; Nelson et al., 2006). Students can learn to prioritize their patient care using the hierarchy in Figure 12.3.

Delegation

Another aspect of cognitive stacking is delegation, which is a component of effective prioritization. Delegation is the process by which a nursing task or activity is assigned from one person, normally a higher authority, to another (Barrow & Sharma, 2022; Clarke, 2021). In nursing, this includes assigning patient care activities to unlicensed, certified assistive personnel, such as certified nurse assistants or patient care technicians.

Students, especially those with minimal work experience prior to entering their educational program, may need practice in developing confidence in their delegation skills. Delegation requires excellent interpersonal relationships and effective communication techniques (Barrow & Sharma, 2022).

The nursing code of ethics (Fowler, 2015) notes that delegation is based on the RN's judgment concerning a

> **BOX 12.1   The Five Rights of Delegation**
>
> 1. Right task
> 2. Right circumstance
> 3. Right person
> 4. Right supervision
> 5. Right direction and communication

From Barrow, J. M., & Sharma, S. (2022). *Nursing five rights of delegation.* NCBI; StatPearls Publishing.

patient's condition, the competence of all members of the nursing team, and the degree of supervision required. Components of delegation include accountability, authority, and responsibility. The delegator always maintains accountability for completion of nursing tasks. Box 12.1 lists the five rights of delegation. There are legal and ethical constraints to delegation. State nurse practice acts and institutional policies and procedures prescribe who can delegate, and related role expectations. Preceptors role-model delegation skills and have ongoing opportunities to discuss appropriate use of delegation with students.

THE END OF THE CLINICAL DAY

Following the daily clinical experience, preceptors and nursing faculty need to meet with students to debrief. During debriefing, faculty or preceptors review patient diagnoses and plans of care to broaden students' understanding of multiple different diagnoses. Debriefing is also an opportune time to facilitate discussion regarding students' social, emotional, physical, and cognitive response in caring for patients (Shellenbarger & Robb, 2016). At the end of the clinical day, the student is able to practice handoff communication skills with the preceptor and receive constructive feedback.

Preceptors and faculty should also meet to discuss their own supervisory experiences and develop goals and strategies for future precepting experiences. Overall, collaborative interaction among the preceptor, faculty, and students throughout a clinical experience will pave the way for a strong nursing workforce.

REFERENCES

American Association of Colleges of Nursing. (2021). *The Essentials: Core competencies for professional nursing education.* https://www.aacnnursing.org/essentials

Barrow, J. M., & Sharma, S. (2022). *Nursing five rights of delegation.* NCBI: StatPearls Publishing. https://www.ncbi.nlm.nih.gov/books/NBK519519/

Clarke, H. (2021). How pre-registration nursing students acquire delegation skills: A systematic literature review. *Nurse Education Today, 106,* 105096. https://doi.org/10.1016/j.nedt.2021.105096

Commission on Collegiate Nursing Education. (2018). *Standards for accreditation of baccalaureate and graduate nursing programs.* https://www.aacnnursing.org/Portals/42/CCNE/PDF/Standards-Final-2018.pdf

Fowler, M. (2015). *Guide to the code of ethics for nurses with interpretive statements: Development, interpretation, and application* (2nd ed.). American Nurses Association.

Fritz, E., Hanson, K., & Hoeft, M. (2020). Pre-licensure nursing students in ambulatory care: Lessons learned. *AAACN Viewpoint, 42*(4), 3–7.

Horning, M. L., Ostrow, L., Beierwaltes, P., Beaudette, J., Schmitz, K., & Fulkerson, J. A. (2020). Service learning within community-engaged research: Facilitating nursing student learning outcomes. *Journal of Professional Nursing, 36*(6), 510–513. https://doi.org/10.1016/j.profnurs.2020.04.005

Institute of Medicine (2010). *The future of nursing: Leading change, advancing health.* http://books.nap.edu/openbook.php?record_id=12956&page=R1

Jarden, R. J., Jones, V., McClunie-Trust, P., Winnington, R., Merrick, E., Shannon, K., Turner, R., Donaldson, A.E. and Macdiarmid, R. (2021). Exploring the experiences and perceptions of students in a graduate entry nursing programme: A qualitative meta-synthesis. *Nurse Education Today, 107,* 105121. https://doi.org/10.1016/j.nedt.2021.105121

Kamolo, E., Vernon, R., & Toffoli, L. (2017). A critical review of preceptor development for nurses working with undergraduate nursing students. *International Journal of Caring Sciences, 10*(2) 1989.

Kantar, L. D. (2021). Teaching domains of clinical instruction from the experiences of preceptors. *Nurse Education in Practice, 52.* https://doi.org/10.1016/j.nepr.2021.103010. 103010.

Kohtz, C., Gowda, C., & Guede, P. (2017). Cognitive stacking. *Nursing, 47*(1), 18–20. https://doi.org/10.1097/01.nurse.0000510758.31326.92

Interprofessional Education Collaborative (2022). IPEC Core Competencies Revision FAQs. https://www.ipecollaborative.org/ipec-ccr-faqs

Luebbers, E. L., Dolansky, M. A., Vehovec, A., & Petty, G. (2017). Implementation and evaluation of a community-based interprofessional learning activity. *Journal of interprofessional care, 31*(1), 91–97. https://doi.org/10.1080/13561820.2016.1237936

McKenna, L., Copnell, B., Butler, A. E., & Lau, R. (2018). Learning style preferences of Australian accelerated postgraduate pre-registration nursing students: A cross-sectional survey. *Nurse education in practice, 28,* 280–284. https://doi.org/10.1016/j.nepr.2017.10.011

Melnyk, B. M., Gallagher-Ford, L., Zellefrow, C., Tucker, S., Thomas, B., Sinnott, L. T., & Tan, A. (2018). The first US study on nurses' evidence-based practice competencies indicates major deficits that threaten healthcare quality, safety, and patient outcomes. *Worldviews on Evidence-Based Nursing, 15*(1), 16–25. https://doi.org/10.1111/wvn.12269

Melnyk, B. M., Tan, A., Hsieh, A. P., & Gallagher-Ford, L. (2021). Evidence-based practice culture and mentorship predict EBP implementation, nurse job satisfaction, and intent to stay: Support for the ARCC© Model. *Worldviews on Evidence-Based Nursing, 18*(4), 272–281. https://doi.org/10.1111/wvn.12524

Nelson, J. L., Kummeth, P. J., Crane, L. J., Mueller, C. L., Olson, C. J., Schatz, T. F., & Wilson, D. M. (2006). Teaching prioritization skills. *Journal for Nurses in Staff Development (JNSD), 22*(4), 172–178. https://doi.org/10.1097/00124645-200607000-00003

Nursing B.S.N. Accreditation | Temple University. (n.d.). www.temple.edu. https://www.temple.edu/academics/degree-programs/nursing-major-hp-nurs-bsnu/nursing-bsn-accreditation

Park, S., Lebovitz, L., & Pincus, K. J. (2019). Addressing preceptor shortages with a novel structure of blended ambulatory care rotations. *Currents in Pharmacy Teaching and Learning, 11*(12), 1248–1253. https://doi.org/10.1016/j.cptl.2019.09.014

Shellenbarger, T., & Robb, M. (2016). Effective mentoring in the clinical setting: Strategies for clinical instructors and preceptors. *AJN, American Journal of Nursing, 116*(4), 64–68. https://doi.org/10.1097/01.NAJ.0000482149.37081.61

Smith, M. M. (2022). Emergency department immersion: A clinical elective. *Journal of Emergency Nursing, 48*(6), 647–649. https://doi.org/10.1016/j.jen.2022.07.011

Temple, A., & Mast, M. E. (2016). Interprofessional education through service learning with undergraduate health administration and nursing students. *The Journal of Health Administration Education, 33*(1), 5.

Wojnar, D. M., & Whelan, E. M. (2017). Preparing nursing students for enhanced roles in primary care: The current state of prelicensure and RN-to-BSN education. *Nursing Outlook, 65*(2), 222–232. https://doi.org/10.1016/j.outlook.2016.10.006

Woodward, K. F., Kett, P. M., Willgerodt, M., Summerside, N., Hart, J., Buchanan, D. T., Cunitz, T. C., Birkey, C., & Zierler, B. K. (2022). Using an academic-practice partnership to enhance ambulatory care nursing skills. *Nurse Education Today, 119*, 105585. https://doi.org/10.1016/j.nedt.2022.105585

Woolforde, L., Mercado, N. R., Pawelczak, M., Callahan, B., & Block, L. (2022). Interprofessional precepting: A nursing–medicine partnership. *Journal for Nurses in Professional Development, 38*(5), 302–307. https://doi.org/10.1097/NND.0000000000000860

13

Onboarding the New Nurse

Carol Ann Shaw, Anna Herbert, Beth Heuer, and Cynthia A. Danford

CHAPTER OBJECTIVES

- Discuss foundational expectations and clinical learning needs to facilitate onboarding
- Identify various roles of the preceptor during onboarding

- Integrate principles of safety and optimize patient/family care within the orientation experience
- Design the precepting experience to create a balance between the art and science of nursing for the orientee

Precepting a new nurse is like constructing a new home. The solid knowledge foundation must be laid, the learning framework must be organized and sturdy, and there must be a final walk-through to ensure every detail is addressed.

The new nurse or orientee is the nurse who has graduated from nursing school, passed the NCLEX exam, and recently started their first job. As a new graduate, nurses often have a very narrow, and overly optimistic, view of nursing. Orientees may also be nurses who have transferred from another care area within the same institution, have experience at another healthcare facility, or are newly assigned from outside agencies (e.g., travel nurses). Each type of new nurse or orientee requires distinctive precepting skills. This chapter focuses on onboarding the new-graduate nurse and the nurse who has experience at another healthcare facility. Through a discussion of universal concepts, concrete techniques, and implementable strategies, a foundation for the precepting experience will be built.

When orienting the new nurse, the preceptor helps the orientee to bridge the gap between what the orientee currently knows to what the orientee needs to know. At the same time, the preceptor must demonstrate how to navigate the complexities of the healthcare system.

There is nothing better than using experiential learning and storytelling to help the learner learn. Consider the vignettes of two preceptors, Emily and Chase (Vignette 1).

LAYING THE FOUNDATION: EXPECTATIONS

The *first shift* is the initial clinical experience where the orientee and preceptor work together, and it sets the tone for the entire onboarding experience. Establishing orientation expectations during the new nurse's first shift will promote a positive orientee–preceptor relationship while ensuring the orientee stays focused on their learning needs. These expectations provide boundaries that offer safety within the learning environment. When orientees feel psychologically safe, they are more likely to engage in and take ownership of their learning. Furthermore, clear expectations decrease uncertainty and anxiety, as well as reduce the risk of conflict between the preceptor and orientee. Expectations help create an environment for collaborative interaction, effective communication, and two-way, constructive feedback.

Specific orientation expectations will be unique to preceptors, care areas, and patient populations. However, broad expectations are universal, and need to be identified for both the preceptor and orientee. During the first shift, the preceptor should express to the orientee the following:

1. "Expect me to give you feedback throughout every shift. This feedback will include what you are doing well and what needs improvement. I expect you to give me feedback on my teaching—what is working and what I can do better. I expect feedback to be part of our daily conversation. Open communication between us is key."

2. "Expect me to provide a comprehensive orientation by seeking out diverse learning opportunities and providing simulated experiences when needed. I expect you to progressively take ownership of your learning and speak up about knowledge and skills you feel you need."

3. "Expect me to be positive, engaged, and supportive. Your transition to practicing independently and safely is paramount. I expect you to be positive, engaged, and enthusiastic with your learning process."

By setting expectations during the first shift and beyond, the preceptor demonstrates that they care and value the orientee's success.

LAYING THE FOUNDATION: SOCIALIZATION

Creating a work environment of trust and support begins with effective relationships between team members. These relationships do not just happen. It is essential for the preceptor to help the orientee make connections so they can quickly feel like a valued member of the team. Working in the role of socializer, the preceptor should introduce the orientee to all team members, facilitate learning experiences with other nurses, and engage them through informal social events. Additionally, the preceptor must familiarize the orientee with the culture of both the unit and the institution.

Socialization is a dynamic and ongoing process that builds resilience and promotes work-life harmony. It ensures the orientee can build relationships with more experienced nurses to help overcome challenges and enhance collaboration and unity. As the orientation progresses, the entire team can help guide and support the orientee's professional growth.

LAYING THE FOUNDATION: COLLABORATION

Effective preceptors recognize that a successful orientation experience depends upon the orientee gradually taking ownership of their learning. This requires a collaborative partnership where prebriefing, debriefing, feedback, and evaluation regularly occur. The orientation experience begins with the preceptor being directive in providing guidance and transitions to a bidirectional interactive process with the orientee. The preceptor uses prebriefing to prepare the orientee and debriefing to process new learning experiences. Providing constructive feedback is essential to knowledge and skill acquisition. The preceptor evaluates the performance of the orientee, what was effective, and what needs to be modified.

Preceptors also utilize soft skills, which are personal traits that include active listening, professionalism, empathy, problem-solving ability, adaptability, and initiative (Figure 13.1) (Laari et al., 2022; Widad & Abdellah, 2022). Collaboration demands use of soft skills, such as flexibility and patience, especially when precepting a challenging learner (see Chapter 17). The onus is on the preceptor to create a positive working relationship and to adapt their precepting style to the varied learning needs of each orientee (Vignette 2). When working with a low-confidence

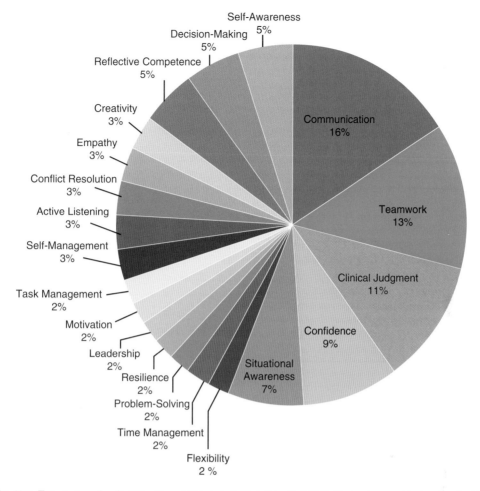

Fig. 13.1 Taxonomy of soft skills. (From Widad, A. & Abdellah, G. (2022). Strategies used to teach soft skills in undergraduate nursing education: A scoping review. *Journal of Professional Nursing: Official Journal of the American Association of Colleges of Nursing, 42*, 209–218.)

learner, the preceptor can provide ongoing encouragement and find ways for the orientee to accomplish small successes. When precepting an error-prone learner, simulations can be used prior to attempting new skills. Those who precept "know-it-all" learners must practice empathy, as this type of learner tends to have low confidence on top of an abundance of fear.

Additionally, the preceptor role requires a bit of detective work, as the orientee may be reticent or may be struggling to identify learning needs. Precepting requires a holistic approach. Taking the time to listen, asking questions, and paying attention to body language and nonverbal expressions can help to address the learning, emotional, mental, and physical needs of the orientee.

New nurses may need to develop strategies for managing a work-life balance when working rotating shifts. In addition, orientees may need guidance about decompressing and seeking support outside of the clinical environment.

BUILDING THE FRAMEWORK: ORIENTATION IS A CONTINUUM

The preceptor holds the blueprints of the orientation process that guide the orientee toward the end point of becoming a confident, competent, and resourceful nurse. Orientation begins with performance of specific, basic skills. Knowledge and skills are scaffolded by adding complexity. The preceptor supports the orientee as

Vignette 2: Building Rapport

*During the first shift, **Emily** worked hard to build a rapport with her orientee. She learned that the orientee moved 8 hours away from her family for this job. She also discovered that the orientee has some fear and uneasiness caused by having to retake the NCLEX exam. Emily knew that to help the orientee feel connected, she would need to socialize her to the unit, the institution, and the city. She introduced the orientee to other healthcare providers on the unit and told her to expect ongoing feedback on her progress. Finally, during the first shift, Emily and the orientee made plans to socialize with several coworkers outside of work.*

*Although nervous to be precepting a more experienced nurse, **Chase** enthusiastically introduced himself to his new orientee. The orientee's response was polite but muted. When assessing the first patient, the orientee told Chase that she knew what she was doing and that he did not have to be in the room. Chase calmly explained, "One of my roles as your preceptor is to ensure you can provide safe care, independently and competently. I will respect and honor your knowledge and skill, and I will observe, evaluate, and provide feedback on your performance."*

TABLE 13.1   Nurse Preceptor Responsibilities: Group Orientation Model

Similar to the nursing school model where a clinical instructor oversees a group of students, hospital settings are taking a new look at the group orientation model. Allowing one preceptor to work with a group of two to four novice nurses moves beyond the 1:1 nurse-preceptor ratio and advances the preceptor role as facilitator and teacher.

Learning or Care Activity	Nurse Preceptor Responsibility
Patient assignment	Carries no direct patient assignment
	Works with two or more orientees
	Creates patient care assignments according to orientee needs and patient acuity
Supervision	Oversees delivery of patient care by orientees
Teaching and learning	Provides both didactic and hands-on learning
	Facilitates patient report and daily debriefing
	Establishes daily and weekly goals with orientees
Evaluation	Provides timely formative and summative evaluation (Chapter 21)
	Monitors competency development
	Provides coaching for competency development
	Revises goals and orientation plan as needed

Adapted from McDermott, C. (2023). Reimagining the preceptor role. *Nursing Administration Quarterly, 47*(3), 227–233.

they build upon their current knowledge. Examples of supporting comments include, "Your time management is improving. It is time to take a full patient assignment," or "I have confidence that you can complete this PICC dressing change on our 2-year-old patient. The process is the same as it was for our 15-year-old patient. I will help you through the challenge of working with a younger, noncompliant patient." Approaching orientation as a continuum affords the orientee an experience where they can develop the knowledge and skills required to care for patients independently and confidently.

ROLES OF THE PRECEPTOR DURING ONBOARDING

Several precepting roles are necessary for an effective orientation. Each of these elements require intentionality, as it is essential to recognize that the best precepting is purposeful. Roles and responsibilities of the preceptor are dependent on the number of orientees and the precepting model used (Table 13.1).

Teaching

The preceptor develops a learning plan for the orientee. This plan guides the preceptor to assess learning gaps and ask for specific assignments or reach out to colleagues who can help the orientee practice needed skills. Repetition allows the orientee to transfer and solidify knowledge and skills. Additionally, the preceptor proposes case studies and "what-if" scenarios, which expand the orientee's learning, reinforce clinical judgment, and create safe spaces to work through uncertainty.

Role-Modeling

The preceptor demonstrates how to be a competent nurse, supportive teammate, and polished professional. By practicing according to institutional policy, the preceptor mitigates short-cuts that could lead to unsafe practice. By providing help and anticipating needs, the preceptor demonstrates a culture of care. By being timely, flexible, and respectful, the preceptor establishes the professionalism that is expected on the unit.

Protecting

The preceptor actively protects the orientee in two ways. First, the preceptor observes the orientee's practice until competency is obtained. This helps protect the orientee

from making a mistake, thus also protecting the patient. Second, the preceptor addresses any lateral incivility or unprofessionalism from colleagues targeted at the orientee.

Debriefing

Debriefing can be informal or formal, occurs regularly, and can be used to identify learning needs and inform practice changes. The preceptor should utilize "I" statements and set the stage for feedback by letting

---

Exemplar: Onboarding the New Nurse in a Pediatric Post-Anesthesia Care Unit (PACU)

Vatula Marie Seward

Caring for children immediately after surgery requires a special skill set. Nurses must pay careful attention to patient safety, airway management, and pain control. For that reason, our Pediatric Post-Anesthesia Care Unit (PACU) hires experienced nurses who already possess strong assessment and organizational skills. Pediatric patients are unique not only due to their developmental stage, anatomy, and psychosocial needs, but their pain management can be intimidating for nurses who are not familiar with weight-based medication dosing. When I am orienting new nurses, we typically start with patients recovering from less-complex surgeries (e.g., adenoidectomies, tympanostomy tube placement, hernia repairs, strabismus surgery, circumcisions, etc.). The care of patients after complex surgeries is gradually introduced.

We had recently hired an experienced nurse who needed orientation to the PACU. Early on, it became clear that she was apprehensive about giving intravenous pain medications to children. During one case the orientee believed that the amount of narcotic pain medication she administered IV was adequate. However, a cycle repeated where the patient complained of pain, IV medication was administered, the patient would fall asleep, the medicine would wear off, and the patient would awaken and complain about having pain again.

As her preceptor, I recognized that we needed "to get ahead of the pain," which meant administering a dose of oral pain medication at the same time the IV narcotic was given. The orientee expressed concern that the patient would be over-medicated and they were uncomfortable with this plan. The orientee needed reassurance, so I suggested that we look up the half-life of both medications. After reviewing the drug formulary, I advised them that it was safe to administer both medications together because while the IV medication would provide immediate relief, it would wear off quickly and the oral medication would provide a delayed,

but sustained therapeutic effect. However, the orientee still was not convinced. They remained hesitant and preferred the medications be given separately.

At this point I gave the orientee two options: 1) The orientee would give the IV pain medication and I would give the oral medication, or 2) we could continue with the orientee's plan to administer them separately. As a note, we agreed that we would not allow the patient to be in pain and that I, as the preceptor, would step in to advocate as needed. The orientee preferred to first administer IV medication and stated they would give the oral medication when needed. The IV medication was given to the patient who quickly fell asleep and was resting comfortably.

At this time, we needed to admit another patient to recovery and I assigned the admission to the orientee. While the orientee was busy admitting the new patient, the first patient's medication began to wear off and they complained of pain. Since the orientee was busy attending to the second patient and could not leave the bedside, I decided to intervene. I gave the first patient both IV and oral medications together as I had previously suggested. After the orientee was able to reassess the first patient, we discussed comprehensive pain management and anticipation of patient care needs. On review of this situation, they finally understood the implications of under-managing post-operative pain.

This was a great learning opportunity for both of us as sometimes "experience" is the best teacher. I learned I could not push the orientee to do something that they were not comfortable with, even if I knew it would work. A new nurse would have simply followed the instructions and trusted their preceptor, but they were not a brand-new nurse. The orientee needed to understand the situation for themself. When they told me "I don't feel comfortable," I realized this could create unnecessary conflict and that I needed to earn their trust.

the orientee know feedback will be provided. The preceptor could say, "Is now a good time to provide you with some feedback? I noticed when you called the provider, you seemed frustrated with the conversation. I think it may have been because you were not sure of the answer to some of her questions. I wonder if it would be helpful for us to practice reporting before calling the provider. Would that help you feel better prepared?"

Goal Setting

The preceptor must work with the orientee to develop short-term and long-term goals. This provides the preceptor with clear benchmarks for assessing knowledge and skills and gauging improvement. Setting daily goals at the beginning of each shift provides a focus for preceptor–orientee collaboration.

Vignette 3: Adjusting the Teaching Approach

Emily was pleased with how her orientee was progressing through orientation. The orientee was detail-oriented, focused, and thoughtful, and was taking more initiative. Then a challenge arose. Near the end of orientation, Emily's orientee had a particularly difficult day involving new orders, an unexpected admission, and a combative patient. The orientee's frustration level rose and Emily knew she needed to debrief. During a short break, Emily began by expressing how well the orientee was doing. She explained that some days are harder than others, but often end up as valuable learning experiences. Emily and the orientee modified their goals for the remainder of the shift and the rest of orientation. Emily's orientee finished orientation on time and was confident to practice independently.

After several shifts together, *Chase* was worried that his orientee was not learning and retaining knowledge and skills as quickly as she needed. During their next shift together, Chase had an informal conversation with his orientee and learned that she is predominately an auditory learner. With this knowledge, Chase began to "narrate the day." He verbalized almost everything he was thinking. While practicing a central line dressing change, he demonstrated the skill on a manikin and verbally explained each step. This was an easy change for him and it made a big difference for his orientee's learning. After adjusting his teaching approach, the orientee showed marked progress. She completed orientation showing competence in her knowledge and skills.

Evaluating

For many preceptors, evaluating the orientee is challenging and stressful. (See Chapter 21, *Evaluation*.) Preceptors may feel it is not their role to evaluate, as a manager or educator also provide formal evaluation. However, preceptors are uniquely positioned to fully evaluate the orientee's progress. For example, the preceptor may informally state, "You did a great job completing that assessment. Next time, I know you can do it independently." When formal, scheduled conversations take place with unit leadership, the preceptor can give formalized feedback such as, "During the last four shifts, the orientee and I have focused on time-management as an area needing improvement. We are collaborating to ensure our patient assignments are appropriate to meet this learning need without being overwhelming." Formal, unscheduled discussions may have to occur when the orientee is not progressing as expected (Vignette 3).

BUILDING THE FRAMEWORK: ENSURING SAFE PRACTICE

Safety and optimizing patient health are central to the preceptor–learner experience (Brown et al., 2019). Safe nursing practice includes: 1) prioritizing care to prevent harm or injury, 2) remaining aware of fundamental principles behind nursing actions, 3) recognizing limitations and when to seek assistance, and 4) following policy and procedures (Wolff et al., 2010). Patient safety can be achieved through the integration of situational awareness, personal integrity, and the art of nursing practice (Figure 13.2).

The time-bound nature of orientation creates an urgency to ensure the orientee has diverse learning experiences. This urgency creates tunnel-vision for the preceptor, who may focus solely on building the orientee's repertoire of skills and inadvertently give less attention to *teaching* about situational awareness, integrity, and the art of nursing practice. By not addressing these learning needs, the preceptor is only teaching part of what the orientee needs to practice safely.

Situational Awareness

Situational awareness refers to a dynamic process where the nurse engages in continuous in-depth assessment

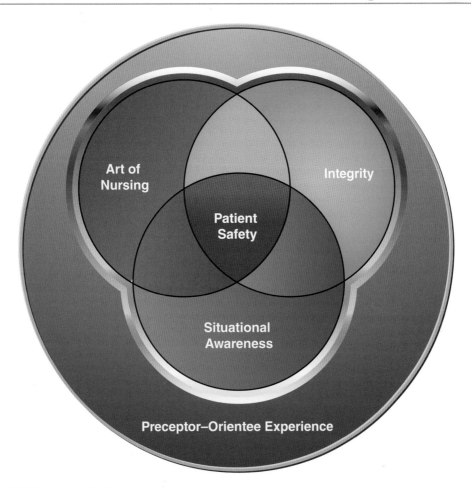

Fig. 13.2 Components of patient safety.

and interpretation of clinical cues related to the patient and their response to their environment. Identification of relevant cues allows for development of individualized care (Sitterding et al., 2012). Situational awareness is a teachable skill guided by the preceptor (Box 13.1). Using situational awareness skills, the nurse can anticipate problems and maintain patient safety.

Integrity

Precepting with integrity means role-modeling ethical behavior with orientees. The nursing code of ethics (Fowler, 2015) includes four main principles: 1) autonomy (respect of individual patient's right to self-determination and decision-making), 2) beneficence (acting in the best interest of others), 3) justice (fairness), and 4) nonmaleficence (doing no harm). Specific behaviors

include following policies, speaking up for safety, and treating patients and colleagues with respect and dignity. A culture of safety includes creating an ethical, blame-free environment where individuals are able to report errors or near misses without fear of reprimand or punishment (Agency for Healthcare Research and Quality, 2019).

THE ART OF NURSING

A balance between the art and science of nursing contributes to safe patient outcomes and is a primary focus during the precepting experience. The science of nursing includes using a systematic, evidence-based approach in providing skilled healthcare. The art of nursing implies the application of holistic and humanistic

BOX 13.1 Teaching Situational Awareness

1. Entering the patient room, the preceptor notices:
   a) the patient's breathing is a bit more labored than yesterday.
   b) the patient's mother seems a little bit more anxious.
   c) the patient is alert, and vital signs are stable.
2. Outside the patient room, the preceptor leads debriefing with the orientee using the following questions:
   a) "Did you notice anything about the patient's breathing?"
   b) "What did you think about the affect of the patient's mother?"
3. Observation of the patient situation and follow-up discussion between the preceptor and orientee help:
   a) translate knowledge and compare present and previous assessment findings.
   b) highlight additional situational details.
   c) integrate findings to ensure safe, comprehensive patient care.

perspectives. The *science* may be considered concrete and direct, whereas the *art* is abstract and less direct. Administering oral medication to a toddler or providing skilled care to an adult are examples of concrete nursing tasks, reflecting the science of nursing. However, safe and effective nursing care results when considering the patient's age, developmental level, overall situation, and

The Final Walk-Through: Bringing It All Together

The preceptor guides the orientee through the continuum of learning by assessing and building basic knowledge and skills. The preceptor then helps the orientee in the development of clinical judgment (see Chapter 8) and time management skills. Providing both simulated and real experiences allows the new nurse to expand their skill sets. To fill in remaining gaps, the preceptor must help the orientee to apply evidence-based practice, encourage self-directed learning through available resources, and participate in professional development (Chapter 16) and self-care (Chapter 18) activities.

Exemplar: Precepting in an End-of-Life Environment
Kristen Starr

One of the challenging aspects of precepting is helping new nurses to experience nursing practice from a patient- and family-centered perspective, instead of focusing on task completion. This is particularly important on the medical oncology inpatient unit, where patients are facing a life-limiting diagnosis. Many patients are actively dealing with end-of-life decisions. Acute hospital stays frequently prompt discussions around changing treatment options or decisions to forgo additional treatment and focus on comfort. At our specialty oncology hospital, nurse-to-patient ratios are generally low specifically to allow nurses time to fully engage with patients and provide support.

When precepting new nurses, I encourage them to spend time conversing and developing a trusting relationship with patients and families. Getting to know who the patient is allows for effective, holistic, and individualized care. *What is important to them? What do they value most in their life? How can our care help them meet their goals?* I also encourage the nurse to do a thorough medical record review to understand the patient's illness journey. *How long have they been fighting cancer? What treatments and procedures have they already been through?* Initially, I assign new nurses to one patient so they have time for relationship-building.

One of the best ways to help a new nurse see the whole patient is for them to participate in a "goals of care" discussion. At our institution, discussions occur at key decision-making points in a patient's cancer journey and may lead to the decision to pursue hospice care instead of further cancer-directed treatment. These discussions typically include the patient, key family members, the oncologist, social workers, and other members of the care team. These conversations are often very emotional and may include both a life review and a review of the cancer course.

While a new nurse may feel that they have little to add to these discussions, participation clearly demonstrates the importance of physical presence and emotional support. I have found care discussions to be important tools in onboarding new nurses, both illustrating the caring side of nursing and letting the new nurse know that it is okay to show emotion with patients. The nurses I have precepted have been grateful for the experience and pointed to these discussions as one of their more impactful learning experiences. In the end, my role as a preceptor is not just to develop a highly skilled nurse, but a holistic care professional who views themself as an integral partner in the patient's oncology journey.

communication needs to tailor the nursing interventions. The nurse's approach and response to situations can make the difference between a positive or negative and safe or unsafe outcome.

REFERENCES

Agency for Healthcare Research and Quality. (2019). September 7. Culture of Safety | PSNet. AHRQ.gov. https://psnet.ahrq.gov/primer/culture-safety

Brown, H., Lisk, L., & Scruth, E. (2019). Applying an ethical approach to building great preceptorships. *Clinical Nurse Specialist*, *33*(6), 250–252. https://doi.org/10.1097/NUR.0000000000000479

Fowler, M. (2015). *Guide to the code of ethics for nurses with interpretive statements: Development, interpretation, and application* (2nd ed.). American Nurses Association.

Laari, L., Anim-Boamah, O., & Boso, C. (2022). Soft skills the matchless traits and skills in nursing practice: An integrative review. *Nursing Practice Today*, *9*(4), 267–278. https://doi.org/10.18502/npt.v9i4.11199

Sitterding, M. C., Broome, M. E., Everett, L. Q., & Ebright, P. (2012). Understanding situation awareness in nursing work: A hybrid concept analysis. ANS. *Advances in Nursing Science*, *35*(1), 77–92. https://doi.org/10.1097/ANS.0b013e3182450158

Widad, A., & Abdellah, G. (2022). Strategies used to teach soft skills in undergraduate nursing education: A scoping review. *Journal of Professional Nursing*, *42*, 209–218. https://doi.org/10.1016/j.profnurs.2022.07.010

Wolff, A., Regan, S., Pesut, B., & Black, J. (2010). Ready for what? An exploration of the meaning of new graduate nurses' readiness for practice. *International Journal of Nursing Education Scholarship*, *7*(1), 1–14. https://doi.org/10.2202/1548-923x.1827

14

Orienting the Advanced Practice Registered Nurse Student

Shayna Dahan, Beth Heuer, and Cynthia A. Danford

CHAPTER OBJECTIVES

- Review safe practice strategies when working with advanced practice registered nurse (APRN) students
- Choose effective scheduling strategies with APRN students to maximize learning and clinical effectiveness
- Describe strategies to progress APRN clinical skills throughout the learning practicum

Orientation lays the framework that a clinical setting is a safe, supportive environment, which is essential for learning (Rooke et al., 2022). Advanced practice registered nurse (APRN) student orientation to the clinical setting involves discussing expectations, assessing current skills, planning for skills development, and reviewing pertinent patient education materials and topics. The preceptor has the opportunity to gather information about the student's knowledge, skills, and attitudes, (Roberts et al., 2020) and to review the student's learning goals. The student is encouraged to become familiar with the clinical setting to ease preparation for their clinical days, seize learning opportunities, and strategize how to further develop their skills. When preceptors and students communicate and develop rapport prior to the onset of the clinical rotation, students feel more welcomed and open to explaining their needs and asking questions.

Ideally, the clinical site orientation should occur *before* the first clinical day. This allows the student time to process the site-specific expectations and prepare themselves, while the preceptor develops an idea of the student's current capabilities and the specific experiences needed. Depending on the clinical setting, an orientation can be formal or informal, and may only need to consist of a brief conversation, virtually or in-person. The preceptor's roadmap for the student clinical experience can be formulated with the information gathered at the orientation. If the student is less experienced and the clinic schedule allows, the student may need to shadow the preceptor while orienting on the first day.

Advanced practice nursing students arrive at their clinical sites with varying levels of knowledge and experiences depending on their progression in the academic program. For example, an APRN student in their final graduate semester may be entering an emergency department (ED) rotation with extensive medical-surgical experience, but without any ED clinical experience. Another APRN student beginning their first clinical experience may have extensive experience as an RN in pediatric surgery, but none in primary care. Both of these students present with important foundational knowledge that can be integrated with new knowledge relevant to the clinical site.

Preceptors will find it helpful to become familiar with the type of APRN program that the student attends. Answers to various questions provide perspective on how to facilitate student learning: Are they a full-time or a part-time student? Are they in a direct-entry-to-practice program where they have no prior nursing experience? What specialty track are they studying? Among nurse practitioner students, a pediatric nurse practitioner (PNP) student may have more pediatric-focused skills and knowledge of early childhood development in comparison to a family nurse practitioner (FNP) student, depending on how much pediatric didactic and clinical the FNP student has completed prior to the rotation. Students in acute care NP programs will bring a degree of acute and critical care experience, but not necessarily in a subspecialty area (e.g., inpatient oncology or neurosurgery). The student directly entering an APRN program from an undergraduate program may only have experience working as a student nurse, but may be highly motivated to learn.

The preceptor should keep an open mind and use orientation time to assess what useful skills the student can immediately implement on the first day of their clinical experience. Orientation starts a process where the student is included as an active member of the care team while providing learning opportunities for skill and knowledge development.

EXPECTATIONS FOR THE ADVANCED PRACTICE REGISTERED NURSE STUDENT

The preceptor and student should discuss reasonable expectations and goals for the clinical experience on day one. Providing students with a brief outline of clinical site information, such as clinical hours, what to do in the event they will be late or absent, dress code requirements (e.g., lab coat), and necessary equipment or supplies may minimize initial anxiety. Other more tailored expectations include presenting the types of skills the student should review prior to their first clinical day. In a specialty setting, discussing frequently seen diagnoses is helpful so that students can prepare appropriately. Realistic and measurable goals should be delineated at the onset of the clinical experience and agreed upon between the preceptor and student. An expectation can be set that by the end of the semester the student will be able to perform a focused sick visit with minimal supervision. Another expectation can be that the student presents a unique case study at interdisciplinary clinical conferences. These expectations are examples of how to

---

Exemplar: Providing Anticipatory Guidance

Cynthia Ann Chew

A nurse practitioner (NP) student in my pediatric primary care clinic was struggling with how to provide anticipatory guidance. Early in the clinical rotation, he expressed that much of the anticipatory guidance provided was "common sense" and worried that he might be insulting families by teaching them what they already knew. After validating his concern, we talked about strategies to address the issue, which included using information gathered in the history to prioritize needs and individualize teaching for the family.

To illustrate this point, the NP student and I compared two patients we had seen earlier in the day for well-child visits. Both were school-aged children. When asked about oral hygiene practices, one child reported brushing teeth twice a day and the other admitted to brushing only a few times a week. For the first patient, a quick statement of praise for their healthy routine and a reminder about the importance of continuing this routine was enough anticipatory guidance. With the second patient, we spent significantly more time discussing the importance of oral hygiene. We also incorporated motivational interviewing techniques to improve compliance with teeth brushing. Utilizing "common sense" in real time helped the student

to understand the nuances of providing anticipatory guidance in an individualized way.

To enhance his learning, the NP student and I incorporated Bright Futures guidelines into each patient's overall treatment and management plan. After reporting on a patient, the NP student would identify anticipatory guidance topics for the patient or family based on the history and assessment. We utilized role-playing when the NP student was unsure about how to discuss a topic with the patient and family. I would state, "Tell me what you're going to teach to the patient." This provided him with the opportunity to practice prior to seeing the patient, and allowed me to provide feedback in a lower stakes environment while boosting his confidence in these teaching skills. We also debriefed after seeing patients so the NP student could reflect on what went well and develop alternative approaches for what could have gone better.

By the end of the clinical rotation, the NP student was automatically integrating an anticipatory guidance plan into the patient report. He independently provided anticipatory guidance that met patient needs in an individualized and meaningful manner.

help students embrace the APRN role and envision ways to meet their learning goals by the end of the clinical experience.

The student should communicate clearly about what they expect and need from the preceptor and during the clinical rotation. Clarifying how much supervision students *perceive* they require will give the preceptor further insight. If the student describes being independent in previous settings, the preceptor may wish to observe the student perform a routine visit or procedure once before allowing them to continue independently. Preceptors should identify, with the student, a preferred learning style, and what worked and did not work in previous clinical experiences.

While the preceptor and student work out the logistics of working together, the third "member" of the learning team, the student's school/university, should not be overlooked. Faculty's expectations for student learning will be clearly outlined in the course syllabus and *must* be shared with the preceptor. Expectations or assignments might include specific skills assessment observations (referred to as "sign-outs" or competencies), simulation experiences, or objective structured clinical examinations (called "OSCEs" [pronounced OS-keys]). Awareness of learning expectations helps with identifying and planning experiences where the student can practice necessary skills. Some schools of nursing require input of clinical case write-ups, Subjective, Objective, Assessment, Plan (SOAP) notes, and case entries into electronic tracking systems that quantify student learning experiences. Students document specific information about cases seen during their clinical day for the purposes of assigned case studies and case entries. Additional documentation for assignments can be time consuming, yet the preceptor can brainstorm with the student about the most efficient way to track case data without interfering with the clinic flow and/or work day. Reviewing the required clinical evaluation tool early in the semester is helpful when providing ongoing feedback on the student's progress throughout the rotation (see Chapter 21) (Box 14.1).

ASSESSING APRN STUDENT SKILLS AND PLANNING FOR DEVELOPMENT

A recommendation for anyone who precepts regularly is to develop an orientation toolkit to help organize

> **BOX 14.1   Key Points: Establishing Expectations**
>
> - Establish basic expectations, including dress code, work hours, and what to do in the event that the student or preceptor must call off or will be late.
> - Gather information about student's skills, previous experiences, and academic program and specialty.
> - Discuss the most common visit types and illnesses treated so students can prepare and refresh their knowledge.
> - Review the student's syllabus and evaluation forms.
> - Provide ongoing feedback.
> - Discuss positive experiences and encounters. In previous clinical experiences, what enhanced student learning? Are students more hands-on and independent, or do they prefer to observe before "jumping in"?
> - Identify student limitations and areas requiring immediate improvement.
> - Review opportunities for further growth.

student learning profiles and checklists of what students need to know to function proficiently. The toolkit can include suggested reading lists and contact information for local resources (Box 14.2). If students do not provide a standardized checklist of specific skills and competencies, preceptors can develop their own list specific to the clinical setting. Selective activities can be used to validate that students can apply key concepts (Nelson & Joswiak, 2020). Knowing the APRN student's current skill level and tracking their progress helps with clarifying their readiness for more advanced learning experiences. Students cannot be expected to learn about every diagnosis and perform every skill at a single practice site. When assessing the student's skills, a goal is to have the student ready to safely practice independently or with minimal guidance by graduation.

At the onset of a clinical experience, a useful baseline skills assessment can be performed in various ways. Preceptors can create a checklist describing the most common skills performed at their clinical site and have the student note how much supervision they need for each skill. For example, the student can note that they need full supervision, moderate, minimal, or no supervision for specific exam techniques. The checklist can then be reviewed mid-semester to assess students' improvement, with the expectation that steady progress will be maintained throughout the clinical rotation.

> ### BOX 14.2 Site Specific Resources and Directives to Guide the NP Student
>
> - Explore evidence-based guidelines and practice parameters used in the specific clinical area (e.g., American Academy of Pediatrics, American Academy of Sleep Medicine, Centers for Disease Control, Society of Critical Care Medicine).
> - Review pertinent assessment skills and developmental expectations.
> - Set the expectation that the student will explore and share new evidence.
> - Develop a small toolkit of essential resources for your practice. Many preceptors develop a folder of essential evidence-based articles for their practice. Students should be expected to review pertinent literature prior to the first clinical experience and throughout the rotation.
> - Consider developing a checklist of skills and experiences that are unique to the clinical setting and challenge students to seek these experiences.
> - Provide a guide detailing commonly used community resources in the local area (e.g., Meals on Wheels, home care agencies, and mental health providers). This can remain a valuable tool for students as they move into the APRN role.
> - Develop a list of objectives for students to meet during the clinical rotation (Appendix N: Examples of Nurse Practitioner Student Learning Needs and Clinical Objectives).
> - Encourage the student to develop their own resource guide to use as a reference as they transition to independent practice.

Taking time throughout the semester to observe and evaluate students' physical assessment skills provides ongoing feedback and allows for guided improvement (Vae et al., 2018) (see Chapter 21 for tips on constructive feedback). Students may feel self-conscious and cautious as they demonstrate new knowledge, which may influence their ability to self-assess how well their skills are developing (Ugland et al., 2018).

APRN students always need assistance in fine-tuning their skills. The tendency to take a few shortcuts may present, yet shortcuts can lead to missing key clinical information (Haugh, 2015). One way to stop the shortcuts is by verifying that students' assessment skills do not drift once they become more independent and are striving to be time-efficient. Observe whether students are assessing heart sounds correctly using both the bell and the diaphragm of the stethoscope. Are they auscultating the abdomen prior to palpation? Do they check cranial nerves appropriately? Whatever the clinical area, regularly re-evaluating whether the student is practicing skills safely and effectively will lead to consistency in practice.

The preceptor can address progress through discussion and direct observation of student performance in the clinical setting. However, taking a full or half day to closely observe student performance may affect clinic flow or timely completion of other patient care responsibilities. This method may need to be modified to short, intermittent observations or spot checking. When students quickly assimilate as contributors to the healthcare team, the preceptor will find more freedom to role model and help refine student performance.

Advanced practice nursing students are typically proficient in RN-specific skills and should be able to perform within this scope of practice from day one without supervision. Examples of RN proficiency include taking vital signs, administering vaccines and medications, and auscultating breath sounds. Some APRN students may be in an entry-to-practice program where they have achieved basic RN knowledge and skills, but lack the clinical experience that a more *seasoned* APRN student will have. These students may require closer supervision initially, but are known to be resilient (Meyer & Shatto, 2018). When compared to traditional students, direct-entry students have a tendency toward using a medical model approach to care, being mechanical, and finding confidence when following routines or guidelines (Lavoie & Clarke, 2022). These seemingly negative behaviors are often a cover-up for initial lack of confidence and resolve with support and experience. In the long run, the outcome for both traditional and direct-entry students is the same (Lavoie & Clarke, 2022).

SKILL EXPECTATIONS FOR NURSE PRACTITIONER STUDENTS

Skill expectations for NP students are highlighted below:

- *History taking and patient/family interview skills* should be conducted using a culturally competent approach. While APRN students have developed basic interviewing skills, direction may be needed to facilitate communication techniques for episodic or well visits, admissions, and acute, chronic, or critical incidents. Time management related to interviewing skills should be refined throughout the clinical rotation.

- *Physical examination skills* should be well-developed. APRN students complete an advanced physical assessment course prior to entering clinical rotations. Mastering skills such as using an ophthalmoscope or otoscope in a small child, intubating, or inserting chest tubes will require additional support and direction.
- *Clinical reasoning and identifying differential diagnoses* is often a challenge for students early in their clinical education. It is important to help students consider not only the most obvious diagnosis but also to discuss other possibilities and develop the rationale for selecting one.
- *Treatment, management, and developing plans of care* are skills mastered later in graduate nursing education. Improvement occurs as clinical exposure increases.
- *Reporting and presentation skills* may initially be unorganized. Students may require direction in fine-tuning a methodical reporting process and in identifying or prioritizing pertinent positive and negative findings (see Chapter 8).
- *Additional skills* based on the clinical setting may require review or refining, including procedures and specialty diagnostic modalities.
- *Documentation* will need to be reviewed. Many students will need help with documenting in the electronic health record (EHR), learning how to be time efficient with documentation, and incorporating documentation into their daily routine (see Chapter 20).
- *Time-management skills and prioritizing* will develop with practice and experience.
- *Billing and coding* will need to be reviewed with each encounter and correlated with documentation (Box 14.3).

PROVIDING PATIENT EDUCATION

Undergraduate nursing education emphasizes patient education skills. Nurses are often proficient in educating the patients and families for whom they provide care. Many APRN students have confidence in teaching patients and can provide patient education at times when the preceptor may be busy multitasking. This is

> **BOX 14.3   Key Points: Assessing Advanced Practice Registered Nurse Student Skills and Planning for Development**
>
> - Create a list of common skills relevant to your clinical site and have students determine whether they need full, moderate, minimal, or no supervision for each skill.
> - Identify skills the student can do independently to utilize the student efficiently and delegate proper assignments and tasks.
> - Identify the skills for which the student needs full and moderate supervision, set measurable learning goals, and make time to teach and practice.
> - Reassess and evaluate student skills throughout the semester to ensure proper technique and safe practice.
> - Provide feedback for improvement throughout the semester.

an opportune time to capitalize on student strengths. Primary care APRN students may provide education on topics such as health promotion, disease prevention, health maintenance, and care specific to disease processes. Acute care APRN students may provide education on topics such as care specific to disease processes, the structure of the team caring for the patient, monitoring (noninvasive and invasive), procedure indications, nutrition, respiratory support, medications, clinical decision-making processes, and more. Preceptors can work closely with the student to expand their patient education skills within their new APRN role, as patient education is integrated into all aspects of patient care.

Students often complete a patient/family education project as an academic assignment and may ask the preceptor for assistance in identifying relevant topics. Specific examples for pediatrics practices can include information on preventing infection, flu shots, Lyme disease protection, treating fever and discomfort, or introducing solid food to infants. In a women's health setting, patient education might include sexual and reproductive health, fitness and nutrition, intimate partner violence, and cancer prevention and screening. Projects may be presented in the form of handouts, trifolds, posters, or bulletin boards. These are value-added products for practice settings that provide students with focused educational experiences.

Exemplar: Building Confidence in Caring for Patients Experiencing Trauma

Kirstyn Kameg and Brayden Kameg

I work as a psychiatric-mental health nurse practitioner (PMHNP) in an outpatient setting treating patients across the lifespan who experience a variety of mental health problems, such as depression, anxiety, and trauma-related issues. While precepting a PMHNP student who was completing her final clinical rotation, I started by having the student spend time shadowing my patient visits. I then allowed the student to take the lead in conducting initial evaluations and follow-up visits and engaged the student in clinical decision-making related to the treatment plan.

Early on, the student disclosed that she did not feel comfortable working with patients who have a history of trauma. She stated, "I often do not know what to say to patients" who are disclosing trauma. She expressed lacking confidence when assessing trauma-related symptoms. I identified the student's concern as a gap in knowledge related to trauma-informed care (TIC).

To help the student gain confidence, I evaluated her current knowledge of trauma assessment and treatment, and principles of TIC. After gaining a better understanding of the student's needs and knowledge deficits, I offered additional resources and readings on TIC, some of which we reviewed together. Next we focused on finding patient encounters where she could refine her skills.

As the semester continued, the student improved her knowledge, yet continued to lack confidence when working with patients with a history of trauma. I modified my approach by further exploring the source of the student's discomfort. The student feared that she might inadvertently trigger or re-traumatize a patient. We spent additional time reviewing TIC principles, which helped the student feel more empowered to treat patients with trauma-related symptoms. By the conclusion of this clinical experience, the student was more capable in her management of patients with trauma-related presentations.

BOX 14.4   Examples of Introductions of Advanced Practice Registered Nurse Students

- This is ___, a registered nurse who is a student at ____ College's/University's graduate/doctoral program. They are learning the (nurse practitioner [NP]/clinical nurse specialist [CNS], etc.,) role, like what I do. Today they are working with me; I will be back in after they have spent some time with you.
- This is ___, an APRN student working with our team. They will begin reviewing your/your child's history and completing the assessment. I will be here to listen and fill in any blanks.
- This is ___, an APRN student from ___College/University. As a registered nurse, they are now getting an advanced degree like the degree I have. They are working with me today and will be beginning your exam.

announcements or welcome posters in the waiting room or examination room (Appendix F: Welcome Poster for Clinical Site). Directly introducing the learner as an *APRN student* emphasizes that the student is already an educated, licensed registered nurse who is presently learning an APRN specialized role. Respectfully avoid referring to the student as *my* student.

Capitalizing on the benefit of working as a preceptor–APRN student team is exemplified with the following introduction: "This NP student will be speaking with and examining you/your child prior our visit. They are highly skilled, and we will be working together to give you the best treatment possible."

Patients and families appreciate reassurance that they are getting the care they would normally receive with the addition of an intelligent, detail-oriented, and motivated student. Another example is: "I have an NP student working with me today. I am going to have them begin asking questions and complete the physical exam, and then I will be back in."

Additionally, the preceptor might explain: "An NP student is working with me today. Together, we are going to begin discussing your history, but I am going to have them take the lead. Please know that I am available to them and to you at all times."

Depending on the clinical setting and the student's level of experience, many preceptors have the student introduce themselves to the patient and caregiver, explain that the preceptor will be in shortly, begin history-taking, and then perform a physical examination (Box 14.4).

INTRODUCING THE NURSE PRACTITIONER STUDENT TO PATIENTS AND FAMILIES

A positive approach when introducing the APRN student to patients and families sets the stage for successful interactions. Introductions can be indirect and direct. Indirect student introductions may include

CONCLUSION

Precepting an APRN student can be an exciting challenge and add new depth and knowledge to one's own clinical experiences. Providing an effective orientation is an essential component of precepting, as it can help the student to "hit the ground running" and lays the foundation to build their skills and competence.

REFERENCES

Haugh, K. H. (2015). Head-to-toe. *Nursing, 45*(12), 58–61. https://doi.org/10.1097/01.nurse.0000473396.43930.9d

Lavoie, P., & Clarke, S. P. (2022). Educators' perceptions of the development of clinical judgment of direct-entry students and experienced RNs enrolled in NP programs. *Journal of Nursing Regulation, 12*(4), 4–15. https://doi.org/10.1016/S2155-8256(22)00011-4

Meyer, G., & Shatto, B. (2018). Resilience and transition to practice in direct entry nursing graduates. *Nurse Education in Practice, 28,* 276–279. https://doi.org/10.1016/j.nepr.2017.10.008

Nelson, D. M., & Joswiak, M. E. (2020). Preceptor teaching tools to support consistency while training novice nurses. *Journal for Nurses in Professional Development, 36*(5), 307–312. https://doi.org/10.1097/nnd.0000000000000672

Roberts, L. R., Champlin, A., Saunders, J. S. D., Pueschel, R. D., & Huerta, G. M. (2020). Meeting preceptor expectations to facilitate optimal nurse practitioner student clinical rotations. *Journal of the American Association of Nurse Practitioners, 32*(5), 400–407. https://doi.org/10.1097/jxx.0000000000000304

Rooke, S., Thevenard, G., Suthendran, S., Jung, S., Tolentino, N., Annandale, J., & Ward, K. (2022). What makes a great preceptor? Nursing students have their say. *Kaitiaki Nursing New Zealand, 28*(4), 7. https://kaitiaki.org.nz/article/what-makes-a-great-preceptor-nursing-students-have-their-say/#ref7

Vae, K. J. U., Engström, M., Mårtensson, G., & Löfmark, A. (2018). Nursing students' and preceptors' experience of assessment during clinical practice: A multilevel repeated-interview study of student–preceptor dyads. *Nurse Education in Practice, 30,* 13–19. https://doi.org/10.1016/j.nepr.2017.11.014

15

Guiding the Nurse Practitioner Student Experience

Beth Heuer, Cynthia A. Danford, Christina Gabele, and Angela Gager

CHAPTER OBJECTIVES

- Describe how to ensure safe practice for advanced practice registered nurse (APRN) students
- Explain time management skills for the clinical day
- Explore scheduling strategies to best manage the student experience
- Identify a structured plan to progress student skills

Preceptors working with nurse practitioner (NP) students engage in time management strategies to allow for effective learning experiences and ensure safe practice, no matter the clinical setting (inpatient or outpatient, with acute or primary care patients). This chapter explores scheduling strategies and fundamentals to help learners progress their clinical skills and get the most from each clinical experience.

ENSURING SAFE PRACTICE

Safe practice is always at the forefront of clinical practice. The entire healthcare team is responsible for keeping the patient, the environment, and each other safe. As students progress through their clinical rotations, learning new skills and procedures, assuming new responsibilities, and embracing a culture of safety lead to prevention of errors. Good communication is foundational to safe practice, preventing errors at critical times, such as patient handoffs. The transition of adult patients from primary care to acute tertiary settings is an example of a complex transition where errors in handoff communication can cause errors and delays in necessary treatment (Keating et al., 2021). Use of a handoff checklist , such as one guided by Situation, Background, Assessment,

Recommendation (SBAR) (Halterman et al., 2019), can aid in communication between staff members, assuring those essential items are not missed, even if there are distractions or interruptions (Box 15.1).

In addition, infection control and risk management should be addressed. Preceptors role-model hand hygiene, donning and doffing personal protective equipment (PPE), sterile and aseptic nontouch technique, and adherence to isolation precautions. Students are attentive to their preceptors' tutelage and augment their learning by observing carefully, following the various practices they are shown, and safely adapting techniques to fit their own individual approach to patient encounters..

Assessing the work environment helps to ensure that there is a culture of safety (Dutra & Guirardello, 2021). Risk management includes assessing the workload for the day, as well as self-care. Errors and missed care can occur more often when providers are stressed, tired, or hungry. It is well known that sleep deprivation can lead to poor health and clinical judgment amongst healthcare providers, and nursing students are no exception (Cho & Steege, 2021; Thomas et al., 2017). The simple measure of taking time for small breaks, including lunch, and even pausing for a moment to take a few short deep breaths is vital to ensuring safe and quality practice (Melnyk et al., 2020).

USING TIME WISELY

Having enough time in the clinical day is always a challenge, and the goal is to work smarter, not harder. Not having enough perceived time or poor time management are both associated with anxiety. When in a state of high anxiety the student's working memory is constrained, which significantly diminishes their abilities to complete tasks and ultimately reduces their effectiveness (Goldsby et al., 2020). While most APRN students have previously worked as registered nurses (RNs) and have some experience in managing the anxiety of a high-pressure clinical environment, they are new to the stresses and time limitations associated with the nurse practitioner (NP) role.

Preparing ahead of time creates a more efficient clinical experience. Students are always expected to come to the clinical site early to review the daily schedule, study the electronic health records (EHRs), and organize a plan for each day. At the end of each day, the preceptor can go over the next clinical day's schedule with the student to allow adequate time for preparation.

Students should make time during each patient encounter to provide health promotion and patient education while also remaining aware of time constraints within the busy clinic environment. By seeing patients who are known to require extra time, support, and education, students can focus their energy on comprehensive patient encounters. Obtaining a comprehensive history of present illness (HPI), past medical history, family history, social history, and review of systems (ROS) on multiple patients will afford the student time to refine their skills.

SCHEDULING STRATEGIES

Scheduling strategies within the clinical setting are discussed to assist in providing experiences for students that optimize the preceptor's time in addition to the student's and other health care provider's time while keeping the day running smoothly.

Observational Experience

Observational experiences are appropriate for all students in both ambulatory and acute care settings. Depending on the student's level of education and experience, preceptors may choose to have students observe the preceptor conducting patient visits and developing associated treatment plans. This strategy is used initially to assist new students in applying didactic material to the clinical setting. This is also a valuable method to orient students of all levels to a new clinical setting and to evaluate the learning needs and skill levels of more experienced students. However, this is *not* an appropriate teaching strategy beyond the first few days.

Appointment Modifications

The strategy of modifying appointments is most appropriate for students in ambulatory settings. For preceptors, the clinical workload typically does not change when students join the team (Heusinkvelt & Tracy, 2020). In the ambulatory care setting, it may be feasible to modify appointments so that the preceptor has adequate time to give students a meaningful educational experience. For example, an appropriate schedule modification may be to remove one appointment in the morning and one or two appointments in the afternoon. An allowance for longer appointment times on the schedule is another option to increase preceptor time and availability to interact with students. Ideally, the preceptor's productivity equation should be adjusted to accommodate necessary schedule changes.

Structured Approach

Structured approaches to learning can be effective in either ambulatory or acute care settings. A structured approach is often best suited for NP students and tailored according to the setting. Patients are carefully selected based on student skills and level of experience. The novice NP student is often able to manage uncomplicated, routine visits for patients with stable chronic conditions. They may also be assigned less complex cases and scheduled admissions in acute care and inpatient settings. Patient encounters can then increase in number and complexity as the student progresses.

A structured approach allows the student ample time to prepare for the patient encounter. Prior to each patient encounter, the student should:
- Review the chart and the reason for the encounter
- Discuss pertinent issues with the preceptor
- Prepare components of anticipatory guidance and health promotion (primary care). Alternatively, develop an anticipated plan of care prior to the patient's arrival (acute care)
- Engage in a formal pre-encounter and postencounter discussion with the preceptor

Structured Approach Example: Acute Care Inpatient and Intensive Care Settings

As a preceptor in the ICU, I review the postoperative schedule to identify possible cases that would be appropriate for the acute care NP student to manage. Once the patient is assigned, I have the student review the patient's chart, discuss pertinent past medical history, and formulate an anticipated postoperative care plan relevant to the surgical procedure. After the patient is admitted to the ICU, together we review the patient's condition and modify the student's anticipated postop plan as necessary.

Structured Approach Example: Primary/Specialty Care

At the beginning of each day, the student and I identify key objectives. We then review the schedule and discuss appropriate patient encounters. Prior to each encounter, we review the patient's chart and key points for the visit. The student independently begins the visit, following through with the history and physical exam. We then meet to discuss the chief complaint and exam findings, followed by formulating a plan of care. After discussing the student encounter, we complete the visit together.

Focused Half-Day

A focused-half day approach can be effective for experiences in both ambulatory and acute care settings. The preceptor chooses one or two patients for the student to focus on for the morning or afternoon schedule while the preceptor manages the remaining patient visits. The encounters are focused so that the student can develop experience with patients of various ages, medical conditions, and presenting complaints. Students can focus on practicing assessment skills and developing treatment plans that match course objectives and student learning goals. The student may use the additional time to perform in-depth medical record reviews and investigate current evidence-based practice guidelines as they develop comprehensive care plans. Time can also be used to complete patient documentation after each visit. This type of scheduling allows an in-depth experience instead of observation or limited exposure to a higher quantity of patients. On busy clinic days, this approach facilitates independent learning balanced with high productivity.

Wave Scheduling

Wave scheduling is most appropriate to use in ambulatory care settings. It can be used in specialty clinics but may not always be appropriate. Specialty clinics that schedule patient visits with multidisciplinary teams might not have the flexibility to schedule in waves, which works best when patients are scheduled in consistent blocks of time. The wave scheduling model allows the preceptor to supervise NP students and manage their typical patient load each day. Within a clinic setting, the wave schedule does not compromise access to care or provider productivity (Lehner & Smith, 2016). In this approach, two or three patients are scheduled in one time block. The student sees one patient while the preceptor completes one or two patient encounters. The remaining time at the end of the block is used for feedback or consultation and completion of the visit with the NP student.

Wave Scheduling Examples

1:00 pm: Two patients scheduled in 30-minute block (student sees one; preceptor completes one)
1:20 pm: Consultation/feedback with NP student (student and preceptor complete patient visit)
1:30 pm: Two patients scheduled in the following 30-minute block (each sees one)

OR

1:00 pm: Three patients scheduled in 30-minute block (student sees one, preceptor completes two)
1:30 pm: Consultation/feedback with NP student (student and preceptor complete patient visit)
1:30 pm: Two or three patients scheduled in the following 30-minute block

"Typical" Clinical Day

Following a "typical" clinical day schedule is effective for NP students in both ambulatory and acute care settings. Caution in using this approach in specialty settings may be needed depending on the complexity of the patent encounter. A consistent approach to a "typical" clinical day can work well with the beginning-to-advanced NP student. The student is establishing more independence, so there is less formal previsit and postvisit discussion between the preceptor and the student. The NP student assesses the patient while the preceptor is with another patient. After the preceptor finishes with the patient, the NP student presents the patient case to the preceptor with the diagnosis and treatment plan outlined. The student and preceptor then reenter the room to complete the visit, which may include validation or modification of the diagnosis and treatment plan. The student follows by implementing the plan with assistance as needed.

Typical Clinical Day Example: Ambulatory Care

I have four clinic rooms and allow the student to enter one room as I go into another to conduct a visit. The student completes the HPI and exam, starts developing a differential diagnosis list and plan, and waits to present the plan to me. The student gives me the report, then we go back to the exam room together. If the student and I have agreed on the plan, the student reviews the plan with the patient/family and provides patient education. While the student *is completing the visit, I start another patient visit. When the student is done with their assigned patient encounter, they start another visit, and so on.*

"Sink or Swim": Moving Toward Independence

The "sink or swim" approach is best suited for a *final* semester student in ambulatory care settings. The student is assigned a variety of patients and sees them independently in preparation for the transition to autonomous APRN clinical practice. The preceptor offers less support, and there is minimal previsit teaching. However, the preceptor is ultimately responsible for decisions and is available for consultation at all times. A postvisit discussion with the preceptor is included in which the patient presentation and treatment plan are discussed and agreed upon.

As students become more autonomous in the advanced practice role, they may become overwhelmed and overfocused on themselves and how they are adjusting (Thrasher & Walker, 2018). Frequent check-ins still remain essential. The preceptor closely monitors student progress and decision-making as they begin to work more independently.

In some acute care settings, the sink-or-swim approach will be more challenging. Often, the student presents to a large team in interprofessional rounds and receives feedback throughout the process. The preceptor is able take a more hands-off approach and allow the student to develop their plan and get feedback from other team members without stepping in. However, the need for supervision is inevitable due to the complexity of care and the involvement of interprofessional teams. Therefore, the preceptor remains available for backup and is ultimately responsible for decisions to the extent that they are usually responsible.

PROGRESSION OF APRN STUDENT SKILLS

Students are expected to develop increased autonomy as the rotation progresses. The following outlines typical APRN student progression of skills in the primary care setting.

- The student shadows the preceptor, who is performing the history and physical (H&P) and discussing a treatment plan with the patient and family.

- The student performs the H&P with the preceptor present to observe and prompt as needed. Together they develop a treatment plan.
- The student performs the H&P with the preceptor, and the preceptor allows the student to develop an independent treatment plan. The preceptor then discusses necessary changes and reviews H&P data that the student has missed.
- The student performs the H&P and independently develops a treatment plan. The student presents the case to the preceptor with the diagnosis and treatment plan outlined. The student and preceptor then reenter the room to evaluate the patient together. The preceptor discusses necessary changes and further H&P data the student may have missed and validates or modifies the diagnosis and plan with the student.

Note: Any rapid change in patient status can lead to the student shifting back to an observational and assisting role as the preceptor takes the lead in managing emergent needs.

ENTRUSTABLE PROFESSIONAL ACTIVITIES

Nursing education has shifted its focus to having students attain specific learner-centered competencies (American Association of Colleges of Nursing [AACN], 2021). Competencies are the knowledge, skills, and attitudes related to performance of specific skills. Entrustable professional activities (EPAs) are professional practice responsibilities that can be entrusted to students once they have attained specific competencies (Meyer et al., 2019; Corrigan et al., 2022; Sarkar et al., 2021). There are marked differences between competencies and EPAs. Competencies describe the students' abilities while EPAs describe the actual tasks. Schools may provide digital support by structuring student electronic portfolios to track individual progress in their attainment of *both* competencies and EPAs. Preceptors will want to entrust students with activities as they show skill progression, and further increase their autonomy with additional learning opportunities. Progression toward independence can be reflected by how well the student prioritizes, manages their time, and follows up on diagnostic testing and other concerning findings. It is up to the preceptor to directly follow up with the student,

> **BOX 15.2 Prompts to Facilitate Student Progression in Treatment Planning**
>
> - What diagnostic testing is needed?
> - What are the diagnostic results?
> - What do the results mean?
> - How do the results change the plan of care?
> - Are further diagnostic tests indicated?
> - What outcomes require ongoing assessment?
> - How will outcomes be measured?

particularly when there are pending patient care needs. Preceptors typically provide prompts to appraise the student's clinical judgment skills, assess their abilities, and guide them through new tasks (Box 15.2).

While steady progression of student skills is expected, preceptors should intermittently reevaluate student physical examination skills to identify any areas of deficiency. Learning a correct physical examination technique or procedure initially is much easier than retraining students who have been doing something incorrectly. Once basic examination skills are mastered, the preceptor may have the opportunity to share advanced skills with students. Advanced skills that may be performed in the clinical setting may include: suturing, arthrocentesis or joint injections, pelvic and breast examinations, or incision and drainage of uncomplicated abscesses. Students should never perform any advanced skill without the preceptor present.

Acute Care Example

The student is working with you in the cardiac ICU. During rounds, the student suggests ordering an echocardiogram to evaluate the cardiac function of the patient they are following. The interdisciplinary team agrees, and an echocardiogram is ordered during rounds. As the preceptor, you want to give the student more autonomy and allow them to progress in patient assessment, follow-up, and management decisions. For example, while the student obtains an H&P on a different patient, you check the electronic health record and see that the echocardiogram results are available. You review the results, noting that function is improving, so you decide to continue with the current treatment plan. You then wait for the student to follow up on the echocardiogram results and present the plan. Did the student follow up? What is their interpretation of the results? Did they discuss the treatment plan based on the results? How long did it take the student to prioritize this over other patient care responsibilities? This exemplifies prioritization and time management in the acute care setting.

CONCLUSION

Time can be limited during clinical rotations. The preceptor will want to facilitate student progression, maximize learning opportunities, and utilize time wisely while maintaining work productivity. Practical approaches such as those included in this chapter help to seamlessly and efficiently reorganize the clinical day and can be beneficial for both the preceptor and the APRN student.

REFERENCES

American Association of Colleges of Nursing. (2021). *The Essentials: Core competencies for professional nursing education.* https://www.aacnnursing.org/Essentials

Cho, H., & Steege, L. M. (2021). Nurse fatigue and nurse, patient safety, and organizational outcomes: A systematic review. *Western Journal of Nursing Research, 43*(12), 1157–1168. https://doi.org/10.1177/0193945921990892

Corrigan, C., Moran, K., Kesten, K., Conrad, D., Manderscheid, A., Beebe, S. L., & Pohl, E. (2022). Entrustable professional activities in clinical education. *Nurse Educator, 47*(5), 261–266. Pubhttps://doi.org/10.1097/nne.0000000000001184

Dutra, C. K. D. R., & Guirardello, E. D. B. (2021). Nurse work environment and its impact on reasons for missed care, safety climate, and job satisfaction: A cross-sectional study. *Journal of Advanced Nursing, 77*, 2398–2406. https://doi.org/10.1111/jan.14764

Goldsby, E., Goldsby, M., Neck, C. B., & Neck, C. P. (2020). Under pressure: Time management, self-leadership, and the nurse manager. *Administrative Sciences, 10*(3). https://doi.org/10.3390/admsci10030038

Halterman, R. S., Gaber, M., Janjua, M. S., Hogan, G. T., & Cartwright, S. M. (2019). Use of a checklist for the postanesthesia care unit patient handoff. *Journal of Perianesthesia Nursing, 34*(4), 834–841. https://doi.org/10.1016/j.jopan.2018.10.007

Heusinkvelt, S. E., & Tracy, M. (2020). Improving nurse practitioner and physician assistant preceptor knowledge, self-efficacy, and willingness in a hospital medicine practice: An online experience. *The Journal of Continuing Education in Nursing, 51*(6), 275–279. https://doi.org/10.3928/00220124-20200514-07

Keating, S., McLeod-Sordjan, R., & Lemp, M. C. (2021). Nurse practitioner handoff communication: A simulation based experience. *Journal of Nursing Education, 60*(8), 476–477. https://doi.org/10.3928/01484834-20210723-03

Lehner, V., & Smith, D. S. (2016). Wave scheduling. *The Journal of Physician Assistant Education, 27*(4), 200–202. https://doi.org/10.1097/jpa.0000000000000094

Melnyk, B. M., Kelly, S. A., Stephens, J., Dhakal, K., McGovern, C., Tucker, S., Hoying, J., McRae, K., Ault, S., Spurlock, E., & Bird, S. B. (2020). Interventions to improve mental health, well-being, physical health, and lifestyle behaviors in physicians and nurses: A systematic review. *American Journal of Health Promotion, 34*(8), 929–941. https://doi.org/10.1177/0890117120920451

Meyer, E. G., Chen, H. C., Uijtdehaage, S., Durning, S. J., & Maggio, L. A. (2019). Scoping review of entrustable professional activities in undergraduate medical education. *Academic Medicine, 94*(7), 1040–1049. https://doi.org/10.1097/acm.0000000000002735

Sarkar, A., Aggarwal, A., Grigoryan, L., Nash, S. G., Mehrotra, N., Zoorob, R. J., & Huang, W. Y. (2021). Improving student confidence with electronic health record order entry. *PRiMER, 5*, 23. https://doi.org/10.22454/primer.2021.619838

Thomas, C. M., McIntosh, C. E., Lamar, R. A., & Allen, R. L. (2017). Sleep deprivation in nursing students: The negative impact for quality and safety. *Journal of Nursing Education and Practice, 7*(5), 87. https://doi.org/10.1097/ANC.0000000000000145

Thrasher, A. B., & Walker, S. E. (2018). Orientation process for newly credentialed athletic trainers in the transition to practice. *Journal of Athletic Training, 53*(3), 292–302. https://doi.org/10.4085/1062-6050-531-16

16

Professional Development for the Preceptor and the Orientee

Audra Rankin

CHAPTER OBJECTIVES

- Explore development of a growth mindset through professional development activities
- Identify components of career development plans

- Explain ways to evaluate the quality of professional development activities

Professional development is an ongoing responsibility for all nurses and nursing students. The preceptor is in a prime position not only to share their expertise with learners and fellow nurses, but also to advance career goals and build professional excellence in themselves and others.

PROFESSIONAL DEVELOPMENT: WHAT IS IT AND WHY IS IT IMPORTANT?

The American Nurses Association defines professional development as a "lifelong process" in which nurses participate actively in learning activities to develop and maintain their continuing competence, enhance their professional practice, and support achievement of their professional goals (King et al., 2021; Yu et al., 2022). These learning opportunities should not be viewed as optional, but rather as an essential exercise in promoting evidence-based practice and quality improvement while influencing change (Shinners & Graebe, 2020).

For nurse preceptors, continuing education and the development of new skills and behaviors updates clinical knowledge and is an important component of modeling best practices. Although often viewed as a personal investment, professional development can benefit both the individual *and* the organization. Nurse preceptors can use development opportunities to positively

influence their own professional work and promote student learning (Phuoung et al., 2020). Organizations thrive when nurses provide the best, most up-to-date evidence-based practice.

"Mindset" is a series of self-beliefs that can influence behaviors, outlook, and mental attitude. A *growth* mindset can set the learner up for professional success and ongoing achievement (Dweck, 2006). Creating a mindset that encourages learner participation in professional activities can be a challenge for some preceptors. A practical way to begin is by focusing on an environment where learning opportunities are viewed as scalable and accessible to everyone. A variety of formal *and* informal learning opportunities in a rich and nurturing clinical environment can help learners develop new skills and knowledge, resulting in increased confidence (Billings, 2019; Neely & Leonardi, 2022).

Reasons for engaging in professional development include meeting personal career goals, fulfilling workplace mandates, or maintaining licensure or certification requirements. Continuing professional education has well-documented benefits related to patient safety and quality of care (Altmiller & Hopkins-Pepe, 2019; Vaismoradi, 2020). Theoretical propositions support that professional development can positively transform individual practice, skills, knowledge, and workplace culture (King, et al., 2021).

GUIDING PROFESSIONAL DEVELOPMENT

Ongoing learning contributes to career or professional development. A career development plan should incorporate personal priorities, current strengths and weaknesses, and short-term and long-term goals (Ziedonis & Ahn, 2019). Professional development is ideally related to the preceptor's work and aligns with clinical practice, organizational needs, and personal development (King et al., 2021). Reviewing aspects of career development planning can be inspiring and provide motivation for both the preceptor and the learner.

A career development plan incorporates motivating factors for the learner and expected outcomes. Motivators can be prompted by concerns, issues, or problems that present in the clinical setting or may align with personal values or interests. A career plan provides a clear and focused path for engaging in meaningful professional learning, connecting new knowledge to a higher purpose and enhancing clinical effectiveness (Keswin, 2022).

Learning opportunities often present in day-to-day professional activities, while other opportunities present unexpectedly. Given competing clinical responsibilities, learners should be guided to prioritize their time effectively. By sharing interesting cases and opportunities, the preceptor can help foster a love and appreciation for lifelong learning. Preceptors should role-model and suggest ongoing professional reading (e.g., journals and professional websites) to augment learning. By role-modeling how professional development can be woven into the daily workflow without significant time and expense, preceptors create a mindset for efficient learning opportunities in fast-paced clinical environments (Bersin et al., 2019).

TYPES OF PROFESSIONAL DEVELOPMENT

Professional development may be self-directed, or formalized through academic, institutional, or organizational learning settings. Professional organizations provide rich and reliable sources for education, skills training, and networking. Many learning opportunities are available at annual meetings and conferences, and through professional organization resources. Educational topics include leadership, research, academic scholarship, mentoring, clinical skills, and advocacy. These organizations support professional development and allow both students and preceptors an opportunity to network with professionals who have common interests (Ziedonis & Ahn, 2019). Encouraging memberships in professional organizations enhances learning and engagement.

All preceptors and learners have individual preferences in how content is delivered. Flexible and creative educational strategies include the use of technology such as video conferencing or social media (Harper et al., 2020). In particular, social media can be used to expand networking possibilities (e.g., live podcasts) and provide opportunities for those with limited resources (Ziedonis & Ahn, 2019). Virtual learning platforms that include breakout rooms and group discussions may be effective formats for delivery of educational content (Harper et al., 2020). Professional development can also occur in the form of microlearning modules, workshops, seminars or symposia, and certificate and degree programs (Phuoung et al., 2020).

EVALUATING PROFESSIONAL DEVELOPMENT OPPORTUNITIES

While many learning opportunities are available, nurses must assess for a good fit between the quality of the learning activity and the outcomes desired. The Kirkpatrick model incorporates four levels of impact to evaluate professional development opportunities: reaction, learning, behavior, and results (Ziedonis & Ahn, 2019) (Figure 16.1). *Reaction* focuses on the learner's satisfaction and motivation. *Learning* reflects changes in knowledge and skills. *Behavior* refers to changes in performance and application of new teaching techniques. *Results* involve change in outcomes for stakeholders, such as students, patients, or the organization (Phuong et al., 2020). A focus on levels of impact will influence acquisition and execution of nursing skills, personal development, and institutional goals. Use of the model leads to validation for participation in professional development. Preceptors and learners can discuss the impact and outcomes anticipated to leverage requests for time off or financial support (Phuong et al., 2020).

Alignment With Institutional Goals

Engagement in professional development can empower an individual to contribute to service and quality improvement, translate new knowledge into practice, and strengthen leadership and role-modeling

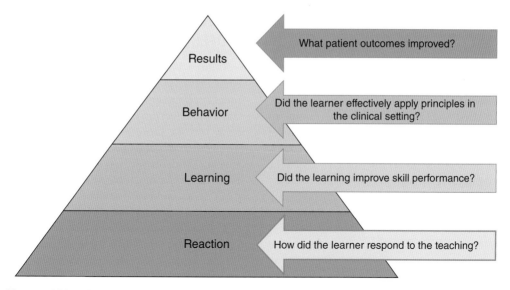

Fig. 16.1 Kirkpatrick model applied to nursing professional development. (Modified from Kirkpatrick, D. L. (1959). Techniques for evaluation training programs. *Journal of the American Society of Training Directors, 13,* 21–26.)

Exemplar: Integrating Professional Development by Engaging APRN students as Health Policy Advocates

Stacia Marie Hays

Advanced practice registered nurse (APRN) students often see advocacy and legislation as "scary" concepts and hesitate to engage in health policy reform. A common barrier to advocacy is anxiety and lack of confidence when engaging with government officials. Breaking down advocacy into smaller steps often alleviates the fear and promotes action. Because of their experiences with barriers to practice and policy constraints (e.g., patient safety), preceptors are in a unique position to guide students in becoming policy advocates.

For the past several years, I have provided anti-trafficking education and training to healthcare providers, of which advocacy and legislative efforts are strong components. One of the initial legislative initiatives was to encourage the State Board of Nursing (SBON) and legislators to mandate anti-trafficking education for all healthcare providers. I had previously engaged two students in policy discussions and they were eager to gain more experience. After some encouragement, they were willing to learn more about human trafficking and participate in a meeting with the executive director and chair of the Board of Nursing.

The first step in our preparations was reviewing the literature and existing policies. Each student took responsibility to research various organizations leading initiatives related to human trafficking education, national educational best practices, SBON educational requirements, and more. To further enhance our knowledge, we completed educational modules provided by the National Association of Pediatric Nurse Practitioners (NAPNAP)

and Advocates for Children in Trafficking (ACT). We then reviewed policy briefs in order to understand how to concisely present information to SBON members. At this point, the students felt confident in their knowledge of human trafficking, were aware of best practices, and were eager to present their information and request that human trafficking education be mandatory.

We decided a 2-minute elevator speech was the ideal format for presenting the information. I encouraged them to identify one fact that would convey the importance of mandating human trafficking education. Together, they chose, "Approximately 80% of victims of human trafficking were seen by a healthcare provider within the year prior to being identified as a victim." I then coached them through weekly sessions to refine and practice their elevator speeches. Within 4 weeks, they were ready to go!

The day of the meeting, we had a final run through of the process and their talking points. With a deep breath, we entered the office of the executive director of the SBON. I witnessed their confidence while they presented their speeches and briefly discussed the importance of mandated education. We left the office, debriefed, and celebrated their hard work and accomplishment. They admitted to being nervous but relied on their preparation and knew the discussions would be successful. They sent a thank-you email to the executive director, who then responded with a request for more information and to meet with them again. Within a year, the SBON mandated human trafficking education for all healthcare licensures.

(King et al., 2021). Professional development opportunities can be aligned with institutional goals and priorities and are an effective way to improve organizational culture. Employees who participate in professional development are more engaged and have a higher retention rate than those that do not participate (Keswin, 2022).

Preceptors need high-quality, up-to-date training to supervise nursing students and orientees. Professional development can enhance the clinical, leadership, and research skills of the preceptor (King et al., 2021). Specialized continuing education can influence salary increases and job promotion (Shinners & Graebe, 2020). When exploring professional development opportunities, preceptors can look for options that blend the needs of their employer with their responsibilities as clinical teachers or adjunct academic faculty. Alignment of professional development goals and opportunities with clinical practice, teaching, and scholarship creates both personal and institutional gains (Ziedonis & Ahn, 2019).

OVERCOMING CHALLENGES WITH PROFESSIONAL DEVELOPMENT

Workforce issues and work–family conflicts can be major obstacles for nurses wanting to engage in professional development (Yu et al., 2022). Although work–life balance has been an ongoing challenge for many nurses, it has become more prominent and concerning since the COVID-19 pandemic. Urgent, often overwhelming clinical care demands have taken precedence over professional development. Nurse preceptors must continue to effectively embrace a mindset of learning as a regular part of their work.

Time constraints, overall lack of interest, learning topics that are seemingly irrelevant, and lack of institutional support can all serve as deterrents to engaging in professional development (Phuong et al., 2020). Improvements in patient care can occur through development of leadership, research, teaching, and clinical

---

Exemplar: Developing the Inquiring Mind

Barbara Giambra

Both graduate and undergraduate nursing programs include education on evidence-based practice, quality improvement, and research. As students or practicing nurses, we strive to improve healthcare through these avenues, but formalizing our ideas to fill knowledge gaps and applying the evidence can be a challenge. Within clinical settings, nurse scientists can mentor nurses through this process. As a nurse scientist, I recently worked with a nurse practitioner (NP) who identified that patients and families did not receive adequate information when tracheostomy placement was recommended for their child. Caregiver education and lifelong implications of managing a tracheostomy were not sufficiently discussed with families so that a more informed decision could be made. This NP thought a preoperative educational intervention for these families would make a positive difference and engaged me, as the nurse scientist, to help.

First, we searched the literature to identify existing interventions. Finding none, we decided a research study was needed. We gathered a multidisciplinary group of providers and, with family input, outlined an intervention for families. The preoperative intervention included detailed and practical information and expectations about caring for a child with a tracheostomy throughout their life. The goal was to facilitate informed decision-making for the family. Next, I encouraged the NP to get buy-in from the providers on the surgical otolaryngology service who place the tracheostomy, and in the intensive care units (ICU) where families were first approached about the surgery. The NP and I talked through these conversations ahead of time to anticipate questions and areas of concern. Ultimately, the NP was able to secure approval from hospital leadership, and plans to implement the intervention moved forward.

I helped the NP design the research study, write the protocol, and navigate the Institutional Review Board process. The study design included identifying criteria for inclusion, choosing validated measures, and finally, planning data analysis. Writing the protocol was an iterative process that included many drafts. This was particularly frustrating for the NP, as the process took time and needed to be balanced with clinical responsibilities. Setting up a standing meeting and using document sharing helped mitigate the challenges. After receiving IRB approval, the NP implemented the study. Over time, the NP gathered the data and together, we analyzed the findings, which included interpretation of both quantitative and qualitative data. I stressed the importance of disseminating the findings. The NP shared the results with the otolaryngology and ICU teams. For wider dissemination, I encouraged the NP to present the study as a poster and a manuscript; I helped with formatting and editing along the way. As a result of this collaborative process, the NP has initiated several more evidence-based and quality-improvement projects, which have resulted in additional improvements for staff, patients, and families.

skills. Protected time to attend professional development, training opportunities within the institution, and mentored interactions can all help reduce challenges (Ziedonis & Ahn, 2019).

CONCLUSION

Professional development has tremendous benefits for the learner, preceptor, and institution. Participation in lifelong learning, and the subsequent application of new skills and knowledge in the clinical setting, models an important behavior for learners and results in an improved learning experience. Reflecting on the needs of the learner, as well as anticipated outcomes, is an important part of identifying professional development opportunities. Learning opportunities can occur in a variety of formats and designs and serve as a valuable resource to network with other professionals (Phuong et al., 2020). Engaging in opportunities that align learning needs and institutional goals is an effective way to foster personal growth, as well as improve outcomes through high-quality care and translation of knowledge (Phuong et al., 2020).

REFERENCES

Altmiller, G., & Hopkins-Pepe, L. (2019). Why quality and safety education for nurses (QSEN) matters in practice. *The Journal of Continuing Education in Nursing, 50*(5), 199–200. https://doi.org/10.3928/00220124-20190416-04

Bersin, J., Zao-Sanders, M. (2019). Making learning a part of everyday work. *Harvard Business Review*, February 19, 2019.

Billings, D. M. (2019). Teaching nurses to make clinical judgments that ensure patient safety. *The Journal of Continuing Education in Nursing, 50*(7), 300–302. https://doi.org/10.3928/00220124-20190612-04

Dweck, C. S. (2006). *Mindset: The new psychology of success.* Random House.

Harper, M., Dougherty, D., & Price, G. (2020). Nursing professional development practice during a pandemic. *The Journal of Continuing Education in Nursing, 51*(8), 349–351. https://doi.org/10.3928/00220124-20200716-02

Keswin, E. (2022). 3 ways to boost retention through professional development. *Harvard Business Review*. https://hbr.org/2022/04/3-ways-to-boost-retention-through-professional-development.

King, R., Taylor, B., Talpur, A., Jackson, C., Manley, K., Ashby, N., Tod, A., Ryan, T., Wood, E., Senek, M., & Robertson, S. (2021). Factors that optimize the impact of continuing professional development in nursing: A rapid evidence review. *Nurse Education Today, 98*(2021), 104652. https://doi.org/10.1016/j.nedt.2020.104652

Neeley, T., & Leonardi, P. (2022). Developing a digital mindset. *Harvard Business Review, 100*(5–6), 50–55.

Phuong, T., Foster, M., & Reio, T. (2020). Faculty development: A systematic review of review studies. *New Horizons in Adult Education & Human Resource Development, 32*(4), 17–36. https://doi.org/10.1002/nha3.20294

Shinners, J., & Graebe, J. (2020). Continuing education as a core component of nursing professional development. *Continuing Education in Nursing, 51*(1), 6–8. https://doi.org/10.3928/00220124-20191217-02

Vaismoradi, M., Tella, S., A. Logan, P., Khakurel, J., & Vizcaya-Moreno, F. (2020). Nurses' adherence to patient safety principles: A systematic review. *International Journal of Environmental Research and Public Health, 17*(6), 2028. https://doi.org/10.3390/ijerph17062028

Yu, X., Huang, Y., & Liu, Y. (2022). Nurses' perceptions of continuing professional development: Qualitative study. *BMC Nursing, 21*, 162. https://doi.org/10.1186/s12912-022-00940-z

Ziedonis & Ahn, D., Ahn, M. (2019). Professional development for clinical faculty in academia. *Psychiatric Clinics of North America, 42*(3). https://doi.org/10.1016/j.psc.2019.05.009

17

Managing Challenging Behaviors With Learners in Clinical Environments

Cynthia A. Danford and Beth Heuer

CHAPTER OBJECTIVES

- Differentiate between challenging learner types
- Identify strategies to help overcome challenges imposed by learners

- Discuss when to initiate a learning plan and when to terminate the preceptor–learner relationship

A successful precepted experience may be thought of as one that goes smoothly, without any challenges or conflicts. Yet, no matter how well-planned and organized a precepted experience, there may be "bumps in the road" that need attention. Even the best plans need modifications along the way due to difficult or challenging behaviors or interactions that unexpectedly arise, especially in fast-paced, unpredictable clinical settings (Burns et al., 2006). Challenges and conflicts can be positive and contribute to learning and growth for everyone in the preceptor–learner–faculty/supervisor triad. Challenges may be defined as problems, issues, or concerns that emerge and disrupt the learner's performance or ability to function safely (Luhanga et al., 2014; Rodger & Juckes, 2021; Roncarolo et al., 2017).

Challenges with learners present in a variety of ways, as a result of overt influences (e.g., unsettling patient, family, provider, or preceptor interactions), and/or covert influences due to internal conflicts or issues. No matter what the cause, the resulting behaviors of the learner may present challenges for the preceptor. What is perceived as a challenging or difficult situation for one preceptor may not be a challenge for others, and may be completely unknown to the learner and even faculty or supervisors.

The goal of this chapter is to describe challenging learner behaviors and present strategies to overcome or minimize challenges that arise. Overcoming obstacles

and troubleshooting challenges occurs with effective communication within the preceptor–learner–faculty/supervisor triad. Preceptors should never have to deal with any challenges or obstacles in isolation. The bottom line for all preceptors is to guide the learner to always provide safe patient care. If safety comes into question as a result of learner behavior or interaction, the issue must be immediately addressed.

WHEN CHALLENGES PRESENT, OR DEFINING THE ISSUE OF CONCERN

Identifying the issue of concern is a first step to resolution of any challenge that presents with a learner. Subtleties or "soft signs" of concern may present before becoming obvious. The preceptor may suspect that something is not right with the learner's interaction or behavior, but is unable to specifically articulate what is concerning. Reflecting on questions such as, "Why am I concerned?" "What is the issue?" or "What is the problem causing concern?" can help frame the presenting challenge.

If naming the issue or concern is not possible, then describing the concern through use of examples can be helpful. Reflecting on several examples may help with defining the concern. If the concern remains unclear, especially when working with a nursing student, presenting examples to the faculty can be helpful in

---

Exemplar: Preceptor–Student Relationship: Identifying When Something Is Wrong

Laura Rauth

I was clinical faculty for an undergraduate nursing course at a large metropolitan university. Groups of six to eight nursing students completed 7-week rotations on hospital units applying the skills and content they were learning in class under my guidance. The consistency of interaction between nursing students in the clinical group and faculty during one 7-week rotation proved vital for a particular student.

When beginning any new clinical rotation, it is not surprising that nursing students are nervous. Clinical faculty and preceptors can minimize or alleviate worries while helping them gain important knowledge and experience. Developing relationships can help ensure students are comfortable discussing various issues with faculty and preceptors. While there are many ways to build a faculty/preceptor–student relationship, my style is to take a few moments each clinical day to spend time with each student and check in with them about school and life outside the classroom. I find this helps to quickly build a valuable relationship, leading to a more confident student who is better prepared for clinical. Relationship building also creates trust and is helpful when providing constructive feedback and guidance. My general observations, such as disheveled appearance, lack of eye contact, shaky hands, change in demeanor, or lack of preparation, all convey helpful information about the student that guide my interactions.

During one clinical rotation I worked with a student who could not wait to come to clinical each week. She was always neat in appearance, organized in her work, and while quiet and reserved, was always willing to participate in group discussions and engage in new experiences. She was the epitome of an enthusiastic learner. However, when clinical week 4 arrived, so did a very different student. She arrived 10 minutes late and was disheveled in appearance. She made no eye contact during our preclinical meeting and appeared pale, withdrawn, and disengaged. She was not prepared for her clinical assignment. I pulled her aside as we began our clinical day and asked if she was okay. I told her she seemed a bit "off" this morning and I was worried about her. She initially denied anything was wrong, commenting that she was unprepared due to having a "late night." An hour later, however, she came to me crying and asking to talk. This student had been sexually assaulted the previous night. She didn't want to miss a clinical day and thought she could "make it through the day," which she quickly learned was not possible. I was able to work with the student and ensure she received the proper support, medical care, and counseling. I firmly believe that without the relationship we had developed and without getting to know her as I did, this young woman may never have opened up and may never have received the care she needed. I could have seen her as an unprepared student who did not prioritize her clinical work over the college experience. However, by building a trusting relationship with her, I was able to help her when she needed it the most. And, had I never asked, I may never have known.

---

strategizing next steps. Some issues of concern or challenging behaviors presented by students include: lack of focus; trouble relating to a patient or family; difficulty communicating with patients, preceptors, or staff; poor decision-making; inability to integrate evidence-based practice; or lack of awareness of boundaries during interactions. Challenging behaviors can be addressed by preceptors, but may require more intense remediation, which is best handled by faculty. Preceptors can work to mitigate challenges, but they are not expected to "fix" all problems. Faculty should be contacted early before issues become unsurmountable.

BALANCING DIRECTION PROVIDED

Once the issue of concern or challenge is defined and a course of action is devised, the preceptor must balance the amount of direction or guidance provided for the learner. Providing too much direction or giving too much help may stall the learner's movement toward independence and inadvertently create learner dependence on the preceptor. Providing too little direction can also inhibit learner progress toward independence, as the learner may be left floundering without the knowledge on how to improve patient and family care.

The amount of direction provided by preceptors can be guided by reflecting on the individual or course learning objectives, the level of the student in the nursing program, past experience of the learner, and the demands of the clinical setting. Reviewing and operationalizing the objectives according to what is realistic in the clinical setting can be a helpful first step. The preceptor needs to regularly revisit the objectives with the learner to evaluate progress.

Exemplar: Reporting Unsafe Graduate Student Practice

Lorraine M. Novosel

One key difference between graduate and undergraduate clinical nursing education is that program faculty are generally not on-site with the graduate student during the clinical experience. Graduate faculty rely heavily on preceptors to not only help a student develop clinical skills but also to inform faculty when issues or concerns arise so that appropriate action may be taken.

Generally, an institutional practice within colleges of nursing is to ensure that faculty make *a minimum* of one on-site clinical visit per clinical rotation to observe and evaluate the student providing care. In my role as a faculty member, I spent nearly 3 hours with a student during an on-site, midterm visit in which I observed three patient encounters. The student was struggling to provide advanced nursing care and I did not feel they were practicing at the level expected for graduate education. I had my concerns, but also knew that it could be challenging to get an honest, accurate picture of a student's abilities during a single visit. I had reviewed the student's written assignments to that point and found them passable, although I still had concerns that the SOAP notes lacked depth.

I asked the preceptor to sit privately with me, as faculty, and the student to review the student's progress. My experience had been that preceptors, more often than not, would report that everything was going well during the rotation. I sense that the majority of preceptors do not want to be perceived as the "bad guys." However, when I asked this preceptor how the student was performing, the preceptor directly said, "[the student] is not safe for practice" and then shared, in a very professional manner, the observations that led to this summation. This

was a first for me, after nearly 20 years of graduate faculty experience.

To their credit, the student maintained composure and did not challenge the preceptor's assessment. This behavior was telling. It became evident the student could not successfully pass the precepted clinical experience that term. Ultimately, the student decided to withdraw from the course and the program. Sadly, the student was in their penultimate clinical course in the final year of the program.

I have found that clinical preceptors favorably rate students' abilities on structured evaluation forms, often more favorably than faculty might observe from their own interactions with the student. There can be an unsettling disconnect between student performance and preceptor and faculty evaluations. How many students have been passed through clinical experiences due to a preceptor's inability or unwillingness to actually say, "*No*, the student is *not* performing well"?

I do not know how previous faculty missed the student's lack of competence. Fortunately, a preceptor stood up and voiced concern. It is important to recognize that not everyone is cut out to be an advanced practice nurse, and that is okay. When thinking of future providers, I want to be reassured that the best, brightest, and most competent will be taking care of me and my family. We need to encourage and support preceptors as they provide honest evaluations. Patient safety must always come first.

Several years after this experience, I learned the student had transferred out of nursing education and received a graduate degree in another health-related discipline. I suspect this was a better fit, and to this day, I wish them well.

When a student continues to rely heavily on the preceptor, it may be prudent for the preceptor to have the student talk with peers regarding the amount of direction others are receiving in the clinical setting. Input that the student receives from peers might heighten their awareness that they are not prepared enough for their clinical day or need to be proactive in learning and taking initiative in providing patient care. Input from peers can be used in future preceptor–learner discussions to strategize a realistic plan promoting learner progression. Seeking information from peers puts some responsibility for learning back on the student and forces the student to re-evaluate their progress toward goals and objectives. Journaling or writing reflections on events and interactions during the clinical

day can help the learner and preceptor focus on specific examples of concern and clarify when too much or too little direction is provided. If the student learner continues to lean on the preceptor for direction without taking some initiative, the preceptor may need to contact the faculty for support.

PRECEPTOR–LEARNER MISMATCH

Effectively matching learners with preceptors is one way to minimize challenges in interactions. An effective match is always the goal; however, it is not always easy or possible. While great effort goes into coordinating clinical experiences with learners and preceptors, the result is not always optimal. Even in the best situations, the preceptor and learner need to continually evaluate what is going well, what needs improvement, and why. By adjusting their approach and interaction with learners, the preceptor can minimize or resolve issues before they escalate. Although the preceptor–learner match may initially be positive, subtle negative nuances can present and, if not addressed, may create an unhealthy tension, leading to an unresolvable division or mismatch. Mismatches can occur for many reasons, from differences in social style or communication style (Chapter 6) to clashes in personality. Other causes of a mismatch include a difference in career goals, especially when the learner is not interested in the preceptor's specialty.

Exemplar: How I Wish My Preceptors Would Have Optimized My Graduate Clinical Experiences

Abiola Akamo Aghakasiri

As a student in a family nurse practitioner (FNP) program, I was quite fortunate to participate in clinical experiences at a variety of care settings. I spent an equal amount of time learning from both nurse practitioners (NPs) and physicians, who provided me with a range of professional experiences. While my expectations were idealistic, I learned to compromise and find value in each clinical opportunity. My preceptors provided me with impactful experiences, although not all of my experiences were positive. Unfortunately, the negative experiences are easier to recall.

During one specialty rotation, I was challenged because the expectations of the rotation and my preceptor's expectations were not clearly identified. Since my FNP program training was in primary care, my preceptors had to be more flexible in their specialty environments to provide me an effective learning opportunity. I wish my preceptor would have worked with me to formulate clinical objectives that would have been mutually beneficial for the practice and for my learning process. I also wish my preceptor would have had a consistent open and approachable demeanor to create a welcoming learning experience. Simply remembering their first learning experience and how intimidating it can be to enter new and unfamiliar settings may help preceptors consider more productive and realistic responses for student learners.

One day, this preceptor apologized for not having the time to review some concepts and mentioned that it is difficult to offer teaching moments when working with a full patient schedule. He expressed frustration, commenting that a solution to having more time for students is typically through preceptor payment, where financial compensation from the school would have allowed him to schedule less patients each day. With an altered schedule, he would have been able to spend more time teaching and mentoring.

Later that same day, this preceptor contacted my university liaison with two concerns. He complained that I should not be "lingering" in the office after the last patient leaves and that I should arrange a different location in the office to complete my charting. I felt uncomfortable that he spoke to the university liaison without first coming to me directly, especially since his expectations were unclear. There were moments prior to this where I felt uncertain of this preceptor's willingness to work with me. After receiving feedback from my university liaison, I felt even less welcomed in this practice. Since the preceptor holds the power in the preceptor–student relationship, they need to remember that they create the tone, set the boundaries for the rotation, and can either enhance or negatively influence the student's experience. Since I did not feel welcomed, I did not feel like my contributions would bring value to the clinical setting. Unfortunately, that was my sentiment for much of that experience.

Another clinical rotation toward the end of my FNP program was challenging in a different way. I was placed in a primary care practice with an experienced NP who was enthusiastic about her patients, informative, helpful with scheduling, offered opportunities to lead patient interactions, and encouraged the clinical judgment process. It felt like this practice was the perfect setting to learn and I immersed myself in the experience. I wish, however, that this preceptor would have been more thoughtful with her responses when giving constructive feedback. Unfortunately, I cannot forget the preceptor telling me, "You know, I just don't think you'll make it." It is difficult to understand the context from which that comment was shared since the preceptor did not provide any rationale or justification. It was hard to not feel as if this comment was a personal attack. From that moment, I felt that I could not trust this person to be my advocate during the learning process. To maintain my confidence, I felt that I had to ignore the comment that I would not "make it," and move forward to learn what I needed to complete my rotation.

Precepting plays a critically important role in educating and socializing new providers to the nursing profession. I hope that those willing to answer the call to precept consider that students want to do a great job. Preceptors need to remember that students are easily influenced by the comments, opinions, feedback, and attitudes of their preceptors, whom they look to as role models.

There may also be incongruence in understanding clinical objectives or differences in work ethic. The end result is frustration, with both preceptor and learner identifying that valuable time has been wasted.

Once a point of tension presents, the preceptor should address the concern with the learner. Justifying the concern provides perspective and input regarding whether the preceptor and learner agree that there is a growing conflict. Once identified, strategies toward resolution of the issue can be considered. Strategies may involve discussing and redefining learner goals and objectives, as well as preceptor expectations of the learner. The communication approach may need to be re-evaluated and adjusted. At any point, it is reasonable for the preceptor to request an early site visit by the faculty or supervisor to mediate preceptor–learner dialogue and help strategize next steps.

TYPES OF CHALLENGING BEHAVIORS AND STRATEGIES TO FACILITATE PROGRESSION

There are many types of challenging behaviors manifested by learners. The key is recognizing behavioral characteristics of the learner so strategies can be taken to help promote learning, effective integration into the clinical setting, and especially, safe practice. The intent is *not* to label the learner but to identify behaviors and characteristics that may be preventing the learner from advancing toward independent practice. Some behaviors or characteristics of learners may require strategies to facilitate effective advancement (Table 17.1). These include being shy or dependent; lacking commitment; being inflexible, overconfident, or a "know-it-all"; lacking preparation; and focusing on extraneous details (Roberts et al., 2020).

The Learner Manifesting Shy or Dependent Behaviors

The shy or dependent learner may present as an individual hesitant to approach the patient or family. They may show little initiative to seek new experiences, lack confidence, and present with excessive hesitation or fear. This learner tends to be comfortable shadowing the preceptor or other healthcare providers. They may be very complimentary of the preceptor, proclaiming that they are "learning so much" and would like to "shadow" or observe longer. All learners, whether from an academic setting or when transitioning to a new role, need to work toward independence in skill performance and in their role. Keeping the goal of independent practice in mind can help the preceptor strategize and prompt the learner to advance in providing care confidently.

Strategies When Precepting the Learner With Shy or Dependent Behaviors

Identifying and capitalizing on the strengths of the shy or dependent learner is a good place to begin. Directing the learner to provide care for a population they are most comfortable with, such as an adolescent or older adult, or patients ready for discharge, can help to boost confidence. Once confidence with a population grows, the learner can be introduced to patients of other ages and complexity. Providing positive reinforcement and reassurance are additional strategies to promote learner growth. Overtly identifying and expressing praise for effective interactions performed by the learner can provide the motivation for the learner to take initiative in future encounters.

Although a clinical day can change quickly, planning and discussing the schedule for the day can provide the learner with some direction and a sense of control. Advanced notice of patient care needs or potential skills required for the day is helpful in guiding the learner's preparation. Being kind but firm, and complimentary but directive will help the learner advance and prevent enabling of dependence on the preceptor.

Preceptors may seek faculty or supervisor involvement when the learner is not advancing in their performance. Most academic facilities have access to skills and simulation labs, which can help increase learner comfort in a controlled setting.

Graduated Approach to Learning

A graduated approach to learning can be very effective when precepting a shy, dependent, or hesitant learner. Three strategies are useful to moving the learner toward independence: setting parameters, weaning, and refocusing.

Setting parameters specific to the learner's objectives provides stages or leveling to help the learner advance in a step-by-step manner. The objectives may need to be regularly reviewed and operationalized so each step is clear and measurable. The specific parameters identified provide an incremental roadmap, challenging the learner to slowly move out of their comfort zone and engage interactively and proactively in patient care. As

TABLE 17.1	Talking Points to Mitigate Challenging Behaviors and Interactions
Challenge	**Talking Point**
Guidance or Direction	• "I (preceptor) feel as though I am giving you too much direction. Can you (student learner) help me evaluate this? It would help if you could talk with your faculty or peers to find out how much direction others are receiving."
Potential Mismatch	• "I am feeling a disconnect between us. It seems our objectives for _____ are different. Let's review and redefine the goals and objectives for today so we are in agreement with how the day should go."
Shy or Dependent Learner	• "Yes, you are ready." • "Today, you (learner) are going to lead this appointment/patient encounter. I (preceptor) will fill in the gaps. I am here for you." • "You (learner) interact very well with _____ (e.g., type of patient). The next patient is similar. I want you to complete the physical examination after I complete the history."
Lacking Commitment	• "I sense you are not committed to this clinical experience and would prefer being somewhere else. Let's talk about ways to make this experience more meaningful." • "It seems you are having difficulty with _____ (e.g., arriving for your clinical experience on time). Can you tell me about that so we can plan accordingly?"
Inflexible	• "You are very good at following ____ protocol, but I fear you are missing some key information. Let me give you some examples." • "You have completed many history and physical exams using a template. Today, I would like you to complete the history without using your template. I will help you." • "You are correct about the next treatment steps according to the algorithm, but I am not convinced that this patient fits the recommended path. Let's talk about other treatment options and discuss why one might be better than another."
Overconfident	• "Let's pause for a moment and evaluate your encounter with Mr. _____." • "Let's talk about how you ruled in ____ (e.g., specific diagnosis). Tell me about other diagnoses you considered and why you ruled those out."
Unprepared	• "I would like you to read up on _____ (e.g., specific topic) and teach me about the latest treatment that is supported by the evidence during your next clinical day." • "I have a few articles that will be helpful for you when caring for patients following _____ (e.g., a traumatic event). Please read these tonight and tell me about the key points tomorrow." • "When you give me report on the next patient, I want you to identify three differential diagnoses, pick the mostly likely diagnosis, and present a relevant plan of care before I go into the patient room to confirm your findings and solidify a plan."
Detail-Focused	• "The report on ____ patient was well-detailed. Let's review what you reported and together determine the key points so you can focus better." • "To help you with time management while taking a history, I am going to come into the patient room after 10 minutes."

an example, the undergraduate student learner may initially require prompting when preparing and administering subcutaneous insulin; subsequent experiences should require less direct instruction.

Setting parameters can also include incorporating a time factor into the learning experience. The preceptor may need to designate time frames within which the learner is expected to complete a task. For example, the nurse practitioner (NP) student may complete a patient history and physical examination in under 5 minutes and perceive that they have been thorough. The preceptor can address pertinent information that is missing from the exam and tell the student they need to spend at least 10 minutes in the room for a comprehensive examination with the patient before reporting to the preceptor.

Weaning is needed when the learner is solely dependent on or clinging to the preceptor. The preceptor engages the learner in collaborative care, where the preceptor initiates a skill or interaction and the learner completes the encounter. In this case, the preceptor may allow the student to shadow or observe history and physical examinations for three patient visits. Then, on the fourth visit, the preceptor completes the full visit but includes the learner by directing them to conduct a pertinent review of systems with the family. As the learner builds confidence, the preceptor may have the learner obtain a full history and part of the physical exam. The process continues until the learner is able to conduct a full history and physical with minimal support. The weaning process allows the preceptor to monitor the learner for competence and then confidently determine learner readiness to take initiative and complete an exam.

Refocusing is useful when the learner becomes distracted or fears that they are not obtaining enough information, thus relying on the preceptor for direction. Refocusing is especially needed when the learner provides excessive detail while reporting to the preceptor. Initially, the detail may be useful to ensure the learner is being thorough, identifying all relevant information, and providing appropriate care. However, obtaining extraneous details is not practical and can disrupt the flow of patient care. When refocusing, the preceptor can initially critique the learner's patient report by identifying pertinent positive and negative information to include or delete. The preceptor can then role-model a concise report on the patient of interest followed by directives to limit future reporting to 5 minutes and include only pertinent information (Chapter 8).

The Learner Manifesting Lack of Commitment

Most learners come to a clinical experience excited to engage and absorb new knowledge. However, some learners may be perceived as lacking commitment or motivation needed for successful career development. This learner may exhibit behaviors such as not asking questions, appearing disinterested, not arriving in a timely manner, announcing they can only be present for a limited amount of time, or lacking follow-through. If the learner is a student, they may be at risk for failing the clinical rotation. The learner lacking commitment is often quickly identified by the preceptor who may become frustrated, especially if valuable time is poorly used. Concerns with lack of commitment need to be addressed with the learner as soon as possible. If in doubt, consultation with faculty or a supervisor should not be delayed.

Strategies When Precepting the Learner Manifesting Lack of Commitment

Discussing the root cause of the behaviors that suggest a lack of commitment is a first step in determining a plan of action; there is often an underlying issue that is affecting the learner's behavior. If the learner is a student, the preceptor may find that the student is not interested in the specialty area, but needs to have the experience to round out their education. The student may also be questioning their career focus. The family nurse practitioner (FNP) student may prefer interacting with adults and know that they never want to provide care for children or frail elderly adults. Such information warrants a discussion on other career options or what needs to occur for them to have success during their present clinical experience. Understanding the learner's perspective may help in tailoring the experience so it is meaningful. Additionally, although not invested in a specific site, the student may need to be reminded that certain skills and experiences can be translated into other healthcare areas.

Providing documented examples that demonstrate the learner's disinterest or exemplify diminishing commitment may be useful as the preceptor discusses concerns with the student. Examples operationalize the issue at hand and can guide development or modification of subsequent objectives or remediation plans. Presenting examples may also help the learner become more aware of how their behaviors are perceived by patients, families, and the healthcare staff, thereby encouraging professional growth.

The Learner Manifesting Inflexible Behaviors

The learner manifesting inflexible behaviors may be perceived as rigid. This learner has established a routine or approach to interacting with patients and families and is not readily adaptable to changes or variations in the patient encounter. In some cases, the learner may also be "book smart" and have difficulty looking beyond the content and guidelines to see the patient and family comprehensively. Other learners may present as rigid and emphatic on following the rules as a means to cover up their insecurities or lack of confidence. Although the intent of the learner is to be well-prepared or over-prepared, being inflexible when applying knowledge can lead to errors, omissions, or unsafe practice. For example, the student who is obtaining a patient history may be overly focused on following a template of questions and miss details or important nonverbal cues by the patient. Interactions between patients or family members and the learner may become compromised, leading to decreased trust. Overall, important learning opportunities may be missed.

Strategies When Precepting the Learner Manifesting Inflexible Behaviors

Identifying and discussing examples of inflexibility can heighten the learner's awareness that they need to consider more than one approach or option and think critically about the rationale for their choices. Discussion of actual or potential scenarios can provide clear insight into the adverse consequences of being inflexible. Hearing about or seeing the effect of being inflexible on the patient and family can have a profound impact on the learner, leading to modifications in their actions. Preceptors can also role-model and encourage flexibility in clinical judgment skills when providing patient care.

The Learner Manifesting Overconfident or "Know-It-All" Behaviors

Many learners are eager to please and excel in performance when working with preceptors. At times the learner's intent to please is manifested as being overconfident or a "know-it-all." Concerning behaviors that present include being quick to react, fast to judge, and hasty to diagnose and treat patients. The learner may interrupt and provide their opinion during discussions on patient care. Decisions may be made based on assumptions or a history and physical that was completed quickly, resulting in omissions. Learners exhibiting these behaviors are at risk for unsafe practice and questionable care decisions. They may miss pertinent history and physical data and, in their haste, omit inclusion of the most updated practice evidence. These learners are at risk for making mistakes or alienating other members of the healthcare team. Additionally, patients and family members may be concerned or offended by the learner's hasty interactions. Some learners may acquire a "know-it-all" perspective and hide behind their knowledge as a means to conceal their insecurities.

Strategies When Precepting the Learner Manifesting Overconfident or "Know-It-All" Behaviors

When learners present as knowing all, preceptors may react by feeling intimidated and exhibit caution, even when direction and guidance is warranted. However, it is the responsibility of the preceptor to identify overconfident learners and create teaching moments. The learner who is acting quickly and making hasty decisions needs guidance to slow their pace and think critically about their actions.

Preceptors can inquire about the rationale for the learner's actions. With advanced practice nurses, preceptors can focus on ruling in and ruling out differential diagnoses or determining the best treatment and management plan. With undergraduate or newer nurses, the preceptor can engage the learner in a discussion about evidence-based clinical policies. With all learners, the preceptor might consider asking probing questions about alternative plans of action. Discussion of learner errors or omissions can provide valuable teachable moments. The preceptor may ask the learner to evaluate the action in question and provide a more appropriate clinical approach.

In an effort to slow the learner's pace and help them to think critically, role reversal is an option. The learner becomes the observer and evaluator of the preceptor's interactions with the patient and family. This exercise gives the learner an opportunity to identify strengths and gaps in the preceptor's approach, compare and contrast their own approach, and facilitate discussion of best practice. The learner who is "fast" in their interactions may benefit from using a timer so that they spend at least five minutes on gathering history data, followed by reflecting and reporting back to the preceptor.

The Learner Manifesting Behaviors Reflecting Lack of Preparation

The learner who is unprepared is at high risk for compromising patient safety and satisfaction. This learner may present with inefficient patient interactions, poor assessment skills, lack of knowledge about the patient population, brief and flippant responses to thought-provoking questions, and a wealth of excuses justifying their actions, inactions, or inabilities. Time management may be compromised due to lack of preparation. An unprepared learner creates a situation where the preceptor's time is poorly utilized. As a result, the preceptor may need to repeat aspects of the patient encounter. If excessive time is lost, individual patient care is slowed and the flow of the unit or clinic may be compromised.

Strategies When Precepting the Learner Manifesting Lack of Preparation

Once it is determined that a learner is unprepared, review of the objectives and expectations for the clinical experience must be reinforced. Measurable parameters should be redefined, with attention to critical skills necessary for adequate preparation. The preceptor may direct the learner to specific policies or articles for review or prompt the learner to independently seek supporting evidence on specific topics, such as treatment recommendations or comparison of medications (Karlstrom et al., 2019). The preceptor can ask the learner to explore the evidence related to a particular treatment and report back instead of providing the rationale for the learner.

A concrete plan will be most beneficial for the learner who is unprepared. This includes establishing a realistic timeframe for follow-up, providing ongoing feedback, and specifying a realistic timeline for expected behavior change. If the learner is deficient in foundational skills such as conducting an assessment, a plan for remediation (in collaboration with the faculty or supervisor) may be the best direction.

The Learner Manifesting Overly Detail-Focused Behaviors

Learners focused on extraneous details often have a need to be thorough and want to avoid missing an important fact, particularly when completing a history and physical examination. They are committed to providing a comprehensive view of the patient and family and often spend an inordinate amount of time with patients and families during encounters. These learners are unable to focus effectively and tend to have poor ability to prioritize. For the advanced practice nursing student, it becomes difficult to distinguish between a focused versus a comprehensive examination. It is possible that some learners err on the side of gathering and reporting on all possible data due to a lack of confidence in their abilities and concern for missing something important that could impact patient safety. Attention to all details can adversely influence time management for the preceptor and the clinical site.

Strategies When Precepting the Learner Manifesting Detail-Focused Behaviors

The learner committed to providing excessive details may not be aware nor fully understand the ramifications of their behavior and thus be resistant to change. Preceptors can help redirect the learner by providing constructive feedback while using relevant examples. When the learner is reporting on a patient, the preceptor can interject by saying, "That is accurate information, but it is not relevant to the present chief complaint." Providing feedback in real time may have a profound impact on some learners and lead the learner to consciously fine-tune their behavior. Setting specific parameters and defining an appropriate time frame is an effective way to force the learner to critically think about priorities when gathering histories, conducting physical examinations, providing patient care, interacting with patients and families, and delivering reports.

Other Challenging Behaviors

Most learners are open to constructive feedback and strive to emulate or model their preceptors with optimal patient care and safety as a priority. However, even the best learners may intermittently present with behaviors that are challenging.

Exemplar: Managing Mistakes by the Registered Nurse Orientee

Tish Gill

I was precepting a new graduate registered nurse (RN) who had passed her NCLEX exam and was in her first week working on the hospital floor. She was in the medication room organizing and familiarizing herself with the equipment and medications on hand. I was at the nurses' station on the phone and when I finished, I went to check on how she was doing. I found her inserting a syringe into a previously opened, single-dose vial of sodium chloride (NaCl) and combining the solution with another opened NaCl single-dose vial on the counter. When I asked what she was doing, she happily replied that there had been several open vials on the counter, which she was combining into one. The RN orientee pointed to the trash can where another empty vial was deposited. It seemed there were perhaps 5 or so milliliters left in each of the opened single-dose vials. In her mind combining the vials would not waste product and also freed up space in the medication room. I gently stopped her, discarded all the open vials, and engaged her in a long conversation about why this was unsafe practice. The RN orientee was concerned that she would lose her job that very day, which she did not. She was new and her clinical judgment skills needed bolstering. As a follow-up to that day, this RN orientee willingly shared her clinical foible as a lesson to other nurses in a staff safety presentation. She was instrumental in making sure that no one left unlabeled or partially used single-dose vials on the counter in the medication room. This ended well for her and the unit. In the end, this nurse became a well-respected, vital part of our team.

TABLE 17.2 Strategies to Minimize Isolated Challenges

Challenging Behavior	Strategy
Interrupting preceptor	• Set parameters • Example: "Give me five minutes to finish my documentation, then I will answer your questions."
Engaging in negative comments about a patient	• Redirect conversation • Opportunity for teachable moment related to equity and disparities
Jumping to conclusions	• Direct to review the patient history and physical exam • Reflect on rationale for actions
Sharing personal experiences as examples for patients and families	• Redirect to incorporate evidence instead of personal anecdotes • Three-way conversation with preceptor, student, and faculty
Exhibiting defensiveness	• Give time for emotions to settle • Revisit the topic and explain the intent of feedback • Provide examples

These may arise from an eagerness to learn, an urgency to seek information, or nervousness or anxiety. Some behaviors or concerns occur in isolation and can be quickly remedied if brought to the learner's attention. Effective communication can contribute to correcting or changing the behavior. Examples of behaviors that may requiring redirection include the learner interrupting the preceptor, making negative comments about patients or families, jumping to conclusions, responding defensively, or inappropriately empathizing with patients and families (Table 17.2).

RED FLAGS WHEN PRECEPTING, OR WHEN TO CONTACT A STUDENT LEARNER'S FACULTY

When preceptors are working with student learners, they need to remember that they are not working alone. Faculty from the academic institution should be readily available as a resource to answer any questions and to provide assistance when troubleshooting issues or concerns

that arise. Preceptors should *never* hesitate to contact faculty. Student learners presenting with "red flags" always warrant a preceptor–faculty conversation (in person or virtually). The preceptor may choose to manage the concern on their own, but if the issue persists, faculty must be contacted. Red flags include safety concerns, unresolved lack of engagement, ongoing lack of preparedness, expressions of apathy related to patients and the healthcare process, and an adverse change or deterioration in progress. The student who is not engaged may fail to incorporate feedback and ignore preceptor input. The student who is unprepared may state they were "too tired" to prepare for their clinical day. Preceptors may be hesitant to report such behaviors, as they are concerned about the consequences for the student. However, identifying and reporting red flag behavior is a professional responsibility of precepting. Reporting red flag behavior early may prevent adverse long-term consequences for the patient, family, nursing school, or institution while allowing the student learner to receive needed remediation or change their course of study without losing face.

When reporting red flag behavior, preceptors should be prepared to discuss details. Regular documentation of student progress or lack of progress can be enhanced with examples. Documentation of student behaviors can occur in the form of reflective journaling or simple, bulleted lists. Preceptors may begin the discussion with faculty by summarizing the concern and providing relevant examples of adverse behaviors that are consistent with the verbal or written concern. Formative or summative evaluations (Chapter 21) are helpful, but some concerns warrant immediate attention and should not wait. Preceptors may determine that an early clinical site visit by faculty is the best option so that faculty can observe concerning behaviors firsthand. Conflict resolution facilitates a healthy work relationship and a realistic remediation approach for the learner.

"FIRING" A LEARNER

Although uncommon, there are instances where a specific precepted experience does *not* work despite multiple attempts to resolve challenges. The tension between the preceptor and student/learner may not be obvious, or both may be very aware of the tension and think that the precepting experience needs to end. Regardless, the decision to end the preceptor–student/learner experience does not occur abruptly. Red flags may have been noted and remediation for various reasons may have already been instituted. The decision to break the preceptor–student/learner relationship and end the clinical experience must be well documented.

Ideally, discontinuing the preceptor–student/learner relationship starts with an open discussion between the preceptor, faculty, and student/learner and must be justified with evidence. Some common reasons for ending a preceptor–student/learner relationship and clinical experience include:

- Unsafe practice
- Compromising the care of the patient or family
- Lack of respect for patients/families, the healthcare setting, and healthcare providers
- Inaccurate or deceptive reporting and documenting
- Lack of insight and understanding of one's own behavior and the behaviors of others
- Inability to follow specific guidelines presented (and reinforced) during the experience

- Inability to follow through or improve practice despite constructive feedback
- Late arrivals and early departures for the clinical day
- Falsification of clinical hours

Once the preceptor has addressed concerns with the student/learner and faculty, the logistics of pulling the student from the clinical site becomes the responsibility of the faculty and university. The preceptor is not responsible for "firing" the student. The preceptor is responsible for protecting patients, families, and the healthcare institution from unsafe practice.

▌CONCLUSION

The preceptor–learner relationship begins with a clean slate. Most relationships begin with a degree of excitement, enthusiasm, and maybe a little angst about the learning opportunities, with the preceptor–learner on neutral ground. Neither preceptor nor learner begin with preconceived notions that challenges may present and manifest in concerning behaviors

---

Exemplar: Firing an APRN Student

Beth Heuer

While providing inpatient and outpatient care at a small rehabilitation hospital, I agreed to precept an advanced practice registered nurse (APRN) student from a local university. The student reached out to me via email, and we scheduled her clinical days for the semester. I provided her with all the basic clinic orientation information, and we exchanged cell phone numbers so that we could contact each other if there were any schedule changes or questions. She presented as a responsible and reliable student. For her first scheduled clinic day, I instructed the student when and where to arrive so that we could chat and prepare for a scheduled morning admission. That morning, she did not text or call and showed up about 40 minutes late while I was busy admitting the patient. I quickly got her up to speed and later (privately) stressed the importance of being on-time and prepared for clinic as her professional responsibility. She arrived on time for clinical day 2, but exhibited a general lack of interest in the patient cases despite my best efforts to keep her engaged and to provide additional education and patient care opportunities. On clinical day 3, she did not show up and did not respond to my text message. She responded to my email several hours later with a cursory apology, saying that she would attend the next scheduled clinical day. I emailed her faculty instructor to discuss the student's progress and

behavior, particularly her lack of engagement and her tardiness on day 1 and her absence on day 3. The instructor and I agreed to talk after every clinic day to discuss the student's progress. The student arrived on time for clinical day 4. We began the day with a gentle but direct discussion on professional etiquette. I asked whether there were any barriers to her attendance and if she was interested in continuing in the rotation. I also informed her that I had communicated with her instructor and would continue to do so. After assuring me that there were no issues and that she wanted to continue, we had a productive clinical day. Then on clinical day 5, she arrived over two hours late and was again unprepared. This led to another discussion with the student and her faculty instructor. Once again, on clinical day 6, she did not show up and only responded to my email later that morning. In consulting with her faculty instructor, we agreed that this student's rotation with me needed to end immediately. Despite my best intentions and efforts, it was time to inform the student that they were not welcome back at this clinical site as the student's inconsistent attendance and seeming lack of interest was disruptive to the patients, their families, and to my regular clinical responsibilities. My hope is that the student learned from this experience and will be accountable in her work moving forward.

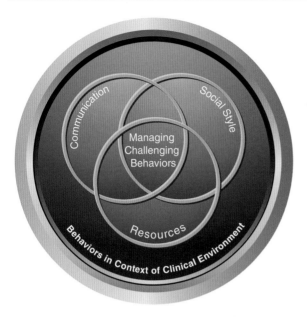

Fig. 17.1 Managing learners with challenging behaviors.

and interactions. Yet, for many reasons, challenging behaviors evolve, and the preceptor–learner relationship may become compromised (Smith & Sweet, 2019). In reviewing strategies to work with learners exhibiting various challenging behaviors, three interconnecting themes emerge and can be used to mitigate challenging behaviors (Figure 17.1): communication, social style, and resources. Preceptors may need to modify their approach to communication depending on their own and the learner's social style while seeking appropriate resources, all of which occurs in the context of a specific clinical environment. Preceptors should always seek out resources such as consultation or guidance related to any learner concerns from faculty, managers, or supervisors; they should never feel isolated when faced with challenging behaviors. As a reminder, providing specific examples of learner

behaviors are helpful when discussing concerns and creating a tailored plan to move forward with learners or their faculty or supervisors.

REFERENCES

Burns, C., Beauchesne, M., Ryan-Krause, P., & Sawin, K. (2006). Mastering the preceptor role: Challenges of clinical teaching. *Journal of Pediatric Health Care: Official Publication of National Association of Pediatric Nurse Associates & Practitioners*, 20(3), 172–183. https://doi.org/10.1016/j.pedhc.2005.10.012.

Karlstrom, M., Anderson, E., Olsen, L., & Moralej, L. (2019). Unsafe student nurse behaviours: The perspectives of expert clinical nurse educators. *Nurse Education in Practice*, 41, 102628. https://doi.org/10.1016/j.nepr.2019.102628.

Luhanga, F., Koren, I., Yonge, O., & Myrick, F. (2014). Strategies for managing unsafe precepted nursing students: A nursing faculty perspective. *Journal of Nursing Education and Practice*, 4(5), 116. http://doi.org/10.5430/jnep.v4n5p116.

Roberts, L. R., Champlin, A., Saunders, J. S., Pueschel, R. D., & Huerta, G. M. (2020). Meeting preceptor expectations to facilitate optimal nurse practitioner student clinical rotations. *Journal of the American Association of Nurse Practitioners*, 32(5), 400–407. https://doi.org/10.1097/JXX.0000000000000304.

Rodger, K. S., & Juckes, K. L. (2021). Managing at risk nursing students: The clinical instructor experience. *Nurse Education Today*, 105, 105036. https://doi.org/10.1016/j.nedt.2021.105036.

Roncarolo, F., Boivin, A., Denis, J. L., Hébert, R., & Lehoux, P. (2017). What do we know about the needs and challenges of health systems? A scoping review of the international literature. *BMC Health Services Research*, 17(1), 636. https://doi.org/10.1186/s12913-017-2585-5.

Smith, J. H., & Sweet, L. (2019). Becoming a nurse preceptor, the challenges and rewards of novice registered nurses in high acuity hospital environments. *Nurse Education in Practice*, 36, 101–107. https://doi.org/10.1016/j.nepr.2019.03.001.

18

Self-Care for the Busy Preceptor

Audra Rankin and Beth Heuer

CHAPTER OBJECTIVES

- Explore ways to manage imposter syndrome and vulnerability in professional practice
- Review strategies for identifying and addressing professional burnout/compassion fatigue
- Describe maintaining boundaries within the preceptor–learner relationship
- Develop tools to manage emotional fatigue during busy clinical days

There is a critical balance between precepting, practicing in clinical settings, meeting other work commitments, and having a life outside of the nursing profession. Preceptor role strain can increase when dealing with multiple stressors, such as administrative responsibilities, hectic or unsupportive work settings, and family demands (Nottingham, 2016). Self-care can mitigate the adverse outcomes resulting from work–life imbalance. Self-care is essential to well-being; it is *not selfish* and instead opens the pathway to being a more compassionate and productive provider and clinical educator (Mills et al., 2015). Nurses have the unfortunate tendency to use self-care as a reactive coping strategy rather than as a proactive, preventive measure (Andrews et al., 2020).

In 2007, the Institute for Healthcare Improvement (IHI) introduced the "triple aim" of healthcare: 1) improving the patient experience of care (including quality and satisfaction), 2) improving the health of populations, and 3) reducing the per capita cost of healthcare (Institute for Healthcare Improvement, n.d.). The American Association of Critical Care Nurses (AACN) further suggested a "quadruple aim," with the fourth goal involving improving the healthcare work environment and *promoting joy* in work (Fitzpatrick et al., 2019). Factors such as leadership support, shared governance, promotion of professional development,

appropriate staffing ratios, timely and positive feedback, and robust communication and collaboration are all factors that can enhance work satisfaction. Advocating for these types of on-site improvements, along with dedicated teaching time for precepting, can help make the preceptor's work more satisfying.

Self-care is not a one-size-fits-all prescription and can mean something different for everyone. Many self-care authors describe 'pillars' of well-being that encompass multiple dimensions of health. Hassed (2011) described the "ESSENCE" of well-being in a mnemonic made up of seven pillars. These pillars are as follows: *Education* (maintaining intellectual curiosity and life-long cognitive stimulation); *Stress management* (engaging in mindfulness, meditation, "finding balance", and restfulness); *Spirituality* (finding meaning in one's life and honoring what brings contentment and gratitude); *Exercise* (developing a routine to keep your heart healthy and your body in motion); *Nutrition* (choosing healthy nourishment versus nutrient-deficient foods because of convenience); *Connectedness* (maintaining and nurturing social and emotional connections), and; *Environment* (surrounding oneself, whether at home or at work, with what creates a sense of peacefulness and content). An investment in self-care can transform a vulnerable preceptor into an empowered preceptor who takes control by preserving self, protecting energy, and creating positivity.

THE VULNERABLE PRECEPTOR

Understanding and Embracing "Imposter Syndrome"

Imposter syndrome, or imposter phenomenon, impacts high-achieving professionals who are unable to acknowledge their own accomplishments. These individuals often experience self-doubt and fear that they will be recognized as an imposter. Early experiences in precepting can leave nurses feeling like imposters. Questions can arise including, "Do I know enough to be teaching someone?" and "What if the learner sees my inexperience?" Imposter syndrome can be found among men and women from a variety of ethnic and racial groups (Bravata et al., 2020) and may be found in groups that lack a sense of belonging (Jeanmonod, 2022). Due to an inability to acknowledge their own success, nurses with imposter syndrome may experience stress, burnout, and job dissatisfaction. Psychological comorbidities can result, including depression, anxiety, poor self-esteem, and social dysfunction (Bravata et al., 2020). Imposter syndrome may impact teaching and professional opportunities, causing nurses to be apprehensive about answering questions or presenting ideas and knowledge formally.

The feeling of imposter syndrome can be fleeting or a more sustained issue for nurse preceptors. Individuals influenced by imposter syndrome may suffer in silence, as the syndrome often manifests as a situational response (Gill, 2020). While self-doubt is a common response, imposter syndrome can also have a positive influence on quality performance. Acknowledging self-doubt leads to a pause in action, allowing for further assessment and validation of clinical decision-making.

Although the consequences of imposter syndrome are well documented, effective interventions to address these feelings require further research. Recognition of the imposter feeling is the first step. A subsequent step is acknowledging successes rather than diminishing them and accepting that no one has all the answers at all times. Nurses often work in high-stake, high-performing environments, where criticism and negative feedback can be common. Learning from constructive feedback, while letting go of personal criticism, can minimize self-doubt. Engaging in activities outside of the workplace and networking enhance peer support and build confidence (Gill, 2020). Precepting is a way of validating one's own experience and moving past imposter syndrome. Learners appreciate when preceptors share specific experiences including how they have learned and grown from their mistakes (Jacqua et al., 2021).

Addressing Burnout/Compassion Fatigue

Common themes described by nurses when precepting new registered nurses (RNs) include "feeling the responsibility" and "having an obligation" to precept (Frankenberger et al., 2021). To find the balance between being a productive patient care provider and an effective clinical teacher, it may be necessary to modify a precepting approach to work smarter, not harder.

By virtue of their role as preceptors, nurses and advanced practice registered nurses (APRNs) are expert clinicians who provide direct patient care. The COVID-19 pandemic magnified the demands in the healthcare system and required even more from already strained nurses. The terms "burnout," "moral distress," and "compassion fatigue" have all been used to describe the emotional exhaustion, depersonalization, and reduced sense of personal accomplishment that is increasingly prevalent among nurses. Exhaustion leads to feelings of inadequacy in one's job performance, with a decrease in both physical and mental health. Compassion fatigue also leads to increased job turnover, absenteeism, poor coworker support, and difficulty recruiting and retaining staff (Lockhart, 2022; Monroe et al., 2021). Box 18.1 lists symptoms associated with compassion fatigue. As more providers leave the nursing profession, there is an increased need within the workforce pipeline and increased demand on those nurses who also precept. When nursing care providers identify with symptoms of compassion fatigue, self-care must increase in priority (Box 18.2).

Because expert preceptors are needed to expand the nursing workforce, minimizing preceptor burnout is a key goal. *Job crafting* presents as a strategy where employees change certain aspects of their jobs in response to job demands (Tims et al., 2012). These strategies should allow the nurse to feel in control of their work setting and responsibilities. Dimensions of job crafting include: 1) decreasing job hindering demands (e.g., saying "no" to additional commitments), 2) increasing social job resources (e.g., asking for

BOX 18.1 Symptoms of Compassion Fatigue

- Anger and irritability, feeling of being "on edge"
- Exhaustion
- Difficulty sleeping
- Reduced sympathy or empathy
- Difficulty making decisions
- Increased use of alcohol or other drugs
- Intrusive thoughts about patients or clients
- Impaired ability to care for patients or clients
- Avoiding any reminders of upsetting experiences with patients
- Reduced satisfaction or enjoyment with work
- Sense of lack of control
- Feeling overwhelmed by the amount of work to be done
- Feeling disconnected from colleagues

Adapted from Substance Abuse and Mental Health Services Administration. (n.d.). *Tips for Healthcare Professionals.* https://store.samhsa.gov/sites/default/files/SAMHSA_Digital_Download/PEP20-01-01-016_508.pdf

BOX 18.2 Developing Resilience

Resilience among nurses results from experience and entails the development of complex skills and knowledge to manage crisis situations and prioritize time and tasks (Cameron & Brownie, 2010). Resilience is:

- Fostered by satisfaction in providing skilled and holistic care
- Enhanced by having a positive attitude or a sense of faith
- Reinforced by the notion of making a difference in patients' and families' lives
- Created through close relationships and sharing of experiences with patients
- Developed among nurses in the workplace through strategies such as debriefing, validating, and self-reflection
- Promoted by support from colleagues, mentors, and a sense of team camaraderie
- Experienced when individuals have emotional intelligence and insight into their ability to recognize stressors
- Generated by integrating strategies (such as humor) to reduce stressors
- Boosted by maintaining exercise, rest, social support, and outside interests

Adapted from Cameron, F., & Brownie, S. (2010). Enhancing resilience in registered aged care nurses. *Australasian Journal on Ageing, 29*(2), 66–71.

help), 3) increasing structural job resources (e.g., utilizing professional development opportunities), and 4) increasing challenging job demands (e.g., taking on a new project that revives one's energy and adds value to work experiences). Job crafting has a positive effect on work-related attitudes and behaviors (Shi et al., 2022). Advocating for healthcare settings to allow for job crafting may help support a culture of well-being (Slowiak & DeLongchap, 2022).

Another way to minimize burnout is by sharing the preceptor role and communicating effectively to maintain continuity with the learner and faculty or administration. Preceptors for students can contribute without feeling overwhelmed by precepting for only one semester per year or for a half-semester or by offering a one-day specialty clinical experience. Scheduling students every day can contribute to preceptor exhaustion. Recognizing a need for a reprieve from precepting and taking a semester off is acceptable and may be necessary.

THE EMPOWERED PRECEPTOR

The Power of Saying "No"

Saying "no" may seem contradictory to a discussion about precepting, especially as *more* preceptors are needed in the ever-changing nursing workforce. This advice is hard to follow when the preceptor feels internal (self-imposed) or external (organizational or institutional) pressure to take on the precepting role. Saying "no" to additional commitments is both acceptable and sometimes necessary. At times, home life, work projects, or exhaustion have to take precedence. The decision to say "no" may be met with initial disappointment by school faculty but will ultimately be respected. A kind "no" is always better than a half-hearted "yes" from an overworked, burned-out preceptor who is unable to provide a good learning experience for the student. It may be harder to say "no" to precepting an RN orientee when precepting is a role expectation or condition tied to career advancement. Saying "no" is one form of self-care. Self-care can also involve setting limits and negotiating for a reduction in other responsibilities (such as quality improvement projects or committee work) to make adequate time for precepting.

Vulnerability, Resilience, and Compassion

In her book *The Gifts of Imperfection*, author Brené Brown (2010) wrote about finding strength in one's own vulnerability. To be vulnerable takes courage and helps to build compassion within oneself and toward others. Those who recognize that they are not perfect and do not have all the answers (but will strive to reasonably find those answers) are more understanding of others who are still growing and learning from mistakes. Recognition helps in establishing deep connections with others, including family, friends, coworkers, patients, and students. Accepting vulnerability may prompt the need to seek employee assistance programming or other professional counseling, which are deep and meaningful forms of self-care.

Nurses are renowned for their compassion for others, yet this trait can add to their vulnerability and diminish their resilience, leading to compassion fatigue. Researchers have investigated the benefit of compassion fatigue resiliency programs within workplaces to raise awareness of the signs of burnout and to develop resilience skills (Deible et al., 2015; Pehlivan & Güner, 2020). Individuals who exhibit resilience: 1) experience significant stress that carries a substantial threat of a negative outcome, 2) access resources (both individual and environmental) that facilitate positive adaptation, and 3) positively adapt or adjust relative to their own developmental life stage (Cusack et al., 2016). Intrinsic factors such as having a positive personality, motivation, confidence, focus, and perceived social support can boost resilience (Saletnik, 2018).

Fostering *self-compassion* is one way to build resilience. The concept of self-compassion is composed of three interrelated aspects: 1) self-kindness, 2) common humanity, and 3) mindfulness (Lefebvre et al., 2020; Neff, 2003). Replacing self-critical talk ("I should have..."; "That was stupid of me") with a kinder inner dialogue ("I am doing my best"; "I can do this") is engaging in self-kindness. Common humanity is embraced when accepting that everyone struggles at times and that struggling is a shared experience. Mindfulness is about acknowledging and accepting thoughts and feelings in the moment, including thoughts of frustration and feelings of emotional exhaustion.

BUILDING AND NURTURING STRONG SUPPORTIVE RELATIONSHIPS

All human beings need to have a sense of belonging. Nurses help patients feel connected throughout periods of health and illness. Nurses excel in caring for others, yet may be less attentive to self-care. Practicing self-care is about attending to one's own health and building connections. Nurturing strong, supportive relationships is part of this practice.

Developing supportive relationships occurs within peer groups, which can include trusted colleagues who provide a listening ear or comfort through silence. Colleagues can also be supportive by providing much needed distraction. In nursing, lack of peer support is significantly related to intent to resign from one's job (Han et al., 2015; Yasin et al., 2020). Other professional peer groups can be found through professional organizations. Many people find comfort in seeking homogenous peer groups. These are people who share commonalities including work environment, personal experiences, and interests. There is also great value in developing heterogeneous relationships with people who provide new perspectives and new energy, thus broadening one's horizons.

Maintain Boundaries

Perceived boundary control is a person's psychological interpretation of how they set limits within their environment (Shi et al., 2022). A person with high perceived boundary control believes they can control the timing, frequency, and direction of how often their personal boundaries are crossed. Job crafting is one way to set boundaries, as it focuses on attaining and optimizing personal or work goals. A person who engages in job crafting asserts a level of control over the projects they take on, such as how frequently they precept.

It can be challenging to maintain boundaries during the precepting day, especially with a novice or dependent student. Preceptor–student boundaries occur within a *power* relationship (Gonzalez & Finnell, 2020). The preceptor has the knowledge and power to assess and determine whether the learner is performing adequately. Conversely, the learner has the power to express their perception that the preceptor is not adequately facilitating their learning needs. Boundaries can be successfully navigated with open and effective communication skills (See Chapter 6).

Working one-on-one with a learner can be an isolating experience. Extrinsic boundaries imposed may feel like being stranded on an island, where the preceptor and learner are working alone to provide patient care, and collaboration with others is minimal. Collaboration can be optimized and boundaries minimized by introducing the learner to colleagues and providing opportunities for formal and informal interactions. The preceptor may also need to independently step away briefly to regroup and reconnect with peers.

Mindfulness

Mindfulness is focused awareness of thoughts, feelings, bodily sensations, and the surrounding environment. The practice of mindfulness facilitates emotional regulation and has a positive impact on stress biomarkers. As a result, it can be an effective tool to combat burnout and emotional exhaustion, allowing nurses to effectively respond to high stress events (Suleiman-Martos et al., 2020).

Mindfulness as a form of stress reduction can decrease exhaustion often associated with fast-paced work environments. Four themes related to mindfulness include: 1) purposefully committing time to explore mindfulness; 2) increasing self-awareness; 3) improving focus and concentration; and 4) developing enhanced coping abilities (Spadara, 2021). The blend of these themes creates a pathway that allows for compassion and self-reflection and can have a positive effect on depression, burnout, and anxiety (Cheli et al., 2020).

There are many guided mindfulness exercises that enhance engagement in the present moment and awareness of thoughts and feelings. Mindfulness is a way of reflecting while doing and paying attention *in the moment*. Deeper self-awareness can help nurses process other people's viewpoints and provide clarity about how perceptions shape actions (Monroe et al., 2020). Preceptors may consider suggesting that engagement in mindfulness practices can increase the learner's patience with themselves and others.

Nurturing Creativity

Creativity is an effective outlet for self-care and is often the inspiration for innovation. Creativity can be described as creating something unique and of value (O'Flynn-Magee et al., 2022), and flourishes when curiosity, imagination, and knowledge interface (Milne, 2020). Nurturing creativity involves making time, engaging in novel experiences, and thinking outside of the box. Engagement in new outside interests can reduce stress responses and facilitate self-care. Thoughtful outlets to express creativity (e.g., art, music, writing, cooking, or dance) create opportunities to relax and recharge (Milne, 2020).

SELF-CARE DURING BUSY CLINICAL DAYS

"Perfectionism is not the same thing as striving to be your best." (Brown, 2010)

Rule number one for busy days (and an excellent general life rule) is to eliminate or minimize perfectionism and be realistic about what can reasonably be accomplished. Setting a realistic example for learners is a way to role-model maintaining boundaries and managing expectations. Interactions between preceptor and learner should enhance and not hinder the work of the clinic. While every case *can* be a teachable moment, not every case *has to be*. There are important tasks that learners can do that, while repetitive, also help build muscle memory and improve speed and competence. Engaging in a small number of focused educational moments can reap great benefits. By focusing on one or two key principles each day, the preceptor can enhance learning without sacrificing productivity.

Another way to stay focused is to clarify expectations up-front. Clear expectations might include: 1) discussing reasonable modifications to achieve a balance between precepting and clinical responsibilities with employers; 2) requesting clarity on institutional goals *for* the learner; and 3) reviewing objectives and progression of skills *with* the learner.

Although challenging during days that are busy and pressured, preceptors need to remember why they love teaching. There is a thrill when a learner suddenly "gets" it and has that "a-ha!" moment (e.g., inserted an IV smoothly on their first try, successfully managed a complicated patient on a ventilator, or interpreted a chest X-ray and came up with the right diagnosis and treatment plan). Those lightbulb moments can be the best moments in clinical precepting, reinforcing why the preceptor goes above and beyond again and again.

Preceptors may feel frustrated during the clinical day, whether lacking time to provide teaching moments, navigating learner difficulties or mistakes, or handling interruptions by the learner when providing patient care. An important component of self-care is acknowledging that *presence* matters (Brown, 2021). Preceptors give of their time and knowledge each day to the best of their ability. They provide care to their own patients and do their best to complete their work as thoroughly as possible. Instead of focusing on what is not completed perfectly, a healthy perspective includes shifting focus to the realization that a bad day is not the end of the world. It can help to soften the harsh edges of a busy day with the learner by asking "What went well?" and "What lessons were learned?"

Gratitude

Gratitude reflects an appreciation of the positive aspects of events, experiences, and circumstances. People who recognize positive outcomes have been shown to have enhanced well-being. A culture of gratitude has been linked to improved physical and psychological health, healthy behaviors, and a sense of hope (Hollingsworth et al., 2022). There are a variety of ways to increase gratitude awareness, such as creating a gratitude list, journaling, or writing letters of thanks. Identifying and sharing instances of gratitude expressed in the workplace improves motivation and strengthens the work culture (Victorson et al., 2021).

Using Reflection and Journaling

Reflection can help to clarify values and priorities, and makes sense of interactions with others, especially instances that create discomfort or anger (Drick, 2014). There are effective ways to engage in reflection to help express feelings and enhance self-awareness. Reflective journaling is a tool commonly recommended by mental health providers to examine boundaries, express feelings, develop clinical judgment skills and coping strategies, and enhance professional growth (Thomson et al., 2022). All that is required for journaling is a method for writing, a few minutes, and a willingness to let thoughts and feelings flow. A journal is an excellent place to document thoughts of gratitude and to reflect on daily accomplishments, whether they are large or small. Over time, a journal becomes tangible evidence of one's growth and accomplishments. Later, rereading a journal offers a chance to reflect on lessons learned and can spark thoughts on future personal and professional growth.

■ CONCLUSION

Successful self-care includes maintaining a work–life balance, having supportive social networks, job crafting to actively manage workload, and proactively accessing counseling either privately or through employee assistance programs. Acknowledging vulnerabilities and embracing self-care and self-compassion can strengthen personal and professional well-being. This reflects an upstream or proactive approach to culture change within the nursing profession.

REFERENCES

Andrews, H., Tierney, S., & Seers, K. (2020). Needing permission: The experience of self-care and self-compassion in nursing: A constructivist grounded theory study. *International Journal of Nursing Studies, 101*(101), 103436. https://doi.org/10.1016/j.ijnurstu.2019.103436

Bravata, D. M., Watts, S. A., Keefer, A. L., Madhusudhan, D. K., Taylor, K. T., Clark, D. M., Nelson, R. S., Cokley, K. O., & Hagg, H. K. (2020). Prevalence, predictors, and treatment of imposter syndrome: A systematic review. *Journal of General Internal Medicine, 35*(4), 1252–1275. https://doi.org/10.1007/s11606-019-05364-1

Brown, B. (2010). *The gifts of imperfection: Let go of who you think you're supposed to be and embrace who you are.* Hazelden Publishing.

Brown, J. (2021). How to care without compromising your well-being. *Nursing Standard, 36*(3), 72–75. https://doi.org/10.7748/ns.36.3.72.s25

Cheli, S., Bartolo, P., & Agostini, A. (2020). Integrating mindfulness into nursing education: A pilot nonrandomized controlled trial. *International Journal of Stress Management, 27*(1), 93–100. http://doi.org/10.1037/str0000126

Deible, S., Fioravanti, M., Tarantino, B., & Cohen, S. (2015). Implementation of an integrative coping and resiliency program for nurses. *Global Advances in Health and Medicine, 4*(1), 28–33. https://doi.org/10.7453/gahmj.2014.057

Drick, C. (2014). Nurturing yourself to enhance your practice. *International Journal of Childbirth Education, 29*(1), 46–51.

Fitzpatrick, B., Bloore, K., & Blake, N. (2019). Joy in work and reducing nurse burnout: From Triple Aim to Quadruple Aim. *AACN Advanced Critical Care, 30*(2), 185–188. https://doi.org/10.4037/aacnacc2019833

Frankenberger, W. D., Roberts, K. E., Hutchins, L., & Froh, E. B. (2021). Experience of burnout among pediatric inpatient nurse preceptors. *Nurse Education Today,* 104862. https://doi.org/10.1016/j.nedt.2021.104862

Gill, P. (2020). Imposter syndrome-why is it so common among nurse researchers and is it really a problem? *Nurse Researcher, 28*(3), 30–36. https://doi.org/10.7748/nr.2020.e1750

Han, K., Trinkoff, A. M., & Gurses, A. P. (2015). Work-related factors, job satisfaction and intent to leave the current job among United States nurses. *Journal of Clinical Nursing*, 24(21–22), 3224–3232. https://doi.org/10.1111/jocn.12987

Hollingsworth, J., & Redden, D. (2022). Tiny habits for gratitude-implications of healthcare education stakeholders. *Frontiers in Public Health*, 10. https://doi.org/10.3389/fpubh.2022.866992

Institute for Healthcare Improvement. (n.d.). *Overview: Triple aim for populations.* https://www.ihi.org/Topics/TripleAim/Pages/Overview.aspx

Jacqua, E. E., Nguyen, V., Park, S., & Hanna, M. (2021). Coping with impostor syndrome. *Family Practice Management*, 28(3) 40–40.

Jeanmonod, R. (2022). Imposter syndrome? Check your biases. *Academic Emergency Medicine*, 29(6), 816–817. https://doi.org/10.1111/acem.14473

Lefebvre, J. I., Montani, F., & Courcy, F. (2020). Self-compassion and resilience at work: A practice-oriented review. *Advances in Developing Human Resources*, 22(4), 452. https://doi.org/10.1177/1523422320949145

Lockhart, L. (2022). How to recognize compassion fatigue. *Nursing Made Incredibly Easy!*, 20(3), 30–33. https://doi.org/10.1097/01.nme.0000824592.38046.62

Mills, J., Wand, T., & Fraser, J. A. (2015). On self-compassion and self-care in nursing: Selfish or essential for compassionate care? *International Journal of Nursing Studies*, 52(4), 791–793. https://doi.org/10.1016/j.ijnurstu.2014.10.009

Milne, J. (2020). What is creativity? *British Journal of Nursing*, 29(12), S4.

Monroe, C., Loresto, F., Horton-Deutsch, S., Kleiner, C., Eron, K., Varney, R., & Grimm, S. (2021). The value of intentional self-care practices: The effects of mindfulness on improving job satisfaction, teamwork, and workplace environments. *Archives of Psychiatric Nursing*, 35(2), 189–194. https://doi.org/10.1016/j.apnu.2020.10.003

Neff, K. (2003). Self-compassion: An alternative conceptualization of a healthy attitude toward oneself. *Self and Identity*, 2(2), 85–101. https://doi.org/10.1080/15298860309032.

Nottingham, S., Barrett, J. L., Mazerolle, S. M., & Eason, C. M. (2016). Examining the role mentorship plays in the development of athletic training preceptors. *Athletic Training Education Journal*, 11(3), 127–137. https://doi.org/10.4085/1103127

O'Flynn-Magee, K., Slemon, A., Mahy, J., & Jenkins, E. (2022). "In touch with my creative side": Supporting self-care among nursing students through arts-based pedagogy. *Quality Advancement in Nursing Education*, 8(1), 1–21. https://doi.org/10.17483/2368-6669.1300

Pehlivan, T., & Güner, P. (2020). Effect of a compassion fatigue resiliency program on nurses' professional quality of life, perceived stress, resilience: A randomized controlled trial. *Journal of Advanced Nursing*, 76(12), 3584–3596. https://doi.org/10.1111/jan.14568

Saletnik, L. (2018). Building personal resilience. *AORN Journal*, 107(2), 175–178. https://doi.org/10.1002/aorn.12067

Shi, Y., Li, D., Zhang, N., Jiang, P., Yuling, D., Xie, J., & Yang, J. (2022). Job crafting and employees' general health: The role of work–nonwork facilitation and perceived boundary control. *BMC Public Health*, 22(1). https://doi.org/10.1186/s12889-022-13569-z

Spadara, K., & Hunker, D. (2021). Experience of an 8-week online mindfulness intervention for nursing students: Qualitative findings. *Nurse Educator*, 46(3), 187–191. https://doi.org/10.1097/NNE.0000000000000881

Substance Abuse and Mental Health Services Administration. (n.d.). *Tips for Healthcare Professionals.* https://store.samhsa.gov/sites/default/files/SAMHSA_Digital_Download/PEP20-01-01-016_508.pdf

Suleiman-Martos, N., Gomez-Urquiza, J., Aguayo-Estremera, R., Canadas-De La Fuente, G. A., De La Fuente-Solana, El, & Albeindin-Garcia, L. (2020). The effect of mindfulness training on burnout syndrome in nursing: A systematic review and meta-analysis. *Journal of Advanced Nursing*, 76, 1124–1140. https://doi.org/10.1111/jan.14318

Thomson, A. E., Smith, N., & Karpa, J. (2022). Strategies used to teach professional boundaries in psychiatric nursing education. *Issues in Mental Health Nursing*, 1–8. https://doi.org/10.1080/01612840.2022.2083737

Tims, M., Bakker, A. B., & Derks, D. (2012). Development and validation of the job crafting scale. *Journal of Vocational Behavior*, 80(1), 173–186. https://doi.org/10.1016/j.jvb.2011.05.009

Victorson, D., Sauer, C., Horowitz, B., & Wolf-Beadle, J. (2021). Development and implementation of a brief healthcare professional support program based in gratitude, mindfulness, self-compassion, and empathy. *The Journal of Nursing Administration*, 51(4), 212–219. https://doi.org/10.1097/nna.0000000000001000

Yasin, Y. M., Kerr, M. S., Wong, C. A., & Bélanger, C. H. (2020). Factors affecting job satisfaction among acute care nurses working in rural and urban settings. *Journal of Advanced Nursing*, 76(9), 2359–2368. https://doi.org/10.1111/jan.14449

19

Managing Barriers in the APRN Clinical Site

Heather Dunn and Maria Lofgren

"There are no immovable barriers to education."
(Irina Bokova)

Clinical sites and academic institutions work together to optimize student learning. Despite best intentions, barriers may interfere with developing and maintaining an effective precepted experience. Perceived barriers to advanced practice registered nurse (APRN) student clinical placements, along with strategies for resolution, will be reviewed in this chapter.

BARRIERS *PRIOR TO* THE CLINICAL EXPERIENCE

Significant barriers to APRN student clinical practicum placements are often encountered before the clinical assignment is obtained. These barriers include preceptor availability, employer support, and difficulty with coordination and communication between the academic institution and the clinical site.

Preceptor Availability

The lack of available clinical sites is a great concern among academic nursing faculty. In a recent National Association of Pediatric Nurse Practitioners survey, 75% of academic respondents reported lack of available clinical sites for their APRN students (Peck & Sonney, 2021). The increasing demand for clinical placements has resulted in a "victim of one's own success" phenomenon, which has caused direct competition among schools of nursing for the limited supply of available preceptors (Forsberg et al., 2015; Hawkins, 2019; Todd et al., 2019). (See Chapter 1 for information on preceptor shortages). Healthcare systems honor a limited number of requests for clinical placements and may receive substantially more requests than they are able to manage due to the work effort and resource allocation necessary to onboard students.

Another barrier may be the presence of multiple learners from different disciplines within each clinical site. Academic medical centers are often accommodating students from organizations educating physician assistants (PAs), medical students, residents, and other healthcare-related disciplines. Practicing APRNs are frequently asked to precept students in other related health disciplines, creating an additional strain on already limited resources (Todd et al., 2019; Webb et al., 2015).

Current standards for nurse practitioner (NP) clinical experiences, as delineated by the National Task Force on Quality Nurse Practitioner Education (NTF), require that clinical placements provide experiences that meet the specialty role and population focus (NTF, 2022). In addition to the limited number of preceptors, *more* clinical sites are needed to meet the consensus model *population-focused* competencies for all NP students (APRN Consensus Work Group & the National Council of State Boards of Nursing APRN Advisory Committee [NCSB], 2008; National Organization of Nurse Practitioner Faculties [NONPF], 2013). For example, family NP (FNP) students may require multiple clinical placements per semester secondary to the range of experiences necessary for this certification (Doherty et al., 2020).

Preceptor Fatigue

Repeated clinical teaching assignments contribute to preceptor fatigue (Forsberg et al., 2015; Lofgren et al., 2021). Layered with the issues of professional burnout and compassion fatigue, preceptor fatigue can decrease the number of preceptors able to work with a student. Precepting students has been reported to lengthen the preceptor's workday and contribute to preceptor fatigue (Hatfield et al., 2022). Data are needed to determine the actual impact on professional productivity that may help support interventions to reduce barriers. Preceptors may choose to decline working with students so that they can take a break and recharge (See Chapter 18). It is expected that academic institutions will respect that preceptors may need a break, and will develop a robust and rotating network of available preceptors.

Employer Support

Lack of employer support can be a highly influential barrier to precepting (Doherty et al., 2020). Often, employers erroneously cite decreased productivity as the reason for not inviting APRN student experiences at the clinical site. The concept of decreased productivity is based on historical data regarding both medical students and APRN students (Amella et al., 2001; Kirz & Larsen, 1986; Pawlson et al., 1980). Evidence regarding the relationship between student presence and clinical productivity is inconclusive. Some researchers report that student presence increases productivity and others report contradictory findings (Cobb et al., 2013; Evans et al., 2018; Hatfield et al., 2022).

Employers that express concern or hesitancy about inviting APRN students for a precepted experience are encouraged to consider potential benefits to the practice.

Preceptor–student reciprocal learning occurs during a clinical practicum and drives the preceptor's knowledge base, clinical judgment skills, and evidence-based practice, which directly benefit patients and the employer (Lafrance, 2018). By the end of the clinical experience, employers may recognize and appreciate the contribution of the APRN student and recruit them for a position on the healthcare team.

Communication and Coordination

Clinical preceptors report a desire for increased communication with faculty that is goal-directed, individualized, and specific to the unique student and clinical site (Burt et al., 2022; Todd et al., 2019). An open circle of communication includes regular dialogue to clarify expectations (Figure 19.1). Checklists specific to the roles of each player in the circle of communication have been developed (Pitts et al., 2019) and are encouraged by professional organizations such as National Organization of Nurse Practitioner Faculties (NONPF) and American Association of Nurse Practitioners (AANP).

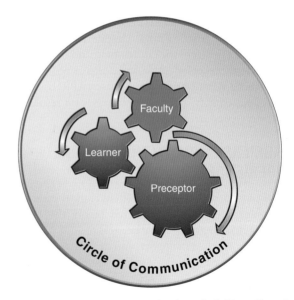

Fig. 19.1 The clinical communication triad. (From Pitts, C., Padden, D., Knestrick, J., & Bigley, M. B. (2019). A checklist for faculty and preceptor to enhance the nurse practitioner student clinical experience. *Journal of the American Association of Nurse Practitioners*, *31*(10), 591–597.)

Exemplar: Minimizing Barriers by Managing Emotional Responses of Learners in Psych-Mental Health Clinical Settings

Marjorie Hart Lehigh

In nursing education, the psychiatric (psych)-mental health rotation for students is unlike any other rotation, as it is often the first time students are exposed to patients behind locked doors, in seclusion rooms, or in restraints. To prepare the student, it is necessary to discuss: 1) characteristics of the unit; 2) diagnoses and potential characteristics of the patients; and 3) measures to maintain safety. We also review questions and concerns to help alleviate student anxiety. Even with all this preparation, situations arise that are unexpected and overwhelming.

It was the first day precepting a nursing student during her psych-mental health rotation. As we entered the locked psychiatric unit and the door closed behind us, the student suddenly looked terrified. She backed up against the wall, immobilized, and was unable to voice what was happening. There were no patients around, so interacting with patients was not a present concern. I made the immediate decision to take her off the unit and find a safe place to talk. Once alone with me, she started crying. After calming down, she told me that as a child, she had to visit her sibling at a locked psychiatric unit and described the visit as a "horrible" experience. She had repressed this experience until we walked into the locked unit and the door closed behind her. Many terrible memories came flooding back, leaving her almost paralyzed. We worked on processing her feelings and talked about the impact of experiences when a family member has a psychiatric illness. We did not go back to the unit that day, to give her the time she needed to process her feelings. She returned the next day, appearing confident and prepared to enter the locked unit. Throughout the rotation she interacted effectively with patients and continued to grow in her ability to understand and share in the feelings of others.

It is crucial to talk about the helpless feeling that comes with being locked on a unit and not having the keys to get out. I assure students and new nurses that an experienced staff member will be available for them at all times and that they will be able to leave the unit when needed. Experiences such as this provide good teaching moments, as students and orientees develop empathy toward patients who are confined and have limited or no control. In the psych-mental health setting, students and orientees gain self-awareness as they increase recognition of their own beliefs, feelings, values, and attitudes. It is important for the preceptor to teach learners that empathy and acceptance are the keys to building therapeutic relationships

BARRIERS DURING THE CLINICAL ROTATION

Once the APRN student clinical placement is secured, new barriers may present. These barriers include: gaining experiences with a diverse patient population, assuring a variety of diagnoses for maximum learning potential, and finding opportunities for a broad range of procedures.

Clinical Site Visits

Academic faculty function in a supporting role during the clinical practicum experiences and should be readily available to support the needs of students and preceptors throughout each clinical experience. There should be frequent check-ins with both the student and the preceptor for bidirectional communication that support clear expectations and set the stage for a range of successful experiences. Preceptors should expect clinical site visits, and if they are not occurring, request to schedule one with the academic faculty member.

Clinical site visits offer an opportunity for enhanced, direct, one-on-one communication with preceptors. The evolution of online programs and the COVID-19 pandemic have resulted in a shift from in-person clinical site visits, yet this is a lost opportunity to share information, reflect and evaluate role expectations, and strengthen the circle of support for the APRN student. Whether clinical site visit communication is face to face, in person, or virtual, they are necessary for the success of the student *and* a requirement by the NTF as an indicator of academic programmatic quality (NTF, 2022).

Direct Supervision Needs

Direct supervision needs coupled with preceptor time constraints are influential factors in APRN decisions to precept (Doherty et al., 2020; Todd et al., 2019).

A small minority of APRN preceptors indicate a preference for precepting first-semester students, who have high direct supervision needs (Webb et al., 2015). Many preceptors believe that first semester students impact productivity negatively, while final semester students positively impact productivity (Todd et al., 2019). When APRN preceptors accept a first-semester student, clear objectives and goals for the student practicum are essential (See Chapter 14). Initial clinical experiences are a stepping stone toward more advanced clinical experiences that ultimately help students form an APRN identity. Clinical practicums

---

Exemplar: Student Who Cannot Manage Time Well in a Busy Women's Health Setting

Elizabeth Mollard

As a women's health nurse practitioner (WHNP) who works in a high-volume, fast-paced clinic setting, I agreed to precept a first semester WHNP student. Starting on the first day, the student arrived at the clinic around the time of the first patient visit instead of arriving early to review patient cases for the day. While obtaining the history, the student spent excessive time gathering information about minor issues and did not ask critical questions related to more pertinent patient concerns. She returned to the clinic about 10 minutes late after her lunch breaks and often missed the first encounter of the afternoon. After the first week of precepting this student, I felt frustrated. My workflow had been significantly slowed, causing me to need to stay after hours to chart.

I quickly recognized that the student needed to work on time management skills and began by setting expectations. I informed the student that they must arrive at least 30 minutes before the day's first encounter and at least 15 minutes before the first encounter after lunch. If these expectations could not be met, the student would have to cancel their clinical experience for the day and risk losing the opportunity to meet required clinical hours. I also provided more specific ideas on how we could improve this student's time management skills, which included reviewing the schedule before the clinic day. The student and I began working together more efficiently by splitting tasks during patient visits; the student would complete the history and I would follow-up with the physical exam and develop a treatment plan. As the student began to build confidence in time management, responsibilities were added each week.

We discussed expected time allotments for each patient encounter. For example, "I expect it will take about 5 minutes to collect a history from Ms. Smith since her chief complaint is straightforward." At the end of each clinic, the student and I would have a quick debriefing session. If the student still had trouble timing the visits, I would use a guiding question such as, "I know that collecting the history for Ms. Smith ended up taking 20 minutes. Can you tell me more about why?"

Although the student was responsive to my feedback, it was still challenging for them to collect all the required patient encounter information in the allotted time. Subsequently, we moved to a wave scheduling model to help the student become more proficient in history-taking skills (See chapter 15). They were then able to gradually add more elements to the patient visit. This approach also allowed me, as preceptor, to manage workflow and adhere to charting demands more efficiently. By the end of the semester, the student could complete 50% of the visits at a reasonable pace. The student and I discussed that conducting half of the visits at a busy clinic was a valuable clinical experience, and that quality should be prioritized in learning over quantity.

My lessons learned included that it is important to set clinic expectations before commencing a preceptor–student relationship. These expectations should include attention to time, such as when the student should arrive at clinic and how long tasks in the clinic day may take. Achieving clinical competence in time management is one way to increase confidence, enhance skills, and minimize potential barriers to learning.

---

for the APRN novice student need not be overly complicated. Student observation coupled with preceptor "think aloud" methods provide valuable insight into the analytical thought process of both the student and preceptor (Lee & Ryan-Wenger, 1997; Logan et al., 2015; Pearson & Hensley, 2019). The clinical case example provides possible questions for a student to explore.

Patient or Family Refusal to Work With Student

Most patients are receptive to student involvement in their care. Occasionally a patient or their family member will refuse student participation. Patients and their families have the right to refuse to have a student perform or be present during medical examinations, just as they have the right to refuse care from any licensed medical or nursing provider. The preceptor can discuss concerns with the patient or the family and reassure them that APRN students are experienced registered nurses. If continued refusal is expressed, the patient is entitled to full and appropriate medical care for their specific condition from a licensed provider. Although reasons for APRN student refusal are lacking, one study on the reasons for patient refusal of care by a medical student included: expressed desire for privacy, perceived inexperience, perception of increased visit duration, and gender and racial biases (Vaughn et al., 2015). Patients are more likely to decline student participation when preceptors are less comfortable discussing student involvement and

Marcella Thomas (fictitious patient) is an 83-year-old, Black, female patient who lives in a long-term care facility secondary to advanced Alzheimer's dementia. Significant past medical history includes HTN, Stage III CKD, and Alzheimer's dementia. She is a full code and was brought to the ED yesterday with reports of congested cough, pleuritic chest pain, increased work of breathing, fatigue, and a fever of 101.6. F Laboratory analysis revealed the following noted abnormalities: WBC 18.4 X10^9/L, BUN 36, and a creatinine 1.67. Arterial blood gas results: 7.31, PCO2 50, PO2 88 on 2 L NC O2, HCO3 29. CXR showed right-sided perihilar consolidation. She was diagnosed with pneumonia in the ED and started on IV antibiotics, given a trial of NIPPV at 12/8 with 50% FiO2, and admitted to the medical floor because the ICU did not have a bed. After admission, her cognition continued to decline, and she became unresponsive. A rapid response was called, the patient was orally intubated, initiated on mechanical ventilation, and transferred to the ICU for higher level care.

Initial question for student to investigate and consider

- What type of pneumonia does Marcella have and why is that your answer?

Probing questions

- What are the classifications of pneumonia?
- What are the diagnostic criteria for the four different classifications of pneumonia (community acquired, healthcare acquired, ventilator-associated, and aspiration)?
- Is she on the appropriate antibiotics for this type of pneumonia? Why or why not?
- What antibiotics would you order?
- What is the anticipated duration of antibiotic therapy for Marcella now that she is on the ventilator and in the ICU?
- What clinical practice guidelines/resources did you use to help you answer the above questions?

ENVIRONMENTAL LIMITATIONS

Physical Space

Perceived lack of physical space, from examination rooms to office space, is a reported barrier for APRN student clinical practicum placement (Hawkins, 2019; Doherty et al., 2020). Flexibility and creativity are often necessary to integrate APRN students into a space-limited clinical setting. Scheduling students on days when fewer providers are present will optimize clinical experiences. Open communication with course faculty and students can facilitate understanding of space limitations within the clinic. Out of courtesy, clinical colleagues should be asked if it is acceptable for students to use their desk space in their absence. Confirming usage of space for students should be mutually agreed upon by clinical management. Students are expected to be respectful of the space provided.

Telehealth is an approach to healthcare visits, and remains a feasible alternative in space-limited practices (Johnson et al., 2022). This clinical approach has spurred learning modifications for preceptor-based education experiences, and has shown to be an effective teaching technique (Gibson et al., 2020; Tyson et al., 2018). See Chapter 11 for more information on precepting using telehealth.

Electronic Health Record Requirements

Access to electronic health records (EHR) is essential for a successful and educational clinical practicum experience. EHRs can contribute to clinical site barriers, necessitating additional training on the student's part and requiring computer support staff to grant access to the system and develop log-in information (Forsberg et al., 2015). When EHR access is unavailable to students, students should document using the standard Subjective, Objective, Assessment, Plan (SOAP) note format. Lack of EHR access is not an excuse for lack of student documentation. In situations where the student is not provided EHR log-in access, students cannot document in the EHR using their preceptor's log-in credentials.

◼ CONCLUSION

Anticipating barriers and expertly managing them will set up the preceptor–student experience for success. When mitigating barriers and identifying opportunities for APRN students, preceptors must remain flexible and creative in developing solutions (Box 19.1).

when consent is obtained while the student is *outside* of the examination room (Tang & Skye, 2009). When patients and families refuse care from APRN students, preceptors need to reassure students that the refusal is not personal.

BOX 19.1 Preceptor Pearls to Minimize Barriers

- Initial advanced practice registered nurse (APRN) student clinical practicums need not be overly complicated. Student observation coupled with simple preceptor "think aloud" methods are valuable.
- Multiple approaches to integrating APRN students into the clinical setting will minimize the barriers associated with clinical precepting.
- Preceptors should request clinical site visits from academic faculty to facilitate communication.
- Time constraints can be managed by spending brief, focused amounts of time with students.

REFERENCES

Amella, E. J., Brown, L., Resnick, B., & McArthur, D. B. (2001). Partners for NP education: The 1999 AANP preceptor and faculty survey. *Journal of the American Academy of Nurse Practitioners, 13*(11), 517–523. https://doi.org/10.1111/j.1745-7599.2001.tb00018.x

APRN Consensus Work Group & the National Council of State Boards of Nursing APRN Advisory Committee. (2008). *Consensus Model for APRN Regulation: Licensure, Accreditation, Certification & Education*. https://www.aacnnursing.org/Portals/42/AcademicNursing/pdf/APRNReport.pdf

Burt, L., Sparbel, K., & Corbridge, S. (2022). Nurse practitioner preceptor resource needs and perceptions of institutional support. *Journal of the American Association of Nurse Practitioners, 34*(2), 348–356. https://doi.org/10.1097/JXX.0000000000000629

Cobb, T., Jeanmonod, D., & Jeanmonod, R. (2013). The impact of working with medical students on resident productivity in the emergency department. *Western Journal of Emergency Medicine, 14*(6), 585–589. https://doi.org/10.5811/westjem.2012.12.12683

Doherty, C. L., Fogg, L., Bigley, M. B., Todd, B., & O'Sullivan, A. L. (2020). Nurse practitioner student clinical placement processes: A national survey of nurse practitioner programs. *Nursing Outlook, 68*(1), 55–61. https://doi.org/10.1016/j.outlook.2019.07.005

Evans, T. C., Wick, K. H., Andrilla, C. H. A., Skaggs, S. A., & Burgin, T. (2018). A method to study the effect of a physician assistant student on preceptor productivity. *Journal of Physician Assistant Education, 29*(4), 205–210. https://doi.org/10.1097/JPA.0000000000000220

Forsberg, I., Swartwout, K., Murphy, M., Danko, K., & Delaney, K. R. (2015). Nurse practitioner education: Greater demand, reduced training opportunities. *Journal of the*

American Association of Nurse Practitioners, 27(2), 66–71. https://doi.org/10.1002/2327-6924.12175

Gibson, N., Arends, R., Voss, J., Marckstadt, S., & Nissen, M. K. (2020). Reinforcing telehealth competence through nurse practitioner student clinical experiences. *Journal of Nursing Education, 59*(7), 413–417. https://doi.org/10.3928/01484834-20200617-12

Hatfield, J., Neal, G., Isbell, T., & Dickey, D. (2022). The effect of a medical student on community preceptor productivity. *Medical Education, 56*(7), 747–753. https://doi.org/10.1111/medu.14733

Hawkins, M. D. (2019). Barriers to preceptor placement for nurse practitioner students. *Journal of Christian Nursing, 36*(1), 48–53. https://doi.org/10.1097/CNJ.0000000000000519

Johnson, D., Gatewood, E., Ling, A., & Kuo, A. C. (2022). Teleprecepting: A timely approach to clinical education during COVID-19. *Journal of the American Association of Nurse Practitioners, 34*(1), 153–159. https://doi.org/10.1097/jxx.0000000000000567

Kirz, H. L., & Larsen, C. (1986). Costs and benefits of medical student training to a health maintenance organization. *JAMA, 256*(6), 734–739.

Lafrance, T. (2018). Exploring the intrinsic benefits of nursing preceptorship: A personal perspective. *Nurse Education in Practice, 33*, 1–3. https://doi.org/10.1016/j.nepr.2018.08.018

Lee, J. E. M., & Ryan-Wenger, N. (1997). The "Think Aloud" seminar for teaching clinical reasoning: A case study of a child with pharyngitis. *Journal of Pediatric Health Care, 11*(3), 101–110. https://doi.org/10.1016/S0891-5245(97)90061-4

Lofgren, M., Dunn, H., Dirks, M., & Reyes, J. (2021). Perspectives, experiences, and opinions precepting advanced practice registered nurse students. *Nursing Outlook.* https://doi.org/10.1016/j.outlook.2021.03.018

Logan, B. L., Kovacs, K. A., & Barry, T. L. (2015). Precepting nurse practitioner students: One medical center's efforts to improve the precepting process. *Journal of the American Association of Nurse Practitioners, 27*(12), 676–682. https://doi.org/10.1002/2327-6924.12265

National Task Force on Quality Nurse Practitioner Education. (2022). *Standards for quality nurse practitioner education, A report of the national task force on quality nurse practitioner education.* (6th ed.). https://cdn.ymaws.com/www.nonpf.org/resource/resmgr/2022/ntfs_/ntfs_final.pdf

Pawlson, L. G., Watkins, R., & Donaldson, M. (1980). The cost of medical student instruction in the practice setting. *Journal of Family Practice, 10*(5), 847–852.

Pearson, T., & Hensley, T. (2019). Positive precepting: Identifying NP student learning levels and needs. *Journal of* the American Association of Nurse Practitioners, 31(2), 131–132. https://doi.org/10.1097/JXX.0000000000000210

Peck, J. L., & Sonney, J. (2021). Exhausted and burned out: COVID-19 emerging impacts threaten the health of the pediatric Advanced Practice Registered Nursing workforce. *Journal of Pediatric Healthcare, 35*(4), 414–424. https://doi.org/10.1016/j.pedhc.2021.04.012

Pitts, C., Padden, D., Knestrick, J., & Bigley, M. B. (2019). A checklist for faculty and preceptor to enhance the nurse practitioner student clinical experience. *Journal of the American Association of Nurse Practitioners, 31*(10), 591–597. https://doi.org/10.1097/JXX.0000000000000310

Tang, T. S., & Skye, E. P. (2009). When patients decline medical student participation: The preceptors' perspective. *Advances in Health Sciences Education, 14*(5), 645–653. https://doi.org/10.1007/s10459-008-9145-z

Todd, B. A., Brom, H., Blunt, E., Dillon, P., Doherty, C., Drayton-Brooks, S., Hung, I., Montgomery, K., Peoples, L., Powell, M., Vanacore, D., Whalen, D., & Aiken, L. (2019).

Precepting nurse practitioner students in the graduate nurse education demonstration: A cross-sectional analysis of the preceptor experience. *Journal of the American Association of Nurse Practitioners, 31*(11), 648–656. https://doi.org/10.1097/JXX.0000000000000301

Tyson, R. L., Brammer, S., & McIntosh, D. (2018). Telehealth in psychiatric nursing education: Lessons from the field. *Journal of the American Psychiatric Nurses Association, 25*(4), 266–271. https://doi.org/10.1177/1078390318807967

Vaughn, J. L., Rickborn, L. R., & Davis, J. A. (2015). Patients' attitudes toward medical student participation across specialties: A systematic review. *Teaching & Learning in Medicine, 27*(3), 245–253. https://doi.org/10.1080/10401334.2015.1044750

Webb, J., Palan Lopez, R., & Guarino, A. J. (2015). Incentives and barriers to precepting nurse practitioner students. *Journal for Nurse Practitioners, 11*(8), 782–789. https://doi.org/10.1016/j.nurpra.2015.06.003

20

Documentation

Beth Heuer

CHAPTER OBJECTIVES

- Review general documentation principles for undergraduate nursing students
- Explore documentation requirements related to advanced practice nursing students
- Provide an overview of Centers for Medicare and Medicaid Services (CMS) Evaluation and

- Management (E&M) guidelines related to documentation and billing
- Discuss additional documentation for preceptors related to educational requirements for learners

Teaching the principles of documentation to nursing and advanced practice nursing students in the clinical setting can be a time-consuming task for preceptors. Yet, accurate documentation is "an essential element of safe, quality, evidence-based nursing practice" (American Nurses Association [ANA], 2010, p. 3). There is truth in the adage that activities such as tasks, observations, or assessments must be documented to verify they were really done. Documentation is often the last piece of a patient care encounter: a record of the care provided during clinical shifts, clinic visits, procedures, and other patient encounters. Documentation is a critical source of information-sharing with the interprofessional team. It is a window to current and past encounters, serving as the record of what happened during patient care interactions. This chapter provides a review of documentation principles for preceptors as they relate to nursing students and advanced practice registered nursing (APRN) students.

Electronic health records (EHRs) are designed to make patient health communication accessible, efficient, and portable. They have the potential to save time and reduce communication errors. They also improve

patient safety by providing essential data entry and allergy alerts to minimize patient care errors, particularly medication errors (McCarthy et al., 2018).

Electronic health records can also serve as a *barrier* for students as they rotate through different clinical sites and navigate different systems (see Chapter 19). Health systems and clinics may use different EHR platforms that require additional staff support to provide onboarding training and develop student log-in profiles (Forsberg et al., 2015). Most large facilities will orient students to the EHR, often through online learning modules, prior to beginning on-site clinical responsibilities. Clinical learning experiences can be delayed if training is not done in a timely fashion. Preceptors should verify that students have EHR access, as appropriate, prior to the start of the rotation and that all necessary training is complete.

Additionally, preceptors should work with leadership in the clinical setting to identify an available space for students to review patient medical records and document care. Students typically require an increased amount of time to complete documentation (Renda et al., 2022), and extended time for charting in clinic rooms or at the patient's bedside is not always feasible.

GENERAL DOCUMENTATION PRINCIPLES

Documentation requires precise language. Students need to document in real clinical situations using accurate and appropriate terminology that reflects the patient's condition. There are critical questions that must be addressed within the narrative. "What happened? What was the exact sequence? What did it look like? What time did it happen? What treatment was provided and what was the response? Who was notified?" This must all be written objectively, without speculation or opinions.

Preceptors can significantly influence aspects of student documentation, as students often emulate the preceptor's words and writing style. One critical aspect of documentation is modeling a neutral tone, without any hint of bias. Preceptors can affect clinical decisions and judgments when documenting in a biased fashion (e.g., "drug-seeking" or "noncompliant"). Stigma can be perpetuated from one healthcare provider to the next, resulting in negative implications for patient care (Martin et al., 2022). The EHR is maintained across a patient's lifetime and transfers from one medical professional to the next (Martin et al., 2022). Thus, any suggestion of bias can flow into the beliefs and attitudes of other nurses or healthcare professionals.

Reviewing and signing-off on new orders and documentation of verbal orders are additional essential learning components, and preceptors may role-model this responsibility for students. The Joint Commission and the Centers for Medicare and Medicaid Services (CMS) have made several important points about medical orders: 1) computerized order entry is preferred because it ensures that orders are directly entered into the EHR; 2) verbal orders can be used when computerized provider order entry is not available, although these verbal orders should be used infrequently; and 3) secure text orders are not currently permitted (Centers for Medicare and Medicaid Services, 2017). Discussing the "checks and balances" in each step of the order process helps to illustrate a team approach to patient care.

Patient medical information serves as retrospective data in quality improvement and research projects. Students may not recognize the importance of their role in documentation as their priority is on patient care. Preceptors can view the student's lack of knowledge as a teaching moment to deepen understanding about the complexity of the nurses' role and the value of EHR documentation. Use of standardized, consistent, non-abbreviated terminology and ICD-10 and billing codes makes medical information searchable when researchers mine for data in chart analyses.

UNDERGRADUATE NURSING STUDENT DOCUMENTATION

Academic learning centers are responsible for educating undergraduate nursing students about documentation (ANA, 2010). Students are taught about their accountability, responsibility, and potential liability associated with charting. They learn the medicolegal risks of poor documentation and become familiar with technologies, digital media, and principles of information access. In the clinical setting, they begin using this knowledge in real time as they access the EHR.

Often, undergraduate students are able to electronically chart vital signs, intakes/outputs, basic nursing assessment findings, and tasks and procedures that they have performed. The simplicity and convenience of electronic charting can, unfortunately, lead to shortcuts. For instance, EHRs may automatically populate with vital signs from the cardiac monitor, blood pressure cuff, glucometer, and other smart technology. Technology does not replace listening to an apical pulse and performing other essential aspects of the assessment. EHRs often have check boxes for body systems where the nurse can document "normal" or "within normal limits," or allow for free texting of pertinent positives. Nursing students must use clinical judgment skills when charting to avoid missing key clinical information.

Typically, prelicensure students do not give medications independently. Clinical instructors or preceptors verify medication preparation, administration, and charting. Preceptors must be familiar with institutional medication administration policies and procedures in relation to nursing students, and be clear about the school or university guidelines for what students are permitted to do. Clinical instructors or preceptors have the ultimate responsibility of reviewing student documentation and signing off on their work at the end of the shift.

Pain documentation is a critical skill, and one that students learn in theory but have no chance to practice until they are in the clinical setting. Documentation includes introduction to whatever pain scale is utilized in the facility, pain assessment prior to and after administration of analgesics, and when the patient is asleep (such as respiratory rate and pattern). While students may not be documenting administration of pain medications or continuous infusions, they should be assessing and reassessing pain in a timely manner, reporting to the nurse or faculty responsible for the patient care, and observing the documentation process (Nelson & Joswiak, 2020).

Use of Block Charting

Preceptors working in critical care areas may be introducing students in real time to the concept of block charting, which may not be a part of their prelicensure education. Block charting is a documentation method used during emergent or critical care periods, when rapid medication titration is necessary (Vizient Newsroom, 2021). This type of documentation is restricted for use in critical and procedural areas, such as a hemodynamic instability event in the ICU. Charting is done in four-hour "blocks" of time. If a patient's emergent situation extends beyond 4 hours and block charting is continued, a new charting "block" period must be started. This time-saving method allows the nurse to provide bedside care without having to document each dose titration. According to The Joint Commission (n.d.), nurses may titrate the prescribed medication in accordance with a medical order. If verbal orders are given, they must be entered into the EHR; this is a requirement for all verbal orders.

The minimum components of block charting include:
- Start and end times for the block charting episode
- Complete, accurate orders for each medication titration
- Maximum rate/dose
- Start and end rate/dose within the block charting period
- Objective parameters reflecting decisions about the titrations

When safe and appropriate, students can observe, participate, and informally document during critical care periods.

Care Planning

Students should strive to write concise, simple care plans that focus on the individual condition and needs of the patient. A majority of students admit that developing nursing diagnoses is the most difficult part of creating a care plan (Salvador et al., 2022). Each student

must review the current care plan for their assigned patients at the start of each shift and consider modifications as appropriate. Preceptors can engage the student in discussion about the care plan, appropriateness of the nursing diagnosis, and progress on short-term and long-term goals. Unless there is a change in patient status, the student nurse may not be making any additions to the patient's established care plan.

APRN STUDENT DOCUMENTATION

For APRN students, the learning associated with documentation focuses more on narrative notes that encompass and tell the story of a patient encounter. Typically, these notes are formed utilizing the SOAP format: Subjective and Objective data, Assessment, and Plan. Nurse practitioner students may write SOAP notes as regular course assignments and often seek advice from the preceptor about language and style. Initially, students need additional guidance to prevent merging subjective and objective data as they learn to make connections between their observations and the assessment and plan (Figure 20.1).

Preceptors should determine with faculty whether students have practiced documentation using simulated patient cases (Graziano et al., 2018). APRN students need to practice the art of proper documentation in real time to develop proficiency and as part of time management skills. Their documentation, however, does not *need* to be a part of the permanent medical record.

APRN Student Charting in Acute Care Settings

There are specific documentation components required for inpatient charting encounters. As providers gain experience, thorough completion of each component becomes easier. Written documentation also affects how encounters are billed. While APRN students learn documentation and billing concepts in their courses, they may not be aware of how to apply the basics once they are in the hospital setting.

A comprehensive review of systems is required as part of the daily encounter. Students should always be reminded to chart on at least eight body systems. Students often make the mistake of combining history with physical exam findings (e.g., after noting that a patient reported being "short of breath," the student documents observations about respiratory distress symptoms and

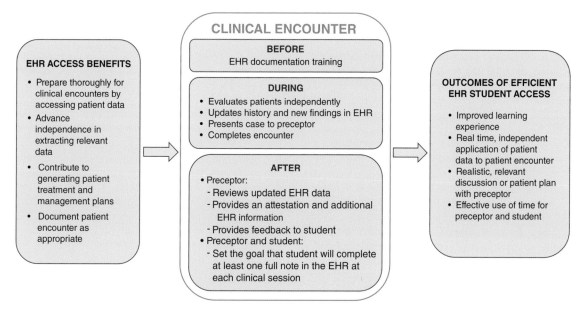

Fig. 20.1 Integrating electronic health records (EHRs) access into advanced practice registered nurse student clinical experience. (Adapted from Altolaguirre, C. V., Reddy, R., Gamaldo, C. E., & Salas, R. M. E. (2023). Developing a standardized EMR workflow for medical students and preceptors. *Health Policy and Technology, 12*(1), 100696.)

lung sounds as part of the chief complaint). Students may need to slow down and be reminded to distinguish between subjective and objective data. Students may also inadvertently omit documenting physical exam findings because they become overly focused on developing the plan of treatment. The treatment plan can be either system-based or problem-based, depending on the site and the individual patient's condition. However, students must be methodical when documenting patient findings and correlating them with the treatment plan.

CMS Evaluation and Management Guidelines for APRN Student Documentation

Medicare and Medicaid payments only cover services provided by physicians, APRNs, and other licensed practitioners. In general, to bill for a service rendered, the billing practitioner must be considered an eligible provider of care (enrolled in Medicare as a provider or credentialed by the insurance carrier). This specific rule led to billing challenges that presented when a student had documented care in the chart. For billing to be approved, preceptors had to rechart aspects of the student documentation.

In January 2020, CMS ruled that APRN preceptors could review and *verify* medical record documentation entered by other licensed healthcare providers and members of the healthcare team, as well as student APRNs (Phillips, n.d.). The rule prevented duplication of effort and allowed students a more active role in documentation of patient care. Reviewing documentation before the end of the day allows for a few valuable teaching moments for the student. Also, the preceptor can add an addendum if any clarification to the EHR is required.

Students can be taught how to chart smarter, not harder. In a study of APRNs who used EHRs, 19.3% of participants reported spending "moderately high" to "excessive" time on EHR documentation at home, and 50% "agreed" or "strongly agreed" EHRs added to their daily frustration (Harris et al., 2018). As a result the authors stressed that workplaces need to decrease or simplify documentation requirements by making the electronic interface more provider-friendly. Preceptors who have developed "smart phrases" or other timesaving documentation tools can share them with learners.

Students must complete their documentation before leaving the clinical site each day. Essential components

Exemplar: Acute Care APRN Student Documentation

Danielle Sebbens

Transitioning from an expert nurse to an advanced practice registered nurse (APRN) student is one of the more challenging adjustments to overcome when beginning graduate school. The discomfort is apparent when jumping from documenting a nursing note to writing a history and physical examination (H&P) or a progress note as a provider.

One stellar student comes to mind when I reflect on my experience precepting APRN students in the acute care setting. As an expert nurse, she was a leader on her unit. Novice nurses asked her about charting, patient care, equipment, and more. She had pride in her knowledge of policies and procedures, and her documentation was used as an exemplar when training new staff. Despite her background, common student documentation mistakes were noted on her first clinical day as an APRN student. She started her H&P with the chief complaint (CC) as a diagnosis, documenting "RSV bronchiolitis" rather than "labored breathing." Similarly, the review of systems (ROS) was based on the student's objective physical exam (PE) findings rather than the caregiver's subjective responses. As we proceeded through the document review, I noted that she alternated subjective and objective descriptions throughout the history of present illness (HPI) and PE. There was no assessment statement included. Finally, the plan of care was a running task list, not organized by system or problem. This provided an excellent opportunity to teach a systematic approach to completing an H&P and documenting the related SOAP note.

After reviewing the H&P in its entirety, we dissected each section. I stated that the CC should be written in the patient's or caregiver's words. She immediately recognized her mistake and changed the wording to "labored breathing." We reviewed the importance of asking questions of the caregiver to elicit the ROS. Again, she identified her error and returned to the caregiver to clarify the ROS. She could articulate that the HPI focuses on subjective information, and the PE focuses on objective findings. But, like many students, she inserted subjective findings into the PE and objective findings into the HPI. She quickly reviewed the expectations and amended the SOAP note to meet the goal. We discussed how the assessment statement helps prioritize important information, formulate a list of differential diagnoses, and eliminate irrelevant data. We worked together to craft a concise assessment statement. A system-based plan of care rounded out her first H&P.

When precepting acute care APRN students, specifically with documentation, I recommend teaching a systematic approach. I explain to students that they will develop a style that works for them over time, but first, they must focus on mastering the basics. With repetition, they develop good habits that prevent them from omitting important details. I acknowledge the growing pains they feel with transitioning from expert nurse to novice APRN student. Coaching with a systematic approach and step-by-step instructions helps students develop independence and confidence in their new role.

BOX 20.1 Prescription Documentation for APRN Students

Preceptors should remember to discuss the issue of prescriptive authority and its influence on clinical practice.

- Encourage Drug Enforcement Agency registration once students receive their license and certification. Encourage discussion with employers about covering this cost.
- Review drug schedules and dose limitations.
- Discuss how to obtain pharmacology, psychopharmacology (if applicable), and controlled substance continuing education (CE) per state/certification requirements.
- For acute care preceptors, discuss the differences between *orders* and *prescriptions*.

of documentation include: notation of pertinent positives and negatives, completion of the review of systems, exam findings, treatment and/or management plans and clinical rationale.

DOCUMENTATION FOR PRECEPTORS

In addition to monitoring and helping with student documentation, preceptors keep up with their own patient charting and *also* keep records about the student's efforts while learning the APRN role. Maintaining records of precepted students may prove to be an invaluable endeavor for a number of reasons. For example, students may reach out to ask for job references. Preceptors should keep records of student clinical hours, procedures supervised, and competencies met. In addition to helping inform the preceptor's evaluation of the student, record-keeping helps validate precepting work efforts. Completed checklists, along with the final (summative) evaluation, are forwarded to faculty as the rotation ends (See Chapter 21). Finally, clinical precepting time may be applied as practice hours for recertification with certifying bodies such as the American Nursing Credentialing Center (ANCC) and the Pediatric Nursing Certification Board (PNCB).

Documenting Prescriptions and Orders in the Clinical Setting for APRN Students

Students may not have EHR access and will not have prescribing and ordering privileges until after graduation, licensing, and credentialing. Preceptors guide students in how to write orders and prescriptions. Nurse practitioner (NP) students should be planning pharmacotherapeutic treatment with preceptor input, choosing medications using best evidence, and calculating dosages, timing, milliliter equivalents (as appropriate), and quantity of medication needed. The preceptor typically writes, electronically enters, and signs orders and prescriptions. The preceptor can demonstrate use of identity authentication procedures for prescribing scheduled drugs. Box 20.1 provides ideas to help the NP student learn about prescription management.

▉ CONCLUSION

EHR access allows undergraduate and APRN students to document patient assessments and care provision in real time. Preceptors have the opportunity to not only role-model unbiased and accurate documentation but also provide feedback so that students are also documenting thoroughly and correctly. Students may require additional guidance in organizing key components of SOAP notes.

REFERENCES

American Nurses Association [ANA]. (2010). *ANA's Principles for Nursing Documentation*. Silver Spring, MD: American Nurses Association. https://www.nursingworld.org/~4af4f2/globalassets/docs/ana/ethics/principles-of-nursing-documentation.pdf

Centers for Medicare and Medicaid Services. (2017). *Memorandum: Texting of patient information among healthcare providers*. Ref: S&C 18-10-ALL. https://www.cms.gov/Medicare/Provider-Enrollment-and-Certification/SurveyCertificationGenInfo/Downloads/Survey-and-Cert-Letter-18-10.pdf

Forsberg, I., Swartwout, K., Murphy, M., Danko, K., & Delaney, K. R. (2015). Nurse practitioner education: Greater demand, reduced training opportunities. *Journal of the American Association of Nurse Practitioners*, 27(2), 66–71. https://doi.org/10.1002/2327-6924.12175

Graziano, S., McKenzie, M., Abbott, J., Buery-Joyner, S., Craig, L., Dalrymple, J., Forstein, D., Hampton, B., Page-Ramsey, S., Pradhan, A., Wolf, A., & Hopkins, L. (2018). Barriers and strategies to engaging our community-based preceptors. *Teaching and Learning in Medicine*, 30(4), 444–450. https://doi.org/10.1080/10401334.2018.1444994

Harris, D. A., Haskell, J., Cooper, E., Crouse, N., & Gardner, R. (2018). Estimating the association between burnout and electronic health record-related stress among advanced practice registered nurses. *Applied Nursing Research*, 43, 36–41. https://doi.org/10.1016/j.apnr.2018.06.014

Martin, K., Bickle, K., & Lok, J. (2022). Investigating the impact of cognitive bias in nursing documentation on decision-making and judgement. *International Journal of Mental Health Nursing*, 31, 897–907. https://doi.org/10.1111/inm.12997

McCarthy, B., Fitzgerald, S., O'Shea, M., Condon, C., Hartnett-Collins, G., Clancy, M., Sheehy, A., Denieffe, S., Bergin, M., & Savage, E. (2018). Electronic nursing documentation interventions to promote or improve patient safety and quality care: A systematic review. *Journal of Nursing Management*, 27(3), 491–501. https://doi.org/10.1111/jonm.12727

Nelson, D. M., & Joswiak, M. E. (2020). Preceptor teaching tools to support consistency while training novice nurses. *Journal for Nurses in Professional Development*, 36(5), 307–312. https://doi.org/10.1097/nnd.0000000000000672

Phillips, S. (n.d.). *CMS Final Rule: NP and PA Preceptor Documentation Updates – Success!* Virginia Council of Nurse Practitioners. https://www.vcnp.net/cms-final-rule-np-and-pa-preceptor-documentation-updates-success

Renda, S., Fingerhood, M., Kverno, K., Slater, T., Gleason, K., & Goodwin, M. (2022). What motivates our practice colleagues to precept the next generation? *The Journal for Nurse Practitioners*, 18(1), 76–80. https://doi.org/10.1016/j.nurpra.2021.09.008

Salvador, J. T., Alqahtani, F. M., Sauce, B. R. J., Alvarez, M. O. C., Rosario, A. B., Reyes, L. D., Mohamed, E. R., Awadh, L. A., Sanchez, K. K. B., Alzaid, M., Agman, D. D., & Schonewille, M. A. P. (2022). Development of student survey on writing nursing care plan: An exploratory sequential mixed-methods study. *Journal of Nursing Management, 30,* O23–O36. https://doi.org/10.1111/jonm.12996

The Joint Commission. (n.d.). Medication Administration - Titration Orders – Documentation During Rapid Titration | Hospital and Hospital Clinics | Medication Management MM. www.jointcommission.org. https://www.jointcommission.org/standards/standard-faqs/

hospital-and-hospital-clinics/medication-management-mm/000002337/

Vizient Newsroom. (2021, July 29). *Joint Commission and block charting during emergencies: Is it right for your hospital?* https://newsroom.vizientinc.com/en-US/releases/joint-commission-and-block-charting-during-emergencies-is-it-right-for-your-hospital

21

Evaluation

Daniel Crawford and Amalia Elizabeth Gedney-Lose

CHAPTER OBJECTIVES

- Describe the role of the preceptor in evaluating the learner in the clinical setting
- Differentiate between formative and summative evaluation
- Adopt effective feedback strategies
- Evaluate strategies for providing difficult feedback

Learners, whether prelicensure or advanced practice students, or orientees in a new nursing role, have an opportunity to apply nursing theory and knowledge, practice psychomotor skills, and develop a professional nursing identity while immersed in the clinical environment. There is tremendous growth during clinical experiences, and evaluation contributes to that growth. Preceptors closely evaluate learners, providing feedback and highlighting areas for improvement. By exposing learners to a variety of patient cases and opportunities for practice and repetition, preceptors help build confidence and competence. Box 21.1 outlines foundational information required for adequate evaluation.

Evaluation is a process of validating competency to ensure safe clinical practice. Effective evaluation, involving constructive criticism and feedback, is an essential component of learning, yet can be an uncomfortable process for a variety of reasons (Box 21.2). When preceptors become skilled in providing constructive criticism, the evaluation experience positively enhances clinical learning. The evaluation process may require different approaches based on the learner's experiences and expectations, thus requiring flexibility by the preceptor. Preceptors need to be aware of learning objectives, specific skills for evaluation, and how to interpret the method of evaluation. This chapter provides an

overview of different types of evaluation and strategies for success when evaluating learners in the clinical setting.

TYPES OF EVALUATION

Evaluation can be divided into two primary types of measures: formative and summative. A well-designed evaluation plan should include both measures. This helps ensure that the learner is progressing as expected and, most importantly, achieves learning outcomes. With both types of evaluation, there are a variety of strategies to verify that an adequate evaluation plan is in place. Using both types of evaluation can help to effectively direct learner progress and avoid later confusion or surprises. Communication regarding evaluations should include preceptors, the learner, and either program faculty or a clinical administrator. Open and ongoing communication encourages learner success and improves the precepting experience.

Formative Evaluation

Formative evaluation measures the learner's *ongoing* progress toward meeting objectives and goals. It is an effective method to help individualize further learning and improve targeted areas of need. Formative

155

evaluation is formational to learning. When done effectively, formative evaluation engages the learner throughout the clinical process and prevents surprises at the time of final evaluation. Lack of progress or failure, while sometimes inevitable, should be discussed with the learner as soon as it is evident.

Formative evaluations can occur formally or informally. Many preceptors unknowingly provide formative evaluation during regular informal communication with learners. Common effective formative evaluation strategies include case presentations or discussions, feedback, interval check-ins ("What went well this week?"; "What could be improved?"), or midterm evaluations. Preceptors should find opportunities during each clinical shift to provide informal feedback. This can be done in a variety of ways, but should always be done in a nonthreatening manner to allow for prompt improvement in skills. An example of informal feedback is when a preceptor observes and comments on general assessment skills (e.g., correcting the learner when auscultating heart and lung sounds over the patient's clothing) in a timely manner. This can be helpful for assessing knowledge, clinical judgment, or diagnostic reasoning skills.

Formative evaluation can serve as a midterm assessment, which is often required by many academic or workplace orientation programs prior to the final (or summative) evaluation. An assessment midway through the clinical experience also allows the preceptor to review the learner's strengths and identify areas for improvement. If a midterm evaluation is not required by the academic or workplace orientation program, preceptors can initiate this on their own to help support learner development and progress toward goals or objectives.

Application of knowledge evolves over the course of the precepted experience, especially as the learner begins to understand and integrate key nursing concepts into a comprehensive patient care plan. Although most learners strive to improve, there may be times when they fail to improve or exhibit potentially dangerous behaviors requiring the need to initiate additional formative evaluation and immediate remediation. The most notable areas of concern are related to safety and ethical patient care practices.

Red flags regarding learner performance may appear (Table 21.1) throughout the course of the clinical rotation or orientation program. Initially, a conversation about the concern should begin with the learner, but if there is no immediate improvement, the evaluation process should be escalated. The preceptor should discuss concerns early with the course faculty or administrator in order to provide additional direction for the learner.

Summative Evaluation

Summative evaluation measures the *final* achievement of learning objectives and goals, developed and provided by the institution or augmented and refined by the preceptor and learner. This type of evaluation typically takes place at the end of a clinical, academic, or workplace orientation experience and carries more weight than formative evaluation. In academic or clinical experiences, summative evaluation is based on the learning objectives outlined by the academic program and are often reflected in a formal evaluation tool. These objectives typically reflect standards for education published by various organizations respective to the learner's academic level (Box 21.3). While evaluation tools may vary by school, they typically are built upon the same standards. In the workplace setting, the standards measured by the summative evaluation often reflect role expectations.

While the evaluation process allows delineation of areas for improvement and growth, it is also used to summarize the learner's progress and accomplishments. Preceptors should anticipate that learners will not typically earn the highest marks or "exceed expectations" on all criteria of the summative evaluation. Each criterion should be candidly assessed. In most cases, evaluation feedback should be communicated from the preceptor directly to the learner. The evaluation is also shared with academic program faculty or administrators.

TABLE 21.1	**Examples of Red Flag Behaviors**		
	Entry Level	**Advanced Level**	**New Hire**
Safety	Unable to identify push rate for parenteral medications	Misses essential components of history and physical assessment	Does not promptly escalate care with concerning changes in patient condition
Standards of Practice	Fails to collect comprehensive data pertinent to the patient's health and condition	Misses opportunities for anticipatory guidance or patient/family education	Does not complete required documentation before shift change
Communication	Unable to present patient cases clearly to peers	Unable to present patient cases clearly during interdisciplinary rounds	Becomes defensive when asked about completed care during patient handoff
Planning	Inconsistently implements the nursing process	Inconsistent identification of differential diagnoses and development of treatment plans	Inappropriate delegation of nursing tasks to nonlicensed staff
Technique	Inattentive to sterile technique when placing an indwelling catheter	Improper technique when performing otoscopic exam	Inadequate rotation of subcutaneous injection sites
Prioritization	Ineffective planning leading to delayed medication administration	Inability to prioritize multiple patient care needs	Inefficient management of timely admissions or discharge

Another type of summative evaluation occurs when the *learner evaluates the site and preceptor*. This type of evaluation is common in the academic setting but may be performed more variably in specific healthcare settings. Learners are typically asked a standardized set of questions that focus on preceptor support for learning and adequacy of the clinical site. Academic programs may forget or choose not to share this information voluntarily with preceptors. It is appropriate for preceptors to ask program faculty for access to the student's evaluation of the precepted experience. In addition to helping the preceptor develop their teaching skills, a summative evaluation can also provide site-specific recommendations to better support future learners.

FEEDBACK

Feedback, as an important aspect of evaluation, helps learners understand gaps in their knowledge and identify areas for performance improvement. Feedback is bidirectional, with the preceptor providing feedback and the learner embracing the feedback as an opportunity for growth. If the feedback process is one-sided, the learner is not held accountable for receiving, accepting, and applying feedback to their learning (Molloy et al., 2020). A positive, trusting relationship with the preceptor positions the learner to be receptive of feedback and engaged in the process (Beaulieu et al., 2019; Lefroy et al., 2015; Molloy et al., 2020). On the other hand, when the preceptor does not provide feedback or follow up on the progress of the learner, the learner can become disengaged and lose motivation.

Using a variety of formal and informal feedback methods consistently during the clinical experience supports learner success during their educational journey. Preceptors are encouraged to provide positive, specific, and timely feedback on a consistent basis. The learner will begin to trust the preceptor when feedback becomes a natural part of daily interactions. Box 21.4 contains a helpful hint for establishing a feedback plan with learners.

Feedback Strategies

The "feedback sandwich" is a method for critiquing performance. Constructive feedback is sandwiched between two pieces of positive or motivational feedback. For example, "Your approach to gathering the patient history was effective. However, I did not hear you ask about employment which relates to how the patient manages his chronic illness in the workplace. The rest of the history sounded very thorough." Sandwiching provides padding around important critique that is meant to support student growth. While it may increase comfort for the preceptor *giving* the feedback, the learner *receiving* the feedback may not process the need for improvement.

Feedback skills can be adapted and used for learners at many different levels, requiring the preceptor to be flexible in their approach. A strategy applicable to various learning levels is the "see one, do one, teach one" method. This allows the preceptor to demonstrate a skill or technique, followed by the learner completing the skill with support and guidance, and culminating in the learner teaching the skill to another individual. Once the learner repeats the skill safely and accurately, the preceptor can determine if the learner can proceed independently.

Providing Difficult Feedback

In addition to using feedback to encourage and foster growth in the learner, the preceptor must also develop skills to provide difficult feedback when expectations are not met or there are safety concerns. Preceptors may

be reluctant to give difficult feedback to learners, even when remediation is necessary (Nielson & Halloran, 2020). Preceptors need to trust their judgment of student performance, and seek support from faculty, administrators, or experienced colleagues when providing difficult but necessary feedback.

Difficult feedback conversations can provoke anxiety in both the preceptor and in the learner. When it is necessary to provide negative feedback, the preceptor should signal good intent and be direct. The learner may have questions or ask for specific examples to clarify the issue of concern. The most effective feedback conversations are two-way, matter of fact, and nonjudgmental in nature (Laskowski-Jones, 2018). Additionally, delivering feedback in a way that is nonpunitive avoids creating a defensive response and is most productive.

Integrating Learner Self-Assessment in the Feedback Process

Self-assessment, resulting from self-reflection, serves as a valuable tool for learners before receiving external feedback from the preceptor. External feedback that is meaningful, positive, constructive, and timely includes: 1) clarification of performance expectations, 2) promotion of self-assessment skills, 3) encouragement of dialogue, and 4) involvement of learners in bridging knowledge gaps (Joyce, 2021).

Integration of learner self-assessment with preceptor input (external feedback) provides useful information in the feedback process. Through self-assessment, learners reflect on their progress toward the attainment of practice competencies (AACN, 2021). See Box 21.5 for a self-assessment strategy that can be referenced throughout the clinical experience.

BOX 21.4 Helpful Hint

Ask the learner how they like to receive feedback. When a learner receives feedback the way they want, in a setting where they are comfortable, they may be more open to listening and processing the information. However, if the learner is openly criticized in front of a patient or peers, it may cause embarrassment, shame, and distrust.

BOX 21.5 Self-Assessment Strategy

A clinical learning contract serves as an agreement between a preceptor and learner. It includes:
- Statement of purpose
- Learning goals and objectives
- Strategies to meet goals
- How goals will be evaluated
- Recommendations from the preceptor

At midterm and the end of the clinical experience, learners should provide a self-assessment of their clinical learning contract to reflect on areas of growth, lessons learned, and areas for further improvement.

One method of providing feedback is to ask the learner to self-assess their performance after specific patient encounters or at the end of the day. This helps to gauge the learner's self-awareness and gives the preceptor a chance to share their impressions (Shellenbarger & Robb, 2016).

The preceptor can request that learners complete a formative self-assessment at midterm or any time prior to final evaluation. Preceptors can then share their midterm evaluation with the learner to identify gaps in perspectives. The AACN Essentials core competencies provide guidance for the preceptor to facilitate learner self-reflection (American Association of Colleges of Nursing, 2021). To promote self-reflection, preceptors can use prompts or reflective activities to engage learners. Examples of prompts linked to the AACN Essentials core and subcompetencies can be found in Table 21.2.

CONCLUSION

Precepting is a rewarding experience that can be further enhanced through formative and summative evaluation. Ongoing feedback helps the learner advance application of foundational knowledge in the clinical setting. Formative evaluation validates ongoing progress while

TABLE 21.2 Examples of Prompts Linked to the AACN Essentials Core and Subcompetencies

Domain	Level	Sucompetency	Prompt
Knowledge for Nursing Practice	Entry	1.2d Examine the influence of personal values in decision-making for nursing practice.	"You seem to be passionate about caring for patients who are underserved. What experiences have you had during your nursing clinical practice or external to nursing that have shaped those perspectives?"
	Advanced	1.3a Demonstrate clinical reasoning.	"The patient we cared for deteriorated quickly and required you to use your clinical judgment on a moment's notice. It is helpful to reflect on your behaviors as you escalated care. Why did you choose to do _____ first, and then do _____? What helped you prioritize the many aspects of that interaction?"
Person-Centered Care	Entry	2.3e Distinguish between normal and abnormal health findings.	"This morning, you documented that the patient was tachycardic. Think about what you know about tachycardia and connect that to potential clinical manifestations you want to assess. Then, I would like you to reassess our patient and present your findings to me."
	Advanced	2.4g Integrate advanced scientific knowledge to guide decision-making.	"In considering how your specialized nursing knowledge affects the care you provide, you need to understand the knowledge and translate that to safe practice. Reflect on some of the common diseases we are managing in the clinical setting and identify how you are integrating knowledge with decision-making to provide evidence-based care."
Interprofessional Partnerships	Entry	6.2b Delegate work to team members based on their roles and competency.	"Delegating work to other members of our team can be challenging. Think about strategies for delegating care appropriately to our team members, and plan to implement these strategies this afternoon."
	Advanced	6.2i Reflect on how one's role and expertise influence team performance.	"We need to work as a team to ensure patients have a smooth transition through our care setting. Consider how you currently support that transition, and ways that you can work together with other members of our team."

From American Association of Colleges of Nursing. (2021). *The Essentials: Core competencies for professional nursing education.* (pp. 27-54). AACN. https://www.aacnnursing.org/Portals/0/PDFs/Publications/Essentials-2021.pdf.

summative evaluation reflects the attainment of learning competencies. The importance of the professional relationship between the preceptor and learner cannot be understated. The relationship should be built on trust and respect to ensure that the learner is poised to receive constructive feedback (Beaulieu et al., 2019; Lefroy et al., 2015).

REFERENCES

American Association of Colleges of Nursing. (2021). The Essentials: Core competencies for professional nursing education (pp. 27–54). AACN. https://www.aacnnursing.org/Portals/0/PDFs/Publications/Essentials-2021.pdf.

Beaulieu, A. M., Kim, B. S., Topor, D. R., & Dickey, C. C. (2019). Seeing is believing: An exploration of what residents value when they receive feedback. *Academic Psychiatry, 43*, 507–511. https://doi.org/10.1007/s40596-019-01071-5

Joyce, P. (2021). Developing physician assistant faculty feedback skills. *Journal of Physician Assistant Education, 32*(3), 154–158. https://doi.org/10.1097/JPA.0000000000000371

Laskowski-Jones, L. (2018). Receiving constructive feedback constructively. *Nursing 2018, 48*(7), 6. https://doi.org/10.1097/.01.NURSE.0000534098.79486.a4

Lefroy, J., Watling, C., Teunissen, P. W., & Brand, P. (2015). Guidelines: The do's, don'ts and don't knows of feedback for clinical education. *Perspectives on Medical Education, 4*, 284–299. https://doi.org/10.1007/s40037-015-0231-7

Molloy, E., Ajjawi, R., Bearman, M., Noble, C., Rudland, J., & Ryan, A. (2020). Challenging feedback myths: Values, learner involvement and promoting effects beyond the immediate task. *Medical Education, 54*, 33–39. https://doi.org/10.1111/medu.13802

Shellenbarger, T., & Robb, M. (2016). Effective mentoring in the clinical setting. *American Journal of Nursing, 116*(4), 64–68. https://doi.org/10.1097/01.NAJ.0000482149.37081.61

22

Moving Into Leadership Roles Beyond Practice

Nanne M. Finis and Larissa Africa

CHAPTER OBJECTIVES

- Identify ways leaders can support team members to begin their professional development journey
- Explore various pathways into leadership roles

- Describe the process for how one would begin a personal leadership journey
- Initiate goal-setting for a personal professional development plan

"*Every nurse is a leader.*" Nursing professionals practice every day within a healthcare system encumbered with chaos, resulting in the need for dynamic leaders. The collective pandemic experience highlighted the need for major improvements in managing patient care with limited resources, communicating with patients and families through interprofessional teams, and preparing a vibrant workforce. Overall, there is a demand for innovation, change, and leadership in today's current system.

As frontline professionals responsible for planning and managing patient care, nurses are central to advancing healthcare. Stakeholders, including patients, families, physicians, and other members of the healthcare team, have high expectations of nurses. They expect nurses to be honest and transparent, and to communicate with a calm, professional, and trusting demeanor. Aligning their work with the mission and values of the organization and representing those values to patients, families, and the public, nurses are uniquely poised to be strong, trusted leaders.

Building effective nursing leaders requires awareness, followed by development of untapped leadership potential. The questions arise: *How do nurses become aware of their leadership potential? How can nurses channel their abilities into leadership roles?* Nurse executives across the spectrum in the healthcare industry agree that no matter the position a nurse holds, the nurse must both *serve* as a

trusted advisor and *have* a trusted advisor as a resource and mentor. Ultimately, it is the personal decision of each nurse to identify their path and how they want to advance. Preceptors play an influential role in providing guidance and role-modeling leadership opportunities.

The current state of nursing presents with many challenges; yet, working together, nurses can create a cohesive, high-functioning, and caring work environment. Nurses can lead by creating committed teams, including partnerships with patients, families, and communities. Preceptors are in unique multifaceted positions, not only as providers of care, but also as team-builders and leaders. Each preceptor is accountable for driving the nursing profession forward with intention and purpose.

LEADERSHIP AND NURSE WELL-BEING

Leaders in nursing are in a prime position to mitigate barriers such as nurse burnout, attrition, and apathy, which are detrimental to the healthcare workforce (Wei, et al., 2020). In the United States today, 54% of nurses and physicians experience symptoms of burnout, including lack of motivation, cynicism, irritability, chronic fatigue, and difficulty with concentration (National Academy of Medicine, 2022). Burnout is a long-standing issue and a fundamental barrier to professional well-being and growth. The COVID-19 pandemic further exacerbated the national burnout problem in nursing due to staff and supply short-ages, higher acuity levels and numbers of patients, and serious healthcare risks to clinicians themselves.

The National Plan for Health Workforce Well-Being from the National Academy of Medicine (2022) inspires collective action focusing on changes needed to improve the well-being of the healthcare workforce. A national initiative is to redesign how healthcare is delivered so that the human connection is strengthened, health equity is achieved, and trust is restored. The vision presented in the *National Plan* is of patients being cared for by a healthy workforce thriving in an environment that fosters their own well-being. In turn, that healthy workforce improves population health, enhances the care experience, reduces costs, and advances health equity.

As the nursing shortage in the United States intensifies, there will be an unprecedented number of opportunities to lead and impact the healthcare landscape. Preceptors already affect the profession as leaders by committing to clinical teaching excellence and by inspiring learners to embrace leadership opportunities.

PROMOTING NURSING LEADERSHIP

Mentoring and radical collaboration are approaches used by nurse leaders to create strategic partnerships and enhance growth opportunities. Mentorship provides a critical pathway for developing leadership skills. However, programs in place for mentoring are often not enough and more opportunities are required for mentorship at all levels of healthcare. Future leaders need exposure to not only academic and clinical knowledge, but to the experiences and wisdom of active leaders. Mentorship allows for a transfer of history and knowledge that is personal and unique (see Chapter 4). "Radical collaboration" refers to a willingness by leaders to step outside the traditional boundaries of the nursing profession to collaborate across disciplines, organizations, and even industries.

The best organizational leaders help their employees develop, plan, and achieve their career goals. Leaders or mentors can provide individualized guidance and support to help employees identify career goals that are directive, meaningful, and motivational (Clark, 2022). Top-ranking organizations support their employees to find the right practice and team culture fit. The following section delineates some starting points for nursing leaders to consider.

STARTING POINTS FOR NURSING LEADERS

Many students and nurses are unsure of their passion and path in nursing. To home in on their passion, learners should reflect on what they enjoy most and least about their current nursing experience, as well as areas of professional curiosity. Preceptors can help learners gain clarity regarding their preferred professional roles and activities to facilitate finding a "right fit." With a clear focus, learners can become actively involved in relevant committees, councils, and professional organizations to acquire leadership experience. Many learners do not have adequate opportunities to engage in new experiences nor work in different areas within nursing. When learners are encouraged to experience new situations, they begin identifying areas of interest that they may wish to explore further. A personalized mentoring approach helps engage learners in their own career planning and helps build their organizational loyalty.

Leaders, preceptors, and mentors may guide learners in the career direction that *they* think is best for them and then take it personally if the learner decides not to follow their advice. The novice's career and leadership aspirations may be vastly different from those envisioned for them by the preceptor or mentor. The preceptor's role is to support learners as they advance *their own* personal career aspirations and goals.

Learning Points to Guide Potential Future Leaders

- Seek opportunities that match the student's strengths
- Be ready to support and encourage
- Reaffirm skills that are currently possessed and gently guide toward skills requiring polishing
- Recognize efforts publicly (in the classroom, office, unit, etc.)
- Celebrate the wins, no matter how small
- Support through any challenges or defeats
- Acknowledge that there are many leadership traits for success—not all leaders are the same and each has their own strength

---

NURSING LEADERSHIP STORIES

Development of nursing leadership skills is a process without a direct, prescribed path as the roles,

---

Exemplar: Nurturing the APRN Clinician Into an APRN Leader

Andrea M. Kline-Tilford

While a top priority for new advanced practice registered nurses (APRNs) is developing strong foundational clinical skills and expertise, fostering leadership skills is equally important. All APRNs are leaders. Many simply require validation or encouragement to recognize that they possess the skills and ability to lead. An essential role of preceptors is identifying and acknowledging the skills and qualities of novice APRNs who they are precepting. Preceptors have the privilege to ignite curiosity into young and early career clinicians.

Reflecting on my own experiences of fostering young leaders, a particular nurse practitioner (NP) stands out in my mind. As a young professional, establishing a clinical base in subspecialty care, it was clear that this NP had a passion for continued growth and impact. As it commonly occurs, I was able to see the leadership potential in the young NP before she was able to see it for herself. The NP slowly became more confident as she engaged in leadership opportunities at local and state levels. As her leadership journey unfolded, door after door magically opened, offering new experiences and opportunities. At times, unique, unsolicited opportunities also presented, yet were not always greeted with the same enthusiasm. She learned that many of the unsolicited experiences resulted in unexpected professional growth and satisfaction. Our responsibility as preceptors is to encourage burgeoning leaders to embrace the unexpected and to believe in their capabilities.

In this NP's case, like many others, reaching toward more advanced levels of leadership prompted questioning and self-doubt. She questioned whether there was a more qualified, confident, experienced leader that could or should fill the gap. We are our own worst critics. This, coupled with the very real "imposter syndrome" (see Chapter 18), are powerful countercurrents to comfortably achieving successful and rewarding leadership roles. Preceptors are instrumental in counterbalancing these forces, reinforcing strengths, highlighting talents, and applauding successes—big and small. I continue to be proud and watch in awe as this NP continues to grow, learn, and influence the NP profession and advocate for the well-being of her patients.

Not all leadership comes with a label or fancy title, though that does not mean that leadership experience is less valuable or impactful. Nursing leaders can make significant impacts locally, regionally, nationally, and internationally. Taking on leadership opportunities one step at a time and remaining open to new possibilities ultimately leads to professional growth and satisfaction.

When precepting students, managing expectations is critical even when exploring leadership experiences. The path is not always smooth; there may be bumps, and sometimes complete retooling is necessary. However, if it were easy to lead and create change, everyone would be doing it! Sometimes, it is important to teach students how to pick themselves up after a fall, brush off, and start again. It took me time to learn that it is okay to be uncomfortable and to get comfortable with being uncomfortable. This is how change and impact are made.

When in a leadership role, it is sometimes necessary to "drive the bus" when all you wanted to do was sit in the back seat. Of course it is not necessary to always do this, but everyone should give it a whirl sometimes. Other key lessons I have learned and teach to those emerging leaders around me include watching other leaders, identifying with their strengths, and developing skills to emulate. Some skills will feel more comfortable than others, and some will take practice. Making notes and engaging in daily affirmations can help prepare for some of the leadership hurdles. Positive self-talk can help prior to new experiences or those that may result in discomfort. If not you, your student, or colleague, then who? It is time to raise ourselves, students, and colleagues up to acknowledge the skills and expertise that APRNs bring to the many tables impacting our profession, patients, and families. Let's prepare and encourage our students and orientees to *drive the bus*!

---

responsibilities, and necessary skills of leaders vary. Nursing leaders often build and expand their skills in a variety of ways and relay recommendations and guidance to aspiring leaders. It is up to those seeking leadership positions to embrace meaningful guidance to advance their abilities. Preceptors can be instrumental in connecting nurses and students with effective nursing leaders, providing exposure to a variety of leadership styles and perspectives. To illustrate a variety of roles, responsibilities, and perspectives, several nursing leaders were interviewed. Reflecting upon their careers as clinicians and nurse leaders, each executive provides motivating perspectives on leadership. Their vision, stories, and words of wisdom are presented to capture the actual essence of nursing leaders. These important insights can help each preceptor prepare for future successes and motivate other learners.

NURSING LEADERSHIP STORIES

Nursing Scholar, Executive, and Influencer

Melissa A. Fitzpatrick

To each of her roles, Melissa Fitzpatrick has brought decades of clinical and executive experience and domain expertise, thought leadership, and strategic guidance to her teams, clients, and partners. She has 35 years of healthcare leadership experience and has held a variety of nursing executive roles at several academic medical centers. She served as editor-in-chief of *Nursing Management* and as chief clinical officer with several technology firms. She is a past national president of the American Association of Critical-Care Nurses and is a Fellow in the American Academy of Nursing. She notes that her nursing background informs all of her efforts and refers to herself as a "nurse's nurse," one with empathy and compassion at the core of her work.

Ms. Fitzpatrick notes that the healthcare industry is currently very volatile and it is a critical time for innovative leadership in nursing. She offers astute guidance gleaned from her extensive experience in many roles, practice settings, and focus areas throughout her nursing career. Some of Ms. Fitzpatrick's key insights and advice about nursing leadership and mentorship are highlighted:

- Nurses should put themselves "out there" and surround themselves with "the best and the brightest."
- Allow for personal growth, without boxing oneself in. Be open and *say yes*!
- Resilience is needed to stay on a nursing career track, especially when working with nonhealthcare leaders supporting the healthcare business.
- "Do well in the clinical role" —gain experience and competence.
- Build a network in many ways. However, professional association involvement is the best approach for discovering opportunities to engage and network with others.
- Utilize executive colleagues, who are often willing to make professional connections and mentor at any stage of a nurse's career.
- Be flexible. *Be* a trusted advisor but also *have* a trusted advisor.
- Nurse leaders need business acumen and diversification of their experience, both of which foster innovation.

- Search out *inaugural roles* in leadership, where there is opportunity to design and shape a new role in academia, professional associations, or on boards.

Ms. Fitzpatrick considers herself lucky to have had three or four inaugural roles throughout her long career. Most recently, she was appointed as the first nurse to serve on the board of a major health system in the Southeast and to chair its quality and patient safety committee. A key to Ms. Fitzpatrick's success across roles, settings, and industries is her ability to use the voice of nursing to inform strategic financial, growth, academic, and community-based conversations.

Industry Expert

Joanne Disch

An industry expert is a nurse who has held many clinical, operational, and administrative roles in healthcare. Dr. Disch, a true industry expert, has held senior leadership roles in almost every type of national organization (e.g., chief nurse executive, interim dean, president of the American Association of Critical-Care Nurses and of the American Academy of Nursing, and chair of the national board of the American Association of Retired Persons [AARP]). She has served on four health system boards (having chaired two of them) and was an original leader of the Quality and Safety Education for Nursing (QSEN) initiative. She has been recognized by numerous organizations for her accomplishments and impact.

Dr. Disch describes what she sees as the skills and responsibilities that come with being an industry expert. She defines a leader as one who works together with others to improve on an identified need. She stresses that every nurse is a leader, and all nurses need to think about leadership across the entire spectrum of their careers. Some of the key concepts that Dr. Disch described as essential in the role of the industry expert are:

- Information is power—and relationships are the keys.
- Nurses must be thoughtful and engage in "boundary spanning," also known as moving outside of one's own "box." As an early career staff nurse, Dr. Disch began lecturing at a school of nursing, which exposed her to other ideas and different ways of thinking.
- What seems at first to be a setback can actually be a stepping stone. She encourages nurses to consider "What can I learn from this and what can I do differently?"

- Core principles that Dr. Disch has learned over her many years in nursing leadership include:
  1. *Embrace paradox* and learn to look at all sides of an issue. Nurse leaders do not limit themselves to superficial analysis and an easy solution to a problem. Instead, they "drill down" on an issue, ask questions, and propose creative alternatives. Leaders try to understand the complexity of an issue, and realize that there may be multiple solutions to a problem. Solutions may be short-term, strategic, and sustainable.
  2. *Understand that ambiguity will be present* in many aspects of a leader's work. Thinking in concrete terms and hard-and-fast "rules" should be avoided. Instead, exploring the complexity in ambiguity allows for a deeper level of thinking, dialogue, and thoughtful decision-making. Nontraditional ways of thinking or ideas may present as solutions.
  3. *Practice creativity at work* to encourage innovative thinking.

Dr. Disch encourages nurses to explore new opportunities to innovate and forge partnerships with administration and nursing faculty. Nursing must continue to focus on academic clinical partnerships and a shared "statement of belief" to answer such questions as: *How can nursing faculty and nursing leaders collaborate and practice together? How can they jointly help make new graduates successful?* Students and nurses should be connected with seasoned nurse leaders who can share their experience and wisdom. Many leaders like Dr. Disch make themselves available as mentors over time and across the spectrum of the nursing profession.

Chief Nursing Officer

Betty Jo Rocchio

Dr. Betty Jo Rocchio currently serves as the Mercy Hospital and Mercy Health Foundation senior vice president and system chief nursing officer. Prior to joining Mercy, Dr. Rocchio held several other health system leadership positions, including chief nurse anesthetist, system director of surgical services, vice president of nursing, and chief nursing officer. According to Dr. Rocchio, "The very best nursing structures and organizations have all three types of leaders: Now, Near, and Far. We need a combination of short-term problem-solving, longer-term thinking, and then truly 'big picture' strategic thinking. We need all three of these kinds of leaders at the table."

Dr. Rocchio offers some practical insights on what attributes leaders need to be successful in today's challenging environment:

- Be adept at change management. Change skills are essential in today's fast-moving environment.
- Leaders must be able to direct transformation and execute an organization's vision and strategy.
- All leaders, from executives to front-line leaders, must be able to educate themselves and then successfully use the science of implementation.

Dr. Rocchio states, "Our approach to mentorship is less about learning nursing tasks. We view it as an opportunity to develop nurses to become a stabilizing factor across our organization." She further offered practical guidance, beginning with her own definition of mentorship.

- Mentorship is a continuous exchange of information that offers consistent learning and growing.
- Nurses must learn lessons from outside of healthcare and individual organizations and bring these critical new insights to nursing leadership.
- A nurse is a mentor and a mentee at the same time.
- Nurse leaders must be transparent and share their ways of thinking as they mentor. As a leader, what is "inside your head" is not always evident in actions or communications. It is those one-to-one transparent conversations that bring clarity to others.
- We must all communicate and engage with our teams, as our goal should be to develop the total nursing workforce to be strong and competent through times of transition.

Dr. Rocchio describes her perspectives regarding onboarding and mentoring of newly graduated nursing staff. She believes that this process requires significant changes in order to meet the demands of today's workforce. The Mercy Health System is shifting from a traditional 90-day residency program to a year-long learning opportunity, based on nursing practice and culture. She notes that "we're missing the mark with nursing students (and this challenge was exacerbated with students trained during the height of the pandemic), and now they are struggling with having sufficient nursing practice and cultural competence." Dr. Rocchio supports a transition to a year-long learning journey for new graduate nurses and proposes that nursing changes the overall concept of *preceptorship* to that of *mentorship*.

The onboarding process in nursing is not about learning "nursing tasks." The role of the nurse has evolved into that of a stabilizing influencer across the organization. Dr. Rocchio uses a football analogy to describe the role of the coach as one who builds a tradition of excellence. The head coach of a team, along with other coaches, contributes to strategy and execution. The role of nurse leaders is to develop and coach players (nurses) to be who the profession needs them to be.

Mercy currently supports a professional practice development center as part of its ministry-wide vision and strategy. It is not just how Mercy onboards and launches new nurses, but how it engages candidates from the very first time they come in contact with Mercy. The relationship with the new nurse starts with their first professional interview. Candidates are assessed to determine how they will fit into the culture. Nurses are offered opportunities to experience many different care settings so that they can find the best fit and culture for themselves. Mercy aims to guide the career lifecycle with its nurses.

According to Dr. Rocchio, career ladders have become as a thing of the past. Development centers instead guide a nurse through the first 5 years of clinical practice and then assist them into new career pursuits, such as nurse anesthetists or other advanced nursing practice roles. Dr. Rocchio believes that there are not enough mentoring opportunities within nursing. Leaders have traditionally sought mentors proactively while finding external opportunities on their own. The profession must get better at helping nurses to develop across the career continuum.

The challenge in today's healthcare climate is finding mentors to help lead the charge of creating and repairing a system under constant change. Unlike some other businesses, healthcare cannot simply shrink or disappear. The community and healthcare organizations depend upon nurses getting it right and remembering that their core mission is excellent patient care. Dr. Rocchio's analogy is that the profession must innovate and build tomorrow's race car, not just make today's horse go faster.

Nurse Scientist

Figaro Loresto

The rise of the nurse scientist role paves yet another opportunity for nurses to engage in research, use their expertise to drive health system changes, and mentor the next generation. The nurse scientist is in a prime position to serve as a resource for others by focusing their interests, formulating research questions, and designing and implementing meaningful clinical projects that impact knowledge in nursing science (Ridge, 2021). In *The Future of Nursing Report 2020–2030*, healthcare organizations are encouraged to leverage nursing expertise in designing, generating, analyzing, and applying data to support initiatives (National Academies of Sciences, Engineering, and Medicine, 2021). The nurse scientist role can help to meet this objective by elevating evidence-based healthcare practices.

Dr. Loresto started as a registered nurse in the emergency department and his long-term goal was to advance his education and explore different roles focused on quality and research. Even before he began his PhD education, Dr. Loresto sought out experiences to expand his knowledge and skills. He took on many roles, from a biostatistician intern to a teaching assistant. He became passionate about designing research, identifying the best ways to use data, and translating science into operations. His curiosity about the processes for accessing data, creating structures in collecting data, and establishing sustainable systems led him to eventually accepting the role of a nurse scientist. Nurse scientists focus on the development, coordination, and management of clinical research studies and have a strong desire to contribute to the overall health sciences literature (Nursing at the NIH Clinical Center, n.d.).

Dr. Loresto wears many hats: assistant professor at a college of nursing, nurse scientist in research, innovation, and professional practice, and RN quality research specialist in nursing education and research. He is extensively published and has presented at many national conferences, sharing his knowledge and expertise.

Dr. Loresto quickly learned that the role of the nurse scientist is expansive. He partners with colleagues and other clinicians *within* and *outside* the organization to achieve outcomes. Nurse scientists mentor other nurses to advance the profession. Dr. Loresto has two types of mentors: a PhD advisor for skill development and nurse leaders in his organization, all of whom provide guidance on how to navigate the healthcare environment. He firmly believes that his mentors contribute greatly to his success, as they serve as his "sounding board," validating his ideas or challenging him to think differently. He states, "As we have been mentored by others, it's also as important to serve as mentors to others who are just beginning their journey." Mentors provide opportunities for growth and open many doors. As others have mentored him, Dr. Loresto mentors other nurses involved with nursing research. He describes that the keys to advancing in a role include: 1) a curiosity to continually learn, 2) a willingness to say "yes" to new opportunities, and 3) a personal investment in finding solutions to problems. As a nurse scientist, he nurtures his curiosity because this leads to innovation. He knows that the priorities of today might not be the same tomorrow, so he is always open to considering new ideas and exploring new methodologies.

Transition to Practice Program Director
Paula Susanne "Susie" Price

Transition to practice programs are an effective strategy to increase competence and confidence among new graduate registered nurses as well as decrease organizational turnover (Goode et al., 2018; Shinners et al., 2021; Spector et al., 2015). There is a recognized need for supporting and developing new advanced practice registered nurses (APRNs). Organizations and programs (e.g., The National Nurse Practitioner Residency & Fellowship Training Consortium [2022] and the American Nurses Credentialing Center's Advanced Practice Provider Fellowship Accreditation™ [2022]) have developed standards aimed at recognizing organizations investing in the development of advanced practice nurses. The focus of the standards highlights the importance of hiring a program director whose responsibilities include program implementation, ongoing management, and monitoring of outcomes (National Nurse Practitioner Residency & Fellowship Training, 2015).

Dr. Price remembers her own experience of transitioning from an expert registered nurse into a novice nurse practitioner (NP), which was a surprisingly uncomfortable experience. There were no residency programs when she started as an NP and her personal experience made her keenly aware that the first year of practice is critical for a successful transition into the NP role. As a result she became a dedicated preceptor to guide novices into their new role.

Dr. Price always wondered why most other healthcare professions (e.g., physical therapy, pharmacy, medicine) had residencies or fellowships, while nursing was often not afforded the support and environment to create an effective role transition. When she was approached about becoming the residency program director for her organization, she was initially hesitant, given that she had not had any previous experience in this area. She

knew that this was an important opportunity to make a difference. Her partner in implementing the residency program provided the mentoring she needed to grow into this new leadership role focusing on areas such as project management and navigating the healthcare environment when implementing a new program.

Individuals serving in the program director role for transition to practice must be familiar with the education design process, which includes development, design, implementation, and evaluation. These leaders must understand how to use outcomes to develop strategies for ongoing development, must be strong communicators, and must possess skills in project management or staff development. As program director, Dr. Price has successfully led the accreditation of the residency program at her organization. She ensures that the residency program is aligned with the standards required for accreditation and uses outcomes to drive the organization's workforce development strategy. She manages the day-to-day operations of the program and provides ongoing support for all who complete the program.

When asked what advice she would give to other nurses, Dr. Price noted, "Be a life-long learner." After working as an NP for many years, she returned to school to earn her doctor of nursing practice (DNP) degree. As a DNP-prepared NP, she was presented with an opportunity to lead organizational change through quality improvement and apply evidence-based practice to impact healthcare. However, no matter how much education, experience, and opportunity one has, she highlighted the importance of always remembering one's "True North." Dr. Price states, "We always have to remember our 'True North' no matter what, and we always have to be our authentic selves if we are to make a difference in our patients' lives." In her mentoring role, Dr. Price takes the opportunity to remind NP residents to be authentic, listen for understanding, and maintain connections with those they serve.

Nurse Entrepreneur
Lisbeth Votruba

Nurses are in a unique position to lead, innovate, and operationalize solutions to improve healthcare systems. Nurse entrepreneurs use their healthcare knowledge as a platform to develop ideas into solutions that address a need or fill a gap in the industry. Nurses can participate in product development, consulting, or private case management (Vannucci & Weinstein, 2017). Others become sought-after industry leaders with national and international recognition, focusing their businesses on health-related areas incorporating information technology and patient data storage or medical devices. Nurse entrepreneurs often see an opportunity to impact clinical practice and care delivery outside of their current practice area and take a calculated risk to make a change.

Ms. Votruba was considered by many to be a rising star at the previous healthcare organization where she was employed. She started her career on a medical-surgical unit, transitioned into critical care, and completed her master's in nursing degree as a nurse practitioner (NP). During her tenure as a staff nurse and early in her career, she precepted new nurses, which fostered her desire to assume leadership roles.

Over time, she became a Magnet™ certification coordinator and was involved in several other system initiatives. However, the turning point for her was when she was denied a promotion. She realized that she had "hit the ceiling" and there was no better time for her to expand her sphere of influence. Her decision to move away from clinical care and pursue her new passion as an innovator was not an easy one. One colleague said to Ms. Votruba, "It's okay to not be clinical. There are others who are in that role and your talents can benefit those who serve in the clinical role." It was the permission she needed to let go of who she thought she was as a professional and to leave clinical practice. Ms. Votruba states, "One does not need to be [in] clinical [areas] in order to impact patients' lives. It took another person for me to recognize that my talents are more valuable in a non-clinical area where I can make a real difference in healthcare."

Nurse entrepreneurs instinctively recognize that there is always room to grow (Daily Nurse, n.d.) and are passionate about creating innovations in nursing (Nneka et al., 2021). Today, as the chief clinical officer for AvaSure, Ms. Votruba is a senior executive responsible for strategic market growth and the clinical innovation roadmap and also supports customer research and quality improvement projects. She embodies the key characteristics of a nurse entrepreneur: compassionate leader, promoter of the nursing profession, and healthcare innovator. She invested in herself by hiring an executive coach to guide both her personal and professional development. As an entrepreneur, Ms. Votruba pioneered the diffusion of new technologies to drive quality care. She is dedicated to advancing dialogue at the state and national policy level, as well as influencing how industry and nurse leaders collaborate to develop and implement technology in rapidly evolving and highly regulated healthcare environments.

Reflecting on her successes, Ms. Votruba shares that her desire to solve problems for others is what opened many doors. She accepted assignments with an open mind and treated them as opportunities to expand her horizon. Networking allowed her to share her expertise and learn from others. She strongly suggests that nurses avoid saying "no" to exciting opportunities as they present.

BUILDING A PROFESSIONAL DEVELOPMENT PLAN

"You must know yourself to grow yourself."
(John C. Maxwell)

A key step to professional development is to set goals focusing on strategies for success. When goal-setting, the key is recognizing potential career opportunities and identifying one's individual **s**trengths, **w**eaknesses, **o**pportunities, and **t**hreats (SWOTs) (Table 22.1). Performing a SWOT analysis can assist in developing a personalized professional development plan (PDP) (Table 22.2). Reviewing PDP progress and making necessary adjustments must occur regularly. Reflecting on the questions that follow helps to tailor a PDP and establish realistic goals:

- What do you like best about your current professional state?
- What do you like least about your current professional state?
- If you were not in your current profession, what would you be doing?
- How would your friends describe you?
- How would your biggest critics describe you?
- Who are the biggest influencers in your life? In your career?
- What motivates you?
- What prevents you from making a change (e.g., time, fear of the unknown, fear of failure)?
- What are you passionate about? What "fills your cup"?
- Where would you like to see yourself 2 years from now?

TABLE 22.1 Personal SWOT Analysis: An Example

Strengths *What are you good at?*	Weaknesses *What are areas for further development?*
• Integrating ideas • Teaching/precepting 1:1 • Presenting to small groups • Organizational skills • Taking a lead on projects • Listening skills	• Networking • Creativity • Giving feedback • Writing for publication • Presenting to a large audience
Opportunities *If you improve on your weaknesses, what opportunities do you see for yourself?*	**Threats** *What are the barriers in achieving those opportunities?*
If I can improve on my weaknesses, I can: • Meet new people outside of my small circle • Find mentors locally and nationally • Find leaders to sponsor me into new opportunities • Provide meaningful feedback to fuel growth in others • Share my knowledge and expertise with a larger audience • Publish and present at conferences	• Time • Self-confidence • Lack of a mentor, preceptor, or sponsor to guide me

TABLE 22.2 Professional Development Plan Sample

OVERARCHING GOAL: BECOME A NATIONAL SUBJECT MATTER EXPERT ABOUT CONGENITAL HEART DISEASES

Year	Goals	Action Items With Specific Timeframes	Measure of Success
Year 1	• Present at a local chapter conference regarding congenital heart disease	• Contact chapter to gather information on local conference within 1 month • Submit an evidence-based abstract to a local conference by due date	• Accepted as a presenter at the local chapter conference
Year 2	• Serve on a local or national board level for a pediatric nursing professional organization	• Gain understanding of the role of a board member within 3 months • Complete SWOT analysis related to board member competencies within 4 months • Pursue nomination for board position within 9 months	Elected to serve on selected board
	• Publish on work related to congenital heart diseases	• Find a mentor to assist with a manuscript within 1 month • Find a coauthor within 2 months • Attend a manuscript writing seminar within 6 months, if available • Complete and submit manuscript within 9 months	Manuscript accepted for publication

Modified from © 2022 Versant Holdings, LLC.

FOSTERING THE PERSONAL LEADERSHIP JOURNEY

The personal leadership journey is ever-evolving, even for the most seasoned leaders, and can be guided by preceptors with expertise in leadership roles. Similar to the nursing process, leaders must:

- **Assess** where they are at this moment in their career
- **Diagnose** the personal strengths, weaknesses, opportunities, and barriers to development

- **Create a plan** for achieving goals
- **Implement** the plan
- **Evaluate** success and opportunities, and recalibrate the strategy as needed (Figure 22.1)

In summary, some steps that preceptors can consider when guiding learners who are aspiring to leadership include:

1. **Gain exposure to leadership roles both inside and outside of the work organization**. This allows the individual to learn about roles with which they might not be familiar. Often nurses have preconceived ideas of what they want to be when they "grow up." Some may aspire to be unit managers, educators, advanced practice nurses, or academicians. However, they may not have in-depth understanding of the roles and accompanying leadership expectations. "Shadowing" individuals who serve in different leadership roles can be informative. There may be value in asking for introductions to others who have nontraditional leadership roles, such as chief nursing informatics officers, nurse entrepreneurs, nurse consultants, or legal nurse specialists. A broad understanding of nursing opportunities will help when formulating a personal professional development plan.

2. **Create a personal professional development plan**. A PDP will assist individuals in gaining insights about present strengths, weaknesses, available opportunities, and barriers (threats) to achievement of personal short-term and long-term goals.

3. **Find a mentor**. Engaging with a mentor was a common theme among the nursing leaders interviewed. Mentors play a critical role in an individual's development. Nurses may engage several mentors based on their areas of interest. Fellow nurses and immediate supervisors may have insights on who can best serve as mentor.

4. **Be a joiner**. Volunteer to serve on unit, hospital, or system-level committees. This creates opportunities for collaboration within the organization. Active participation in professional organizations can showcase leadership skills and provide opportunities at local, state, or national levels.

5. **Build a network**. A professional network may be within or outside of the work environment. Participation in professional organizations will build a wider and stronger external network. Contacts within hospital institutions or clinics can help individuals develop leadership skills and competencies and serve as a sounding board for new ideas. In building a network, some contacts may serve as a mentor and others can act as a sponsor. While a mentor guides, advises, and provides feedback on development, a sponsor can use their influence to pull the burgeoning leader forward and elevate them into other roles.

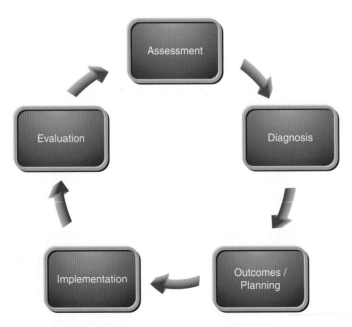

Fig. 22.1 The leadership journey process.

REFERENCES

American Nurses Credentialing Center. (2022). *2023 Advanced practice provider fellowship accreditation application manual.* American Nurses Credentialing Center.

Clark, D. (2022, October 11). How to help an employee figure out their career goals. *Harvard Business Review.* https://hbr.org/2022/10/how-to-help-an-employee-figure-out-their-career-goals?utm_source=Sailthru&utm_medium=email&utm_campaign=Issue:%202022-10-11%20HR%20Dive:%20Talent%20%5Bissue:45172%5D&utm_term=HR%20Dive:%20Talent

Daily Nurse®. The Pulse of Nursing. (n.d.). Entrepreneur/Nurse entrepreneur. https://dailynurse.com/entrepreneur-nurse-entrepreneur/

Goode, C. J., Glassman, K. S., Ponte, P. R., Krugman, M., & Peterman, T. (2018). Requiring a nurse residency for newly licensed registered nurses. *Nursing Outlook, 66*(3), 329–332. https://doi.org/10.1016/j.outlook.2018.04.004

National Academy of Medicine. (2022). *National plan for health workforce well-being.* The National Academies Press. https://doi.org/10.17226/26744

National Academies of Sciences, Engineering, and Medicine [NASEM]. (2021). *The future of nursing 2020–2030: Charting a path to achieve health equity.* National Academies Press. https://doi.org/10.17226/25982

National Nurse Practitioner Residency, & Fellowship Training, Consortium. (2015). National nurse practitioner residency and fellowship training consortium accreditation preparation 2016–2017 Self-study guide. https://www.nppostgradtraining.com/wp-content/uploads/2020/03/Exhibit26SelfStudyGuide_R030420.pdf

Nneka, E. U., Joseph, C. O., Vincent, N. U., Ogbonnaya, N. P., Anarado, A., & Peace, N. I. (2021). The drive process model of entrepreneurship: A grounded theory of nurses' perception of entrepreneurship in nursing. *International Journal of Africa Nursing Sciences, 15,* 100377. https://doi.org/10.1016/j.ijans.2021.100377

Nursing at the NIH Clinical Center (n.d.). *Clinical Research Nurse Roles.* https://clinicalcenter.nih.gov/nursing/careers/roles.html

Ridge, R. A. (2021). Leveraging the nurse scientist role through entrepreneurial innovation. *Nursing Management, 52*(4), 32–38. https://doi.org/10.1097/01.numa.0000737620.13138.e1

Shinners, J., Africa, L., Mallory, C., & Durham, H. (2021). Versant's nurse residency program: A retrospective review. *Nursing Economics, 39*(5), 239–246.

Spector, N., Blegen, Mary A., Silvestre, J., Barnsteiner, J., Lynn, M. R., Ulrich, B., Fogg, L., & Alexander, M. (2015). Transition to practice study in hospital settings. *Journal of Nursing Regulation, 5*(4), 24–38. https://doi.org/10.1016/s2155-8256(15)30031-4

Vannucci, M. J., & Weinstein, S. M. (2017). The nurse entrepreneur: Empowerment needs, challenges, and self-care practices. *Nursing: Research and Reviews, 7,* 57–66. https://doi.org/10.2147/nrr.s98407

Wei, H., King, A., Jiang, Y., Sewell, K. A., & Lake, D. M. (2020). The impact of nurse leadership styles on nurse burnout: A systematic literature review. *Nurse Leader, 18*(5), 439–450. https://doi.org/10.1016/j.mnl.2020.04.002

23

Precepting in Global Health Experiences

B. Elias Snyder and Charlotte Nwogwugwu

CHAPTER OBJECTIVES

- Describe principles of global health and how they influence precepting nurse learners
- Prepare nurse learners before, during, and after global experiences

- Apply scope of practice considerations within the context of the host country

---

Global health experiences are enriching and meaningful learning opportunities. They provide a venue for students and preceptors to step out of their comfort zones and into experiences that can transform not only their perspectives on nursing and healthcare but can change who they are as individuals. Participating in global health work is a privilege and must be approached with a high level of self-awareness, skill, humility, and preparation. Global health practitioners approach their work with conscious humility, curiosity, and a lens of reciprocity whereby they intentionally seek to both learn and share effective interventions that promote health, equity, and justice around the globe.

GUIDING PRINCIPLES FOR GLOBAL HEALTH

Centering on Equity and Justice

The richness of global experiences is in large part due to interactions with people from varying backgrounds and cultures. Creating a successful experience for both the learner and preceptor involves attention to "inner work." Inner work contributes to personal growth and can be explained as bringing awareness to one's perspective of bias, race, and prejudice through

self-reflection. It is often the first step in promoting equity, justice, and healing (Magee, 2019). Another dimension of inner work involves identifying one's *intersectional identities*, described as the rich tapestry of one's individuality (e.g., ancestry, family stories, gender, religion, and cultures). By understanding diverse inner dimensions, nurses can find effective connection points with others, no matter how different they may seem. To explain further,

> *"While preparing to experience the richness of other cultures, one must stop and ask, Who am I? How am I entering this space? How do I hold privilege and power? When those answers have been discovered, then one can commit their actions to authentically center equity and justice."*
>
> **(Conyers, personal communication, September 5, 2023)**

Participation in the global experience allows learners to continue their inner-work reflections while practicing "outer work" during clinical fieldwork. Independent journaling and active discussion can facilitate deeper understanding and appreciation for variations in culture. Appropriate journaling or discussion prompts include social justice and social determinants of health issues, experiences with cultural humility and cross-cultural collaboration, and awareness on the impact of inner bias.

Decolonizing Global Health

While global health initiatives have reduced the burden of many diseases over the last century, they have also created a number of adverse effects. The mission of global health is to "reduce or eliminate inequities" (Abimbola and Pai, 2020). A potentially harmful outcome may result when assuming that "something is better than nothing" as learners undertake health initiatives within global communities. Because global experiences with learners can do more harm than good, a decolonizing approach can be adopted to guide the experience.

Decolonization of global health removes all forms of hierarchy and views all individuals as equal participants. Advocates work against "saviorism" and "mission" trips, which imply that some people need saving and others have all the solutions. Intentionally embracing a philosophy of solidarity reinforces humility and equitable collaboration. The emphasis is on deep relationships with people and communities instead of "pop-in and pop-out" global health projects. A strengths-based approach recognizing protective and support factors within communities is more effective and productive than falling into a "deficit thinking trap" where only problems are identified. Finally, partnerships are viewed through a lens of reciprocal learning between learner, preceptor, and patient/community to improve equity, justice, and health. These approaches lead to generative relationships that benefit all those involved. (See Resources at the end of the chapter).

Strengths-Based Approach

Traditionally, global health professionals have often approached communities with a "deficit-based" outlook, focusing on what is lacking or what needs "fixing." However, in the spirit of decolonizing global health, adopting a strengths-based approach works more effectively. Focusing on strengths acknowledges the resilience, ingenuity, and assets inherent in global communities, rather than merely identifying gaps or shortcomings.

A strengths-based approach calls for a paradigm shift in how global health workers perceive and engage with communities. Instead of asking, "What is missing here?" the question becomes, "What is working well here, and how can we amplify it?" This perspective invites a more equitable partnership between global health professionals and

community members, recognizing that both parties bring valuable expertise to the table. Identifying problems is part of this work and facilitates collaboration with local partners. However, the problems should not overshadow the strength within the community.

For example, consider a community where consistent electricity might not be available. A deficit-based approach might focus solely on this lack of infrastructure, missing out on the resilience and ingenuity that community members have shown by creating alternative sources of energy. Recognizing these community-developed solutions not only respects local innovation but also provides a foundation on which to build sustainable initiatives.

Preceptors preparing learners for fieldwork in global health should instill a strengths-based perspective as a core principle of engagement. Application of this approach is integral to clinical practice and can be emphasized through learner–patient/family interactions, preceptor–learner discussions, predeparture briefings, and reflective journaling. Moreover, preceptors can encourage students to actively seek out and identify community strengths as part of their fieldwork, ensuring these insights inform any proposed interventions or projects. Learners also benefit from discussions with local community members and leaders about observed and perceived strengths.

The Pitfalls of a Deficit-Based Outlook

A deficit-based approach, although often well-intentioned, can inadvertently perpetuate harmful stereotypes and reinforce power imbalances. It risks overshadowing the capabilities and resources that communities have developed over time to meet their unique challenges. Additionally, this outlook can contribute to a "savior complex," where external experts assume they have the solutions to local problems, undermining local knowledge and agency. Preceptors are in a position to discuss identified deficits with learners and, more importantly, redirect learners toward a more productive and respectful strengths-based approach.

PREPARING FOR A GLOBAL EXPERIENCE

Embarking on a global health experience is not something to be taken lightly. Students must be adequately prepared, not just in terms of academic knowledge but also in their understanding of the cultural, linguistic, and social intricacies of their host country. Several pillars of preparatory work can guide students in becoming well-rounded global citizens while minimizing the pitfalls of bias and cultural insensitivity (Box 23.1).

Partnering with organizations and sites involves aligning goals to facilitate long-term reciprocal relationships. Preceptors should work collaboratively with the host institution to identify the needs of the organization/community and ensure that the community needs align with the academic goals of the global experience. As invited guests, the goals of the community should be the first priority.

Logistics

With an emphasis on safety, careful consideration needs to be given to lodging, transportation, meals, and communication. Before arrival, faculty and preceptors need to address whether students/learners will share rooms or have individual rooms. Rooming assignments should be considered carefully, with appropriate accommodations for students with specific needs, such as those who are transgender or gender nonconforming. Accommodations for those with special dietary needs should also be identified. Learners should obtain predeparture vaccinations and any necessary medications for personal needs or possible illnesses.

Safety is a priority and must be addressed prior to as well as throughout the experience. Safety contacts must be identified both home and abroad. A mechanism for group communication (such as WhatsApp) should be established to maintain connections when the group is separated. Safe and reliable in-country transportation must be arranged. On-site considerations such as access to adequate drinking water need to be recognized. Issues surrounding planetary health should be respected by considering, for example, the impact of plastic on the environment.

Culture and Language Preparations

Predeparture exposure to the selected culture can contribute to a successful global health experience. A cultural facilitator can be invited to answer questions about culture, safety, and provide language courses. In addition, participating in local cultural events or festivals can prepare learners to engage with a culture different from their own. Such experiences can serve as a microcosm of the larger experience awaiting them, giving them a preview of the music, food, traditions, and social dynamics they might encounter. Because nursing focuses on holistic care, these cultural events can introduce the learner to pertinent social determinants of health and protective factors within the community.

BOX 23.1 Predeparture Preparations

Inner Work, Bias, and Cultural Humility
- Inner work: Encourage students to engage in introspective practices that help them identify their internal biases against different cultures, communities, practices, etc.
- Cultural humility: Support students, faculty, and preceptors to regularly acknowledge what they do and do not know and humbly ask questions about culture, traditions, and practices with genuine curiosity and respect.

Safety for All
- Sign up for alerts from governmental or trusted news agencies.
- Ensure local facilitators and hosts can reach you at all times.
- Understand cultural norms such as perceptions and laws around lesbian, gay, bisexual, transgender, questioning, intersex, asexual, and two-spirit (LGBTQIA2S+); gender nonconforming individuals; race; and skin color.
- Determine appropriateness for healthcare providers of opposite genders to care for patients.
- Ensure a chaperone is present when needed.

Language
- A basic understanding of the local language(s) can build rapport and trust within host communities; language classes should be considered.
- Numerous languages and dialects coexist in diverse societies; the preferred language(s) of the host country, setting, or population should be respectfully utilized.

Engage Local Facilitators
- Local facilitators can educate preceptors and students about local languages, cultures, safety, belief systems, etc., before, during, and after the trip.

Geopolitics and History
- Educate students with accurate information about the specific location to understand the political, social, and environmental context of the area.
- Work with your local facilitator to identify readings, films, and art to help gain a comprehensive understanding of the host country.

Social Media
- Set clear rules and expectations around the appropriate use of social media.
- Have students sign an "appropriate use of social media" contract.
- Remind students that unintended harm can be caused by inappropriate social media use.

A common assumption among learners from English-speaking countries is that their language will be universally understood, which is not only culturally insensitive but also impractical. Preceptors are responsible for addressing language and communication nuances, not only in global field experiences but also local areas, such as rural communities, where English is not the primary language. Misconceptions can hinder effective communication and compromise the quality of healthcare delivery.

Consider the example of some English-speaking African nations. Many of these countries are linguistically diverse, boasting a multitude of languages. In Nigeria, for instance, there are over 500 languages spoken, and in South Africa, there are 11 official languages. While English may be the language of government and higher education, it is not necessarily the language spoken at home or in rural communities.

Becoming familiar with the local language is not just about facilitating communication; it is also a mark of respect for the host community. It shows a willingness to engage with the culture and people on their own terms, rather than imposing an external framework. As invited guests, putting in the effort to learn some local words and greetings shows a great deal of respect. This is particularly important in healthcare settings where trust and mutual respect are paramount for effective treatment and care.

Briefings on Politics and History

In any international experience, the political and historical contexts cannot be ignored. Preceptors and learners need to be aware of whether the country they will be working in is experiencing political unrest, economic instability, or social tensions. Such factors can significantly affect the safety and feasibility of the project. Briefings on the current political climate, along with historical context, should be part of the predeparture preparation. This knowledge is invaluable for risk assessment and contingency planning and can help learners navigate potential challenges more effectively. Political and historical contexts can also provide insight into how a country operates and offer a richer understanding of why things are the way they are. This information informs the health, safety, and well-being of both visitors and residents alike.

Political and social climates can change rapidly. What might seem like a stable situation during the predeparture conferences can swiftly evolve into a volatile one. Learners need to be prepared for such eventualities and trained in how to adapt their plans and actions accordingly. This calls for ongoing updates even after the initial briefings, right up until the time of departure and potentially throughout the duration of the field experience.

Methods to Keep Abreast of Changes

In preparation for a global experience, preceptors should be attentive to providing regular updates related to the country's situation, establishing local contacts, monitoring social media and developing emergency protocols. Regular updates may come from trusted news sources and governmental advisories to keep learners updated on any significant changes in the political climate (e.g., U.S. State Department STEP Program; International SOS). A network of local contacts can be established to provide real-time updates and nuanced insights that mainstream news might miss. Social media offers timely information, but should be used cautiously and corroborated with more local authoritative sources. Finally, a set of contingency plans should be in place so learners can respond effectively if emergencies present.

Other contextual factors like geography, weather conditions, and local customs should also be included in predeparture materials. Knowledge about the area's environmental conditions can help learners pack appropriately and take necessary health precautions. Similarly, understanding local customs, religious beliefs, and social norms can help learners interact respectfully and effectively with the local community.

Examples of resources for learners include:

- Country briefs: A comprehensive guide detailing all essential information about the country;
- Academic articles: Scholarly perspectives on the region's healthcare system, culture, and more;
- Travel advisories: Trusted news sources or government-issued advisories to provide safety guidelines and other important information;
- Local literature and art: Works by local authors and artists to offer unique insights into the culture and mindset of the people, as well as music, art, and dance.

Professionalism and Dress Codes

Professional attire in global health field experiences is not merely a question of aesthetics; it is a critical component of effective and respectful engagement with diverse communities. Professional attire can vary greatly depending on the cultural and social norms of the host country.

Educators and preceptors should institute a foundational dress code policy for all global health field experiences. Guidelines should be straightforward and include either business casual attire or clinical scrubs along with comfortable footwear. Informal attire may be appropriate for some specific projects. Policies must be adapted and refined based on the specific cultural and climatic contexts of the host country.

Learners must understand how different types of clothing are perceived within the host community. This extends beyond simple questions of formality and delves into local gender norms. Speaking with local leaders and community members before the trip can provide clearer insight instead of relying solely on reading about the cultural norms. For example, in some cultures, women wearing trousers might be considered inappropriate or disrespectful. Awareness of the norms can help in making clothing choices that are both professional and culturally sensitive. Proactively protecting and respecting the identities of students who do not fit into traditional male/female gender categories requires careful consideration. This is particularly necessary in countries that do not officially recognize nonbinary genders. Depending on the cultural and religious norms within a community, additional considerations related to dress code include the appropriateness of head or shoulder coverings or whether shorts may be worn.

DURING THE TRIP: ADVICE ON THE GROUND

During the global health experience, learners integrate all the predeparture work into practice. Preceptors can remind learners to engage in active self-awareness activities throughout the trip to continually evaluate not just what they are gaining from the experience, but also how their attitudes and behaviors may affect those around them. Because cultural and social norms can differ significantly, especially in a foreign host country, what may seem like a harmless action or casual statement could be interpreted very differently by others. In many cases, partners or locals in the host country may not feel comfortable sharing their concerns or grievances openly with the preceptor or learners. Instead, they

may discuss these issues privately among themselves or keep them quiet. Therefore, preceptors and facilitators must be acutely attuned to the social cues and regularly seek feedback from learners and partners. Critical skills include paying attention to not only what is being said, but also to nonverbal communication and changes in group dynamics.

Sample Daily Agenda

While each trip is different, implementing the following agenda with regular question prompts may be helpful:
- **Morning check-ins over breakfast**
  - How is everyone feeling? Is anyone sick?
  - Is there anything we may need to modify today?
- **Review the objectives for the day**
  - Where are we going? What are we doing? What is the schedule?
  - Any clothing considerations or special materials that will be needed?
  - What should we focus on or pay close attention to?
- **Activities of the day**
- **Unstructured time for rest, exploring, visiting local markets, etc.**
- **Debrief and dinner**
  - "Rose, bud, and thorn" discussion prompt: What was a highlight, challenge, and growth opportunity or new experience from the day?
  - Interpersonal check-ins: Is there anything the group needs to discuss or work through?
  - Next day preparation: What is happening tomorrow? What time should we wake up and be ready to go in the morning?

Daily debriefing sessions should be intentionally designed to explore both emotional and analytical responses to the day's events. Questions could focus on comparing and contrasting healthcare practices and community structures between the home and the host country. This encourages learners to think critically about different models of care, governance, and community strengths. Discussion questions may include
- What unique approaches or resources have been deployed to handle day-to-day challenges?
- How might students or learners incorporate these strengths or techniques into their own future practice or community involvement when they return home?

Framing the experience as an opportunity for reciprocal learning, not just a one-way imparting of skills or

---

Exemplar: Unauthorized Photography During a Global Health Field Experience

B. Elias Snyder, PhD, FNP-C, ACHPN

Charlotte Nwogwugwu, DrPH, MPH, MSN-PMHNP, HIV PCP, CPH-BC

During recent preparations for a student trip, we convened for a predeparture session. This gathering was not optional; every student participating in the trip had to attend. Our primary objective was to ensure that each participant understood the plan for the trip and, more crucially, the deeper cultural etiquettes we wanted them to uphold.

We embarked on the vital topic of cultural humility—the ability to maintain an introspective view and openness to learning about other cultures, while recognizing that one's home culture is not the universal norm. As part of this conversation, we discussed the importance of gaining permission before photographing individuals. It is not just a matter of respect, but of recognizing the autonomy of other individuals, especially in foreign cultures where power and privilege dynamics may be blurred or underrecognized.

Drawing from history, we highlighted the disturbing trend by some Western and European travelers who perceive Indigenous peoples as "articles of interest," frequently snapping photos without seeking or receiving consent. Such actions, especially when magnified by the platform of social media, are deeply disrespectful and can perpetuate harmful stereotypes and misconceptions.

Providing a more direct and grounded perspective, we invited a local expert and consultant to the session. He delved into the specific community issues tied to such thoughtless behaviors, ensuring our students heard firsthand about the implications of their actions in the places they would be visiting. He shared how some people in Tanzania expressed that they have often felt like "animals on a safari" when visitors take pictures of them without consent.

While in Tanzania, our students displayed an admirable level of respect and maturity, ensuring photographs were taken judiciously and ethically. For our concluding cultural experience—a safari—we explained that we would be moving through areas in a safari vehicle and would not have the opportunity to engage directly with community members as we had at other sites. We emphasized that no photographs of individuals were allowed. Unbeknownst to us at the time, one student defied this directive. We only discovered this after our return home when a photo taken of a group of Maasai people was shared. The realization was a stark reminder that, despite our best efforts, the challenge of educating on cultural respect is ongoing.

To address the situation, we, as group leaders, initially met to discuss the issue and create a plan. We then met with the student to discuss our concerns. The student seemed a little surprised by the interaction and did not seem to understand the significance of her actions. We reiterated what we discussed in the predeparture meetings regarding appropriate use of photos. We explained the potential harm that taking such a photo could have and asked questions to understand why she decided to take the photo without obtaining consent. We re-emphasized that while such actions may seem benign, there is a potential for harm to be caused. In retrospect, it would also have been interesting to hear more about the student's perspective before we addressed our concerns. Our lesson learned was to be proactive and have all students sign a photo use agreement before embarking on global experiences.

---

knowledge, can help learners take ownership of their growth.

When planning global trips, remember to include periods of unstructured activities. Global health experiences can be overwhelming; therefore, downtime to relax, process the experience, explore, and build group cohesion can be regenerating. Scheduled time for journaling and reflection are additional recommendations, along with one-on-one check-ins with the preceptor.

POST-TRIP INTEGRATION

Because global health experiences can be transformative, post-trip integration should not be overlooked.

The return from intense fieldwork to familiar settings can sometimes create cognitive dissonance. A post-trip debrief offers a structured setting in which to process and integrate newly acquired knowledge and attitudes into future practice.

The post-trip period is an opportunity for more extensive reflection. While immersed in the global health experience, the pace and intensity may not allow time for deep contemplation. Once home, learners can reflect on not only how the trip impacted them personally, but also how their actions and presence impacted the community they visited. Some learners and preceptors may also have a difficult time adjusting to life back at home, thus reconnecting to debrief with the group can be helpful.

Preceptors and learners are encouraged to "bookend" the trip. This means building intentional time *before* the trip to prepare and arrange logistics at home, as well as building in time *after* the trip to rest and integrate the experience.

OTHER CONSIDERATIONS

Utilizing Social Media With Caution

Social media can be a powerful tool for learning about different cultures, but it comes with its own set of limitations. For example, "poverty porn" refers to the act of sharing images and stories of poverty to generate an emotional response or gain. This representation can severely distort one's understanding of a country or culture and inadvertently perpetuate harmful stereotypes, causing "representation harm" or even a "colonial savior" mindset. Learners should be trained to critically assess the information they consume online, focusing on credible sources that offer balanced perspectives.

Some universities that offer global experiences have a policy whereby students, faculty, and preceptors are not permitted to post any identifiable information or imagery to social media without explicit, informed consent from those involved. A thorough explanation of the content of the post and potential impacts needs to be clearly expressed without any coercion, even subtle or unintended. This includes any identifiable posts with children, as they cannot provide informed consent. Learners, preceptors, and faculty should consider the question, "Would it be appropriate to post this if it were about patients and communities in my home country?" This question can be a tool that is part of a larger conversation.

As an example, there is an all-too-familiar story about the nursing student who went to Africa and "delivered a baby." The student was a part of the action, helped the birthing mother, cut the umbilical cord, and then posted all about it on social media and received accolades from friends and family back home. However, the student did not seek permission, thus violating the privacy of the birthing mother. Learners can be guided in discussion about the appropriateness of such posts and strategize what they would do differently.

The use of social media and photography during the global health experience should not be an afterthought. It requires active planning and ethical consideration to ensure that the shared content enhances understanding, respects the dignity of all individuals involved, and aligns with the educational goals. Discussing these issues contributes to a more ethical and impactful learning experience.

Culture Shock

No learner, regardless of background or previous international experience, is wholly insulated from the challenges posed by culture shock, which is a natural response to being in an unfamiliar environment. The phenomenon can be disorienting, and its effects can impact the quality of the educational experience. There are strategies that can be employed to lessen the disorientation. Faculty and preceptors can provide preorientation sessions or preparatory materials that explicitly discuss culture shock and relevant coping strategies.

Understanding that culture shock is a process with identifiable stages can empower learners to navigate more effectively. Stages of culture shock are categorized as follows:

- The honeymoon stage: In this initial period, learners may be enamored by the newness of their environment. Everything may seem fascinating; the focus is often on the similarities between cultures rather than the differences.
- Rejection or frustration stage: As the novelty wears off, learners may become more acutely aware of the differences between their home and host countries. This can result in feelings of irritation, frustration, or even anger toward either culture.
- Regression stage: During this stage, there is a tendency to idealize one's home culture while demeaning the new environment. Learners may withdraw or seek out the company of those from their own culture as a form of comfort.
- Acceptance/negotiation stage: Eventually, learners begin to develop a more balanced perspective. They start to adapt, either by adopting local customs or finding a way to maintain their own cultural identity while respecting those of the host country.
- New-self stage: In the final stage, learners integrate the cultural experience into their identity. They emerge as more-rounded individuals with a greater appreciation for diversity and a nuanced understanding of global health challenges (Arya, 2017; Pedersen, 1995).

PRACTICAL PRECEPTING AND SCOPE OF PRACTICE CONSIDERATIONS

Preceptors must familiarize themselves with the skill level of the learners as well as the scopes of practice in both the home and host countries. In some settings, it is not uncommon for learners and preceptors to be in situations that push them to the edge of their skills and practice limits. In low-resourced settings, a learner may be pulled into an emergency or may become involved in a health or non-health-related situation. In their role, nurses and aspiring nurses exemplify compassion as a superpower. Nurses show profound empathy for their patients and go above and beyond to help them. Honoring this compassion and desire to help in combination with the realities of one's skill levels and scope of practice, is a difficult endeavor but a critical part of global work.

In some countries, the scope of practice allows a nurse to independently tend to a birth. However, a learner's or preceptor's level of training and scope of practice may not allow them to perform this procedure in their home country. An ethical dilemma exists when it is acceptable in the host country for a nurse to deliver a baby but not acceptable in the nurse's home country. Situations like this can be approached by first asking the question, "Is this skill within the learner or preceptor's level of training?" If the answer is no, the skill should *not* be performed. If the answer is yes, then referring to the local practice standards and discussing the procedure with leaders from the host country should occur.

As a reminder, the International Council of Nurses (ICN) Code of Ethics (2021) promotes the practice of safe, person-centered care that emphasizes human rights. The safety of patients and families must be prioritized over the experience of the student in all settings and situations.

More Than Just Helping Learners Build Clinical Skills

The perception that global health experiences are synonymous with "mission trips" is flawed. This is not always the case, but it is a common occurrence. Partnering in the global community is more than simply "doing tasks"; the experience should remain learner-focused, upholding the principles of safety, professionalism, and ethics at all times. Global experiences are meant to holistically change students, not just improve their clinical skills. The very act of venturing into an unfamiliar place is a learning experience. Preceptors function as experience facilitators in the learning process. Facilitation is a skill that can be learned and refined over time. When precepting students on global experiences, it may be helpful to review facilitation skills or seek mentoring from colleagues with experience in this area.

Preceptor and Host Site Considerations

Opportunities may arise when students are precepted by clinicians from the host country. Pairing the correct preceptor with a student needs to be done carefully and intentionally. Since countries vary in nursing training and scope of practice, awareness of these differences creates a respectful learning environment. For nurse practitioner (NP) students, role variations may be particularly challenging, as some countries do not recognize the NP role but may have roles with similar levels of training. For example, in Tanzania, clinical officers, assistant medical officers, and medical doctors are all appropriate preceptors for NP students. The student's faculty member should have a good understanding of the various types of clinicians, their levels of training, and scopes of practice in a particular country to ensure the preceptor–student pair is appropriate. Part of the process of arranging a global clinical experience for students is ensuring that the experience meets the requirements of the accrediting bodies and academic institutions in the home country.

A Note on Licensure

Preceptors need to understand and plan to meet the nursing professional licensure requirements in the host country. If a nurse is practicing or precepting a student, they should be licensed to practice in that country and setting. The board or council of nursing for each country can provide information about obtaining licensure.

WORKING WITH GLOBAL COMMUNITIES AT HOME

Global health travel can be expensive for both learners and preceptors. However, it is not necessary to leave your home country to work with global communities. The United Nations Refugee Agency (UNHCR) estimates that there are over 100 million people in the world who are displaced from their home countries (UNHCR, 2023). Many cities have organizations that support refugees, asylum seekers, immigrants, and migrants, who are often in need of nursing services. Working with global communities at home is an effective way to provide support and learning experiences.

Many of the same skills and considerations previously discussed also apply to global experiences in the home setting. Learners and preceptors should begin with and reflect on inner work throughout the process. In addition, training in trauma-informed care should take place *before* working with individuals who lack resources after leaving their home country. For example, preceptors can consider being trained to conduct forensic evaluations (see Chapter 24) for refugees and asylum seekers (Desmyth et al., 2021). Though challenging work, global experiences can change lives and offer opportunities for both learners and preceptors when providing care for people seeking asylum (see Resources).

RESOURCES

Multiple resources are available for preceptors, students, and faculty to review prior to a global experience. Many of these resources highlight inclusiveness and respect for variations in culture.

Organizations for Working With Displaced Persons
- Physicians for Human Rights: https://phr.org
- Asylum Medicine Training Initiative: https://asylummedtraining.org/
- Society of Asylum Medicine: https://asylummedicine.com/

University of Michigan Inclusive Teaching
- https://sites.lsa.umich.edu/inclusive-teaching/
- Includes teaching points regarding implicit bias, examining power/privilege, and more, to help students deepen their inner awareness.

Global Health History/Colonialism
- Manjapra, K. (2020). *Colonialism in global perspective.* Cambridge University Press.
- Packard, R. M. (2016). *A history of global health interventions into the lives of other peoples.* Baltimore Johns Hopkins University Press.

Inner Bias, Inner Work, Equity, and Justice
- Akparewa, N.E. (2021) *The clinicians guide to microaggressions and unconscious bias: Racial justice in healthcare.* Blurb, Incorporated, 2021.
- Hooks, B. (2013). *Teaching community: A pedagogy of hope.* Taylor and Francis.
- Irving, D. (2014). *Waking up White and finding myself in the story of race.* Elephant Room Press.

- Magee, R. V. (2021). *Inner work of racial justice: Healing ourselves and transforming our communities through mindfulness.* Penguin.
- Menakem, R. (2017). *My grandmother's hands: Racialized trauma and the pathway to mending our hearts and bodies.* Central Recovery Press.
- Paseo Circles of Identity (2001). https://www.schoolreforminitiative.org/download/the-paseo-or-circles-of-identity/

Decolonizing Global Health: Resources for Designing, Implementing, and Evaluating Global Health Experiences
- Abimbola, S., & Pai, M. (2020). Will global health survive its decolonisation? *The Lancet, 396*(10263), 1627–1628. https://doi.org/10.1016/S0140-6736(20)32417-X
- Jumbam, D.T. (2020). How (not) to write about global health. *BMJ Global Health, 5*, e003164. https://gh.bmj.com/content/5/7/e003164.long
- Khan, T., Abimbola, S., Kyobutungi, C., & Pai, M. (2022). How we classify countries and people—and why it matters. *BMJ Global Health, 7*(6), e009704. https://doi.org/10.1136/bmjgh-2022-009704

Activities on Cultural Humility and Understanding
- Trainings and other activities and strategies to develop cultural humility. Equity and Inclusion. (n.d.). Inclusion.uoregon.edu. https://inclusion.uoregon.edu/trainings-and-other-activities-and-strategies-develop-cultural-humility

REFERENCES

Abimbola, S., & Pai, M. (2020). Will global health survive its decolonization? *The Lancet, 396*(10263), 1627–1628. https://doi.org/10.1016/S0140-6736(20)32417-X

Arya, A. N. (2017). *Preparing for International Health Experiences.* CRC Press.

Desmyth, K., Eagar, S., Jones, M., Schmidt, L., & Williams, J. (2021). Refugee health nursing. *Journal of Advanced Nursing, 77*(10). https://doi.org/10.1111/jan.14910

Magee, R. V. (2019). *The inner work of racial justice: Healing ourselves and transforming our communities through mindfulness.* Tarcherperigee, an imprint of Penguin Random House LLC.

Pedersen, P. (1995). *The five stages of culture shock: Critical incidents around the world.* Greenwood Press.

UNHCR, the UN Refugee Agency. (2023). *Global Trends.* UNHCR US, www.unhcr.org/us/global-trends

24

Precepting in Specialty Settings

Cynthia A. Danford and Beth Heuer

CHAPTER OBJECTIVES

- Explore the role of the preceptor working within specialized settings and populations: school nursing; forensic nursing; patients who may be victims of human trafficking; Indigenous populations

- Address the preceptor's role in advising or guiding scholarly projects
- Describe mentoring responsibilities when working with novice nursing faculty

---

Nurse preceptors are called upon to share their knowledge and experience with undergraduate and graduate nursing students and orientees. Preceptors in specialty settings require a high level of dedication and expertise, and additional skills may be needed. This chapter will describe precepting and mentoring in several specialized settings and among various populations.

SCHOOL NURSING

Jess Gordon, Patricia Nicole Anders, and Shayla Dressler

The school nurse preceptor is critical to the success of nurses who have recently graduated and nurses new to the field of school nursing. Although preceptors may not overtly consider framing their approach with a theoretical lens, consideration of Jean Watson's Theory of Human Caring provides a practical perspective on precepting in a community school setting. The theory of human caring is based on ten "carative" factors which integrate modern medicine with nursing care (Watson et al., 2020):

1. Forming selfless, human-centered value systems
2. Instilling faith and hope
3. Cultivating sensitivity with self and others
4. Developing trusting and helping relationships
5. Promoting expression of one's feelings

6. Using problem-solving and decision-making skills
7. Promoting a teaching-learning environment
8. Creating a nurturing environment
9. Focusing on meeting individualized human needs
10. Holistically respecting and embracing the individual's viewpoints

These carative factors are foundational to supporting youth in today's school systems, particularly those youth living in precarious home environments or exposed to vulnerable situations. Building a child's or adolescent's self-esteem and confidence is often a nursing priority requiring attention before or during interactions to enhance physical and mental health acutely or long term. Integrating Watson's carative factors with the care needed in community, school-based environments is part of the preceptor-learner interaction (Box 24.1). The goal for the new school nurse is to emerge as an independent nurse who is able to enrich the optimal health and safety of students and their families.

The School Setting: A New Landscape for Nurses

Precepting a new school nurse is not a linear process due to the multifaceted roles of the school nurse. In particular, school nurses practice autonomously and may not have the same level of support as those in the controlled

---

BOX 24.1   **Carative Behaviors of the Preceptor**

- Integrates their personal values with caring and sensitivity to enhance the learner's self-confidence and foster their tailored approach to patient care.
- Develops a trusting relationship with the learner through expressions of both positive and negative feelings.
- Understands the learning needs of the new nurse through review of social experiences, knowledge, personal belief systems, and clinical skills.
- Models evidence-based care and problem-solving by utilizing best practice guidelines and maintaining an up-to-date knowledge of health conditions to optimize care.
- Demonstrates self-awareness and provides culturally sensitive care.

---

environment of the hospital or clinic. Preceptors can help support the learner by introducing school policies and procedures, as well as state laws addressing health screening and immunization requirements. School nurses must understand their scope of practice and what is legally obligated in this unique setting.

There can be a steep learning curve for many nurses when transitioning from other nursing specialties to school nursing due to variations in structure and autonomy. Many school nurses do not work directly on-site with another licensed healthcare provider. This creates unique challenges for the learner. Some school nurses struggle to organize and prioritize essential functions of the role with this varying level of autonomy.

When precepting a nurse who has never worked in the school setting, it helps to understand their nursing background and prior experience. Orientees often benefit from having backgrounds in hospital- and office-based pediatrics. Those with professional experience in a pediatric emergency department may think quickly and possess the self-confidence that they can handle medical emergencies in the school setting.

Preparing for a New School Year

The onboarding process must be structured and outline the learner's responsibilities and expectations, which evolve throughout the school year. Preceptors introduce various tasks that need to be addressed prior to the arrival of students. New nurses require training on how to review and prioritize student health reports outlining medication needs, management plans (including asthma plans, seizure plans and "sick day" plans for children with diabetes), and health alerts for children with chronic medical conditions. Immunization compliance reports must be reviewed and new orientees must understand the state-mandated immunization requirements for school attendance. The Centers for Disease Control and Prevention (CDC) vaccine schedule and any vaccine requirement summaries from individual State Departments of Health are indispensable tools.

Orientees require a brief tour of the school health room and a review of any medications that have been dropped off by parents. School districts may utilize an Individual Health Plan (IHP) file that contains a tailored health plan for each student. The first day of orientation includes reviewing *what* a health plan is, *why* each student has a health plan, *what* emergency medications are utilized, and *what* medical information needs to be in place for each student on or before the first day of school. The orientee must be familiar with the latest clinical guidelines for treatment of life-threatening conditions including: 1) asthma, 2) cardiac disorders, 3) seizures, 4) life-threatening allergies, and 5) diabetes.

Medication Administration Preparation

Students requiring medications during school hours must have a Medication Administration Record (MAR). These records are typically transcribed or entered by the school nurse from an "Authorization for Medication Administration" form completed by the student's primary care or specialty provider annually and signed by the parent/guardian. Forms must match the corresponding prescription label or over-the-counter label of the provided medications. In most school districts, the completed medication authorization, IHP, and medications (in the original over-the-counter or prescription container) are brought to the office by a parent/guardian and documented. At that time, the medication authorization and the label/packaging are reconciled. If they match, medication information is transcribed onto the MAR. If they do not match, the school nurse cannot accept the medication or the forms, and the parent must have the healthcare provider correct the discrepancy.

Preceptors can break up the intensity of the onboarding process with hands-on teaching experiences. As part of medication training, orientees can practice with multiple bags with simulated medication authorization forms (created *with* and *without* errors) and simulated prescription labels on medications to recognize discrepancies.

School nurses must notify parents when there is an error on the prescriber's medication authorization form that the provider must correct. Once accepted (whether an emergency medication or daily medication), the school nurse is legally required to administer the medication. Controlled substances (including attention deficit hyperactivity disorder [ADHD] stimulant medications and seizure medications such as Midazolam or Diazepam) must be counted with the parent and another staff member and then counted weekly with a staff member and the school nurse. Any discrepancies must be reported to school administration and may necessitate calling the police.

Collaborating to Understand Student Medical Needs

Preceptors and orientees can work together to review and anticipate student needs. Follow-up contact with family may be needed when students are out of compliance with immunizations or to review new or existing health conditions. Pertinent questions related to health conditions include: Is the condition life-threatening? Does the condition require emergency medication at school? What medications does the student take at home and when? When was the last significant illness exacerbation or hospitalization? What medical needs must be met while the student is at school (Box: Maintaining Health in the School Environment)?

Emphasize to new orientees that school nurses provide holistic and collaborative care with students and their families. Families need to feel supported and confident that they are "heard" when it comes to their child's health needs. Meeting with a family at the beginning of the school year will help establish clear communication and a collaborative partnership. With some families, it can be overwhelming to have a child with a new medical diagnosis. The school nurse helps guide the family to secure necessary medical orders and complete an IHP for the child.

Training by the School Nurse in Primary and Secondary Educational Settings

School nurses may have variations in their role depending on the school district and the type of school setting, whether primary (elementary or middle school) or secondary (high school) (Boxes 24.2 and 24.3). Nurses are often assigned to multiple schools as part of their work for the school district, which may require training of other paraprofessionals, teachers, and office staff. Therefore, school nurses must provide necessary

MAINTAINING HEALTH IN THE SCHOOL ENVIRONMENT

Caerissa Fawkes

- School nurses are challenged to balance the management of acute care needs (e.g., injuries, episodic care of ill students, chronic illness exacerbations), and maintenance of school-based health measures (e.g., communicable disease prevention, vision, hearing, and body mass index [BMI] screening). State-mandated health measures are necessary to guide the well-being of all students and communities. School nurses advocate for students to maintain access to basic healthcare. However, children may be living with untreated health conditions and lack an established healthcare provider for wellness checks and episodic care. School nurses must help manage each student's needs with limited resources, while still providing equitable and necessary supports to facilitate optimal learning experiences. The nurse may be the only healthcare provider in the school environment that can provide and translate health information in a way that is applicable and understandable for students and staff.
- Preceptors should guide the school nurse orientee in thinking holistically about student health needs and community resources that are available for support. This includes a focus on individual wellness needs and necessary accommodations to facilitate learning. Setting up students for long-term sustainable health behaviors benefits not only the students but also the families and community.

BOX 24.2 Special Considerations for the School Nurse in Primary School Settings (Elementary and Middle School)

- To promote student independence, school nurses provide ongoing/supplementary education and guidance for students with newly diagnosed chronic diseases such as diabetes.
- Effective and frequent communication with families is required when there are care plan changes and evolving healthcare needs.
- Recognizing signs and symptoms of abuse and neglect in younger students that may not have adequate language and emotional skills to communicate their experience requires special attention by the school nurse.

BOX 24.3 **Special Considerations for the School Nurse in Secondary School Settings (High School)**

- School nurses play an integral role in identifying and managing adolescent sexual health and mental health needs.
- Students with chronic conditions require continued assessment to support increased independence in self-care.
- Local laws regarding the age of consent for various aspects of medical care need to be considered in the health management of adolescents.

health-related training at the beginning of each school year. Paraprofessionals can be trained to manage simple injuries, monitor daily medication, provide some noninvasive aspects of diabetic care, and follow-up on required immunizations. Teachers may require hands-on training to administer epinephrine, provide first aid, and give medications on field trips. Office staff can be utilized for medication administration when needed and as per state law.

Conclusion

Onboarding a new school nurse is not just about medications, health plans, and immunizations. It is about keeping students and staff safe. The school nurse completes monthly checks of the automated external defibrillators (AEDs) and emergency-use naloxone. Additionally, school nurses require resources such as school building maps, phone lists, and translation service information.

The job of a school nurse preceptor continues even after the onboarding requirements and a 90-day new employee evaluation are completed. Onboarding a new school nurse requires strategizing and building self-confidence in the knowledge that the new orientee will often be the sole medical decision-maker in emergency situations at the school.

FORENSIC NURSING

Heather M. Tripp

Forensic nursing, the care of patients who have experienced interpersonal violence or crime, is still a relatively new specialty. Precepting nurses new to this field can be a complex and challenging experience. For many forensic nursing programs, real-time clinical experiences requiring forensic nursing expertise can be intermittent and unpredictable. Consistent immersion experiences are often unavailable. More commonly, forensic clinical experiences are often fragmented over several months, possibly with multiple preceptors.

Forensic Nursing Training

Various learning modalities are used to address the challenge of the direct patient care experience when preparing forensic nurses. As an example, one large healthcare system provides an orientation that includes a 40-hour online didactic course addressing the care of the patient who has experienced a sexual assault or sexual abuse. Additional modules address other types of victimization such as human trafficking and intimate partner violence. New learners are also individually mentored with experienced, full-time staff for a minimum of six to seven times during the orientation phase to review the online material as well as content specific to state law, hospital policies, and best practice. Nurses are encouraged to schedule as much on-call time as possible during orientation to increase the likelihood that they will be called in to work with a preceptor for forensic examination experience.

Simulated Forensic Examinations

Simulated forensic examinations are performed with persons trained as standardized patients also known as "forensic teaching associates." Preceptors, nurses, and standardized patients collaborate to simulate a patient's experience following sexual and physical violence. New forensic nurses often have concerns about what to say to a patient who has just experienced a significant trauma. Simulated patient examinations offer unique opportunities for learning in a psychologically safe environment. Standardized patients allow nurses to practice and develop skills such as collecting evidence, conducting trauma-informed physical assessments, and providing emotional support. These skills are reinforced through reflection and debriefing (See Chapters 10 and 13).

Forensic Resource Nurse Preceptor

Once orientation is completed, new nurses are offered continuous support and reassurance as they independently provide patient care. A 24-hour on-call forensic resource nurse is readily available to provide both clinical and emotional support. The forensic resource nurse preceptor is available by phone to guide nurses through clinical decision-making and reinforce best practices while also debriefing after difficult or emotionally charged cases. Preceptors provide a supportive and trauma-informed approach, helping forensic nurses to feel valued and less anxious about their difficult work.

Precepting Through a Trauma-Informed Lens

Trauma-informed care (TIC) is at the heart of forensic nursing. Nurses trained in trauma-informed care recognize that repeated interactions with systems can often retraumatize patients. Core principles of TIC include: 1) maintaining patient and staff physical and psychological safety; 2) developing transparent and trusting relationships; 3) providing peer support; 4) collaborating with staff and patients for shared decision-making; 5) recognizing and building on strengths to enhance resilience and healing; and 6) addressing cultural humility, historical trauma, and response to stereotypes (Center for Health Care Strategies, 2021) (Figure 24.1).

Trauma-informed care provides nurses with a framework for optimal patient care while also ensuring that their own mental health and well-being is explicitly addressed. Preceptors in forensic nursing need to be proficient at applying trauma-informed care and advocating for change at a systems-level (Box 24.4).

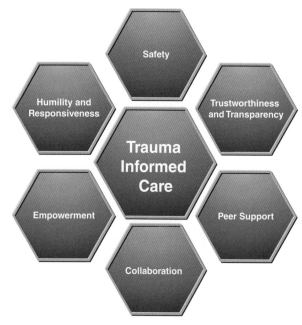

Figure 24.1 Trauma-Informed Care Core Principles. From SAMHSA's Concept of Trauma and Guidance for a Trauma-Informed Approach.

BOX 24.4 Systems Approach to Trauma-Informed Care

For trauma-informed care to be effective, healthcare organizations must adopt a trauma informed care (TIC) model based on a systems level.

- **Public health approach**
  - Recognize and respond to the ubiquitous nature of the trauma experience within the population (including the healthcare workforce)
  - Screen using a "universal precautions"-type process
  - Recognize community members as valuable stakeholders
  - Normalize discussions between clinicians and patients regarding social determinants of health
  - Use peer support models to increase access to care
- **Organizational approach**
  - Combine trauma-informed practice with systemic support for the greatest outcome (e.g., policy change, resolving larger workplace issues)
  - Shift the organizational culture from "What is wrong with you?" to the preferred "What happened to you?"

- Access resources and maximize buy-in from every level of leadership to sustain a TIC model
- **Workforce approach**
  - Recognize that secondary trauma can be associated with staff turnover, missed work, depression, medical errors, and suboptimal care
  - Unaddressed staff trauma is also negatively related to patient outcomes (e.g., patient self-reports of satisfaction and recovery times, treatment adherence)
  - Address systemic inequalities (e.g., gender, race)
  - Provide access to self-care and mental health resources
- **Education approach**
  - Train all members of the organization to recognize and respond appropriately to trauma
  - Incorporate trauma-informed education into health professions curriculums
  - Provide ongoing education with support from organization and leadership for sustainability

Using a TIC lens, specialized training facilitates the nurse's ability to respond appropriately to victims of abuse, exploitation, and violence. Forensic nurses must recognize patient behaviors that result from trauma, while being aware of their own internal reactions. Preceptors in forensic nursing are tasked with not only modeling trauma-informed patient care, but with modeling self-awareness and personal coping skills through a trauma informed lens (Box: Words Matter).

There are opportunities for the preceptor to illustrate how healthcare providers can work for and against trauma-informed care. Awareness of the effect of one's demeanor during patient interactions can allow for greater sensitivity and responsiveness, thus reducing risk for retraumatization. For instance, healthcare providers may approach the patient in a routine manner

when performing physical assessments and obtaining vital signs. This may be perceived by the patient as a lack of respect for personal autonomy. Such lack of respect, knowingly or unknowingly, is harmful for those who have experienced physical, emotional, or sexual abuse. Anxiety can escalate, making patients less likely to seek follow-up care. During forensic nursing exams, patients are empowered to make choices that enhance their feelings of safety. For example, when oral, vaginal, or rectal swabs must be collected for evidence, the nurse can include the patient in the process, thereby fostering a sense of control.

Nurses new to the forensic nursing specialty are expected to become proficient in identifying traumatic responses such as irritability, anger, depression, and symptoms of physical stress (National Institute of

WORDS MATTER

Gabriella Anderson

Patients often present to an acute care setting following a traumatic event. The coordination of patient care can be directly influenced by appropriate use of *trauma-informed language*. Trauma-informed language uses support, empathy, and respect for an individual's boundaries and personal experiences to create a secure environment. Patients may be less likely to agree to a suggested plan of care if they perceive that they are not being heard or their concerns are being dismissed. By consciously choosing words and tone, healthcare providers create a collaborative approach for better patient outcomes.

The *four R's of trauma-informed care* include realizing, recognizing, responding, and resisting retraumatization.

- **Realizing:**
  - Realizing what trauma is and how it affects individuals, families, and communities.
  - Acknowledging that a patient's behavior may be due to a traumatic event.
  - Understanding that these behaviors may be a learned coping strategy.
- **Recognizing:**
  - Recognizing signs of trauma.
  - Following a traumatic event, "acting out" behaviors may include: lying, fighting, arguing, substance abuse, inability to control emotions, and high-risk sexual behaviors.
  - Following a traumatic event, "acting in" behaviors may include: generalized lack of trust, depression, self-harm, and isolation.

- Every patient is different. There is no "normal" behavior for a patient to have following a traumatic event. A patient may display laughing, screaming, or crying, all within the same visit. This does not mean that their event was any less traumatizing or stressful.
- **Responding:**
  - Utilize a calm, patient-centered approach.
  - Focus on providing empathy and support. For example, instead of saying "What's wrong?" say "How can I help you?" This helps a caregiver validate a patient's feelings and experiences while offering support.
- **Resisting Retraumatization:**
  - Being mindful of word and action choice to avoid retraumatizing a patient.
  - Identify and acknowledge triggers which may potentially create discomfort.
  - Avoid comparing the patient's traumatic event with something you have personally experienced; practice self-awareness.
  - Focus on consent and empowerment. Allow a patient control in their plan of care. Discuss the assessment process in advance and allow the patient to consent prior to physical contact.
  - Prioritize transparency. Having difficult conversations can be challenging, but honesty and openness with a patient will help create rapport.

Data from Substance Abuse and Mental Health Services Administration (2014). *SAMHSA's concept of trauma and guidance for a trauma-informed approach*. HHS Publication No. (SMA) 14-4884.

Mental Health, 2020). These responses are protective and often outside of the person's conscious control. Preceptors normalize these reactions and feelings for both the patient as well as the new nurse. As a result, forensic nurses are also at risk for secondary and vicarious trauma. Preceptors should encourage new forensic nurses to self-reflect on warning signs of compassion fatigue and burnout and to identify activities that support health and well-being while building resiliency (See Chapter 18).

FORENSIC NURSING: TRIAL PREPARATION

Jennifer Beigie

Responsibilities of forensic nurses include examining patients, assessing injuries, collecting evidence, and providing testimony in court. These nurses are well-versed in institutional policies and procedures and have the skills to navigate the legal system and follow appropriate chain of custody. Chain of custody refers to the order and manner that evidence is handled during an investigation (Longley, 2022).

Forensic nurses can be subpoenaed by both the prosecuting and defense attorneys and provide unbiased factual and expert testimony related to the care during patient encounters. In preparation for the trial, forensic nurses review medical record documentation including injury assessment and photography. Additionally, they are encouraged to develop an updated resume or curriculum vitae (CV) representative of their current credentials and forensic expertise.

Institutional leadership meets with the forensic nurse who has been subpoenaed to confirm they are prepared and feel confident to testify in court. Preparation also includes reviewing potential questions that may be asked during testimony.

Sample Questions for Trial Preparation
Establishing Credibility

- Please state your name and spell it for the court reporter.
- Who is your current employer?
- How long have you held your current position?
- What are your responsibilities as a registered nurse (RN)?
- How long have you been a RN?
- Describe your formal education.
- Do you hold professional certifications?
- Do you have specialized training in the assessment of sexual abuse patients?

Explanation of Forensic Nursing

- What is a forensic nurse?
- What are your responsibilities as a forensic nurse? Describe your training.
- How many forensic examinations have you completed?
- What services does your current employer offer for sexually abused patients?

Explanation of the Case

- Once you receive a consultation, what is your process as a forensic nurse to complete your examinations?
- Describe your physical findings in this case. In addition to the nurse being prepared to speak about the forensic examination process, they also need to explain how injuries are documented. The forensic nurse must be able to describe the injuries using laymen's terminology. The forensic nurse is also encouraged to reach out to the prosecuting attorney to discuss any additional questions that will be asked during testimony (Exemplar: Easing Pre-Trial Jitters, and Exemplar: Domestic Violence Case and Trial Preparation).

THE ROLE OF THE PRECEPTOR IN TRIAL PREPARATION

Michelle Levay and Kelly Calvey

When working with new forensic nurses, preceptors can emphasize that preparation for a trial does not begin when a subpoena is received. The process begins when the forensic nurse first encounters a patient who is a victim of domestic violence, sexual assault, child abuse, neglect, or human trafficking. Forensic nurses provide expert care while ensuring that documentation is accurate and complete. Every patient's medical record is a legal document that may provide evidence in a trial.

Maintain Current Forensic Nursing Practice

The qualifications of the forensic nurse may be called into question during a trial. To demonstrate competence, both

(Continued)

new and experienced forensic nurses must develop and maintain clinical expertise. Actions to develop competency include:
- Display understanding of the forensic nurse scope of practice.
- Review hospital policies and standard operating procedures.
- Review the state and local nurse practice act.
- Participate in continuing education and additional training through the International Association of Forensic Nursing.
- Review articles in peer-reviewed journals such as:
  - *Journal of Forensic Nursing*
  - *Journal of Emergency Nursing*
  - *Journal of Forensic and Legal Medicine*
  - *Nurse Education Today*
  - *Journal of Trauma Nursing*
  - *Forensic Science International: Synergy*
  - *International Emergency Nursing*
- Consider certification as a Sexual Assault Nurse Examiner – Adult or Pediatric (SANE-A and/or SANE-P)

Tips for Trial Preparation
Before the trial:
- Review the patient's medical record to establish clarity about documented patient findings.
- Utilize all available resources such as photographs, laboratory values, and x-ray findings.
- Practice responding to questions with a forensic nurse experienced in trial testimony.
- Prepare to speak not only with the prosecuting attorney but also the defense attorney.

Court etiquette:
- First impressions matter: dress professionally and arrive early.
- Avoid talking with anyone: waiting rooms may be occupied by families of the patient or defendant.
- Turn off cell phones prior to entering the courtroom.

Court testimony:
- Answer questions with a simple yes or no.
- Avoid elaborate responses unless specifically asked.
- Address the jury when speaking.
- Clarify the forensic nursing process to help the jury make an informed decision, as members of the jury are often not familiar with forensic nursing.
- Directly describe the facts of the incident and injury (or lack of injuries) addressed in the documentation. Remember the forensic nurse is not an "eyewitness" to the crime.

Exemplar: Easing Pre-Trial Jitters

Jennifer Beigie

I recently guided trial preparation with one of the forensic nurses who had been with our team for over 2 years but had never testified in court. While they had been subpoenaed multiple times, those previous cases had never gone to trial. This nurse discussed feeling anxious about providing testimony. I reassured them that trial preparation would increase their readiness to testify. I also coached the nurse to display confidence in their clinical expertise and testimony. We reviewed all documentation related to the patient's multiple injuries, including over 50 photographs. We spent time reviewing each photograph and I ensured the forensic nurse was able to describe each injury using nonmedical language. I reminded the nurse that we are usually factual witnesses and therefore present only the facts without additional detail. Finally, I reviewed trial day logistics (e.g., parking and how to enter the courthouse) to alleviate some of the nurse's anxiety about what to expect.

This nurse did testify and called me afterward saying that our trial preparation was beneficial, and the courtroom experience was not as scary as they had expected. They felt confident answering questions and were proud that their testimony helped the patient seek justice.

HUMAN TRAFFICKING

Michele Reali-Sorrell

Human trafficking is a criminal act in which a person is coerced or compelled to provide services or labor or engage in commercial sex acts (The United States Department of Justice, 2023). Victims of human trafficking may come from all types of backgrounds, however, those who are poor and vulnerable are often targeted (Centers for Disease Control, 2018).

Among healthcare providers, knowledge about the issue of human trafficking is evolving. More recently attention to human trafficking is being integrated into undergraduate nursing and other healthcare provider

---

Exemplar: Domestic Violence Case and Trial Preparation

Michelle Levay and Kelly Calvey

The police were called to the scene of the incident where a young adult female was physically assaulted by her partner. She was transported to the local hospital emergency department (ED) by ambulance. The patient requested to be seen by a sexual assault nurse examiner (SANE) and the ED provided an immediate referral. After a traumatic event where all control is lost, the goal of the SANE encounter is to give the patient the control to make informed decisions.

On arrival to the patient's private room, I introduced myself, explained my role as a forensic nurse and described the services that I could offer. I obtained a thorough history of the event and completed a head-to-toe assessment. Sadly, the patient shared that there was a history of abuse by her partner and the violence was escalating. We discussed the cycle of abuse, the risk to the patient's health and well-being, resources for help, and a safety plan. I followed up with careful documentation of the encounter.

The primary responsibility for a forensic nurse is to assess and treat the patient. In addition, there is a possibility that the case can go to trial. Receiving a subpoena to appear in court can be overwhelming, but forensic nurses view participation in a trial as an extension of the care provided to patients. The forensic nurse may experience doubt and ask the questions: "Is my documentation an accurate reflection of the history of the event?" or "Will my testimony help or hurt the patient's case?" I found the best way to alleviate anxiety was to extensively prepare to testify. I reviewed the documentation, photos, and body map in the patient's medical record. Additionally, I needed to utilize all the resources at my disposal, which included studying the orientation material on trial preparation, meeting with experts within the Forensic Nursing department, and talking with the prosecutor. In preparing for the case, I knew I would be expected to answer questions about the documentation, describe the SANE/forensic nursing process and standard of care, and explain the rationale for the line of questioning during the patient encounter. Forensic nurses are taught to be methodical in the collection of patient information and evidence, but it can be challenging to articulate this in layman's terms to a jury. The time I spent reviewing my training material and consulting with SANE experts increased my confidence during testimony and cross-examination.

In summary, testifying in court was a pivotal moment for me as a forensic nurse. The fear of the unknown was taken away through preparation, much handholding, studying, and practice. A forensic nurse's documentation and testimony alone is not going to win or lose a case, but it will help to provide supplemental evidence. Nurses should be prepared to deliver a testimony that is direct, easy to understand, and, above all else, unbiased.

---

education (Bono-Neri & Toney-Butler, 2023; Lee et al., 2021; McAmis et al., 2022), yet there remains a gap in translation of knowledge to practice. As a result, victims of human trafficking are not always identified when seeking healthcare. Many victims have retrospectively reported that they presented to a healthcare provider or emergency department but were never screened for trafficking (Lederer & Wetzel, 2014).

The preceptor's role is to help educate nurses and others on the red flags of trafficking. Patient screening for trafficking allows for appropriate channels to be followed to address safety and well-being, as well as to provide available resources (Macy et al., 2021) (Appendix U). Additionally, preceptors should stress the responsibility for mandated reporting and guide novices through this process. Ongoing support and debriefing with the new nurse allow the preceptor to reinforce sensitive documentation and enhance patient safety and privacy.

Warning Signs of Trafficking

Warning signs of trafficking can be similar to those exhibited by victims of other abuse or violence. The patient may:

- Exhibit signs of physical injury or abuse;
- Engage in substance abuse or identify an addiction;
- Provide a scripted or inconsistent story that does not coincide with behavior or presenting injuries;
- Require frequent emergency department visits;
- Present with sexually transmitted infections (STI);
- Demonstrate fearful or nervous behavior with the person accompanying them;
- Allow the accompanying person to speak for them and answer questions;
- Reveal they are uninsured without citizenship documentation;
- Disclose that they live at their place of business;
- Divulge they are not in control of their own finances.

RESPECTING DIFFERENCES: INDIGENOUS PEOPLES

Cynthia A. Danford and Beth Heuer

Preceptors are on the forefront of teaching nursing students and other learners about equitable healthcare and respect for life for all individuals no matter their background, history, or life experiences. Equitable healthcare, with attention to ethnicity, culture, and social determinants of health (SDOH) contributes to better mental and physical health outcomes (Ford-Gilboe et al., 2018). Assumptions should be avoided based on physical appearance and cultural background.

Cultural safety is an approach to minimize inequities by recognizing that culture is integral to health and well-being. Within cultural context, healthcare must be respectful and nondiscriminatory. Providing culturally safe healthcare involves engaging the learner in reflexivity (Dawson et al., 2022). Reflexivity builds from basic and critical reflection (Figure 24.2) and provides a structure for preceptor–learner engagement and a means to develop respect for differences within and between cultures.

Attention to cultural safety and use of reflexivity is particularly important when working with Indigenous peoples. Health disparities in Indigenous peoples continue to grow and are expected to increase as the population increases exponentially (Australian Institute of Health and Welfare, 2022; Government of Canada, 2023; Pan American Health Organization PAHO, 2019; Small-Rodriguez & Akee, 2021; WHO, 2023). High incidence of diabetes, maternal and infant mortality, alcoholism, and mental health issues put Indigenous peoples at risk for poor health outcomes and a shorter lifespan (WHO, 2023). Making assumptions and stereotyping related to such health risks is counterproductive and must be avoided (Hyett et al., 2019). Preceptors need to model how to make gentle queries and clarify observations to avoid misunderstandings (WHO, 2023). (Exemplar: The Importance of Language When Preparing Students to Engage With Indigenous Peoples)

Understanding the perspective of Indigenous peoples is complex and involves an interplay between social and emotional well-being within the context of the environment (Dudgeon et al., 2022; Gee et al., 2014; Figure 24.3). This model depicts connections to country; spirit, spirituality and ancestors; culture; community; family and kinship; physical body and actions; mind and emotions. These connections are informed by social, political, cultural, and historical determinants and are experienced and expressed in various ways (Dudgeon et al., 2022).

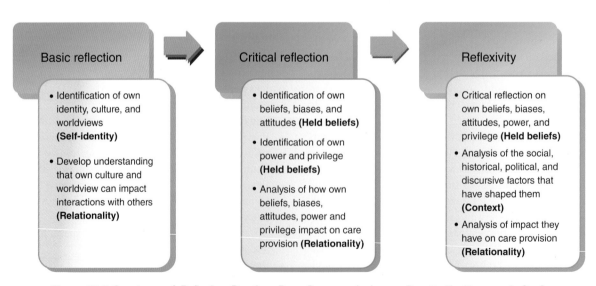

Figure 24.2 Spectrum of Reflexive Practice. From Dawson, J., Laccos-Barrett, K., Hammond, C., & Rumbold, A. (2022). Reflexive practice as an approach to improve healthcare delivery for Indigenous Peoples: A systematic critical synthesis and exploration of the cultural safety education literature. *International Journal of Environmental Research and Public Health, 19*(11), 6691.

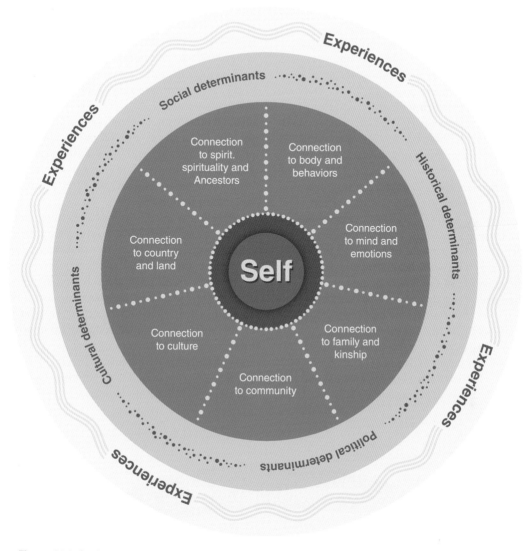

Figure 24.3 Social and Emotional Well-Being Model. From Gee G., Dudgeon P., Schultz C., Hart A., & Kelly K. (2014). Aboriginal and Torres Strait Islander social and emotional wellbeing. In P. Dudgeon, H. Milroy, & R. Walker (Eds.), *Working together: Aboriginal and Torres Strait Islander mental health and wellbeing principles and practice* (pp. 55–68). ACT: Commonwealth of Australia.

Classroom education can create a positive change in knowledge and attitudes about working with Indigenous peoples, but it is unclear whether didactic content alone can help students develop cultural capability in their clinical practice (Mills et al., 2018). Clinical nursing experiences serving Indigenous peoples can help learners develop cultural humility and create positive insights about the culture and health interventions (Cameron & Mitchell, 2022) (Box: Culturally Sensitive Tips When Working With Indigenous Peoples). Non-Indigenous preceptors or educators must, however, approach teaching from a place of cultural humility, without claiming knowledge of Indigenous people's perspectives (Francis-Cracknell et al., 2022). Preceptors should be prepared to provide additional support to learners, who may have strong emotional responses as they begin understanding the past and present harms experienced by Indigenous peoples.

Exploring differences between and within Indigenous peoples with learners can help dispel assumptions and thereby identify individualized approaches to achieve effective health outcomes. Preceptors should comprehensively review proximal, intermediate, and distal barriers with learners when caring for Indigenous peoples (Nguyen et al. 2020). These barriers are interconnected and can have a comprehensive impact on health outcomes (Figure 24.4).

Proximal barriers can geographically impinge on a patient's ability to navigate transportation from rural areas to healthcare facilities and limit accessibility to online health resources. Educationally, language and literacy deficits can contribute to hesitancy in seeking healthcare, interacting with healthcare providers, and leaving the comforts of the family home environment. Bias in the form of negative stereotypes contributes to disregard of social determinants of health and culturally inappropriate services. This contributes further to hesitancy in providing effective healthcare with Indigenous peoples and creates delays in diagnoses and treatment.

Intermediate barriers such as unemployment and low income preclude access to key healthcare services. These intermediate factors can exaggerate proximal barriers and perpetuate a cycle of further delaying healthcare. Additionally, many Indigenous peoples prefer traditional and holistic medicine over Western medicine, which is not a strong focus in formalized education systems.

Distal barriers have a profound effect on both proximal and intermediate barriers. Colonialism (Chapter 23) resulted in Indigenous peoples needing to relocate from their traditional lands to reservations, which often have poor infrastructures and block business and healthcare growth opportunities. The result has been social stratification, isolation, and racism, all of which perpetuate inequitable healthcare.

Preceptors can address inequities and guide learners to plan meaningful healthcare experiences in collaboration with the communities they serve. Refocusing on positive attributes and taking a positive approach to healthcare can minimize the stereotyping and marginalization of Indigenous peoples that has resulted from adopting a deficit-based perspective (Hyett et al., 2019). Health disparities can be reduced by improving cultural resources as well as mitigating the effects of stigma and power/financial inequities (Subica & Link, 2022). (Figure 24.5) (Exemplar: Promoting Culturally Safe Care Among Indigenous Peoples).

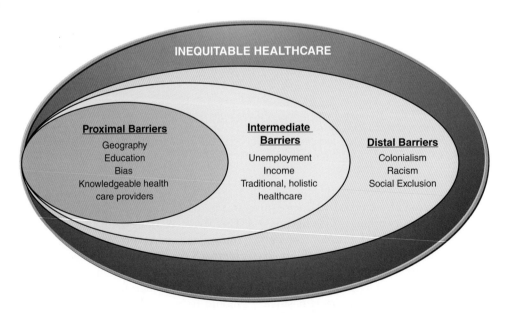

Figure 24.4 Barriers to Equitable Healthcare.

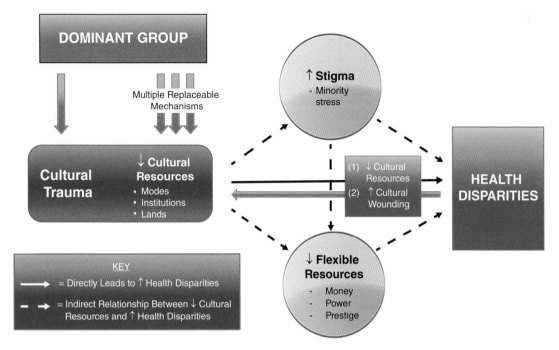

Figure 24.5 Cultural Trauma Conceptual Model. Adapted from Subica, A. M., & Link, B. G. (2022). Cultural trauma as a fundamental cause of health disparities. *Social Science & Medicine, 292*, 114574.

Exemplar: The Importance of Language When Preparing Students to Engage With Indigenous Peoples

Sara Williams

I worked as a registered nurse in the emergency department at rural hospital with a neighboring Indigenous community. Being an Indigenous woman and having worked in the Indigenous health sector for the last 8 years, I was familiar with the language and terminology used by the community.

During the shift, one of the onboarding nurses triaged an Indigenous man in his mid-50s. While reviewing the nurse's charting, I noted that she referred to him as an "active IV drug user." I looked in the waiting room and thought to myself, this individual doesn't look like he uses IV drugs. I didn't want to make assumptions, so I asked the triage nurse if he disclosed that information to her. The nurse responded

that he stated he "uses the needle." I took the opportunity to educate her that many Indigenous people often refer to being on insulin as "using the needle." She suddenly understood the patient's comments and recalled that he had type 2 diabetes. I proceeded to educate her on a study indicating that First Nations people are at high risk of developing type 2 diabetes mellitus at some point in their lifetime (Ruth et al., 2023; Turin et al., 2016).

This situation was an example of what can happen when cultural humility is lacking, and inaccurate assumptions are made. Taking time to explore the patient's and family's understanding of their health situation and becoming familiar with cultural language can reduce barriers to care.

CULTURALLY SENSITIVE TIPS FOR LEARNERS WHEN WORKING WITH INDIGENOUS PEOPLES

Sara Williams

- Identify reputable cultural safety and trauma-informed care training resources for learners.
- Encourage the learner to submerge themselves with the community they are servicing in a respectful way. This may include being flexible with scheduling clinical hours, as ceremonies or community events may take place outside of traditional hours.
- Role-model appropriate interactions, use of language, and cultural humility.

- Share your personal learning journey about working within an Indigenous community.
- Remind the learner to avoid making assumptions about patients from Indigenous communities.
- Understand and respect the patient's need for self-determination.
- Understand that the learner might struggle with guilt when first learning about Indigenous history and encourage them to navigate these emotions in a positive way.

Exemplar: Promoting Culturally Safe Care Among Indigenous Peoples

Shelley Spurr

Nursing educators recognize that a culturally safe approach results in higher-quality care and improved patient outcomes. Culturally safe care is grounded in cultural humility, antiracism, and trauma-informed practice (Culturally Safe and Inclusive Practice, 2021). Implementation of these principles with Indigenous peoples remains a challenge for nurse preceptors in clinical practice.

The importance of implementing culturally safe care became apparent while I was precepting an undergraduate student nurse assigned to care for a 16-year-old Indigenous youth who lived in a remote Indigenous community. The adolescent was admitted for a tonsillectomy, experienced significant postoperative respiratory complications, and spent 3 days in the intensive care unit. The surgeon documented that the respiratory complications were due to morbid obesity, as the patient weighed 300 pounds.

During report, the nurses who worked the night shift were disrespectful and commented negatively on the adolescent's size, placing blame on the parents and the community for this health issue. The student nurse did not speak up on behalf of the patient but approached me immediately after report, upset with what they heard. Although the student nurse had learned that racism can occur within healthcare, this was their first experience hearing inappropriate comments during report and they lacked the confidence to address this issue.

I spoke privately with the student nurse, allowing time for them to vent and process what they heard during report. I asked the student what could have been done differently and they identified that they wanted to address the nurses immediately but did not feel comfortable. We discussed that all nurses have the responsibility to speak up against racism and advocate for appropriate and equitable care; being silent condones the behavior. We reviewed principles of culturally safe nursing care which included: providing healthcare that is free from discrimination and racism; respecting and meeting the unique holistic needs of Indigenous peoples; and recognizing the importance of collaborating with Indigenous peoples in the provision of their health (National Collaborating Centre for Indigenous Health, 2019). I explained that the cause of obesity is extremely complex for Indigenous peoples and is directly linked to the ongoing impact of colonization and systemic racism.

After our discussion, the student nurse provided care for the adolescent and advocated for a dietary consult before discharge. The student worked to build a respectful relationship which included the adolescent's preferences related to connecting with appropriate cultural and community resources. This student also indicated feeling more prepared to address inappropriate staff comments in the future.

Suggestions for nurse preceptors to consider in the promotion of culturally safe care for Indigenous peoples include the following.

1. Principles of cultural safety in clinical practice must be reiterated with student nurses.
2. Patient and family advocacy is the responsibility of all nurses.
3. The impact of colonization and racism on the increasing health disparities among Indigenous populations must be acknowledged.
4. Student nurses require support to engage in collaborative and respectful relationships with Indigenous patients that advocate for culturally appropriate resources and traditional approaches to healthcare.

STUDENT SCHOLARLY PROJECTS

Cynthia A. Danford

Precepting nursing students involves partnership with an academic institution (Hinch et al., 2020) and implies working with students to apply didactic content while establishing effective skills for clinical practice. The end goal is building a workforce of nurses that can provide optimal evidence-based healthcare. An integral part of academic curricula and an ongoing role of nurses includes development of evidence-based practice strategies to improve healthcare. Whether entry- or advanced-level, all nursing students are expected to meet The Essentials competency to advance the scholarship of nursing (AACN, 2021). While entry-level nurses are expected to apply evidence during clinical practica and thereafter, advanced-level nurses are expected to "discern appropriate applications of quality improvement, research, and evaluation methodologies" (p. 37), collaborate to advance their scholarship, and disseminate their scholarship to others (AACN, 2021).

Scholarly Project Roles and Responsibilities

Nurses in clinical settings are asked to participate on Doctor of Nursing Practice (DNP)/ Master of Science in Nursing (MSN) student committees and to serve as preceptors as students develop their scholarly projects. Often the expertise in a particular specialty area is what compels the student to seek partnership with a nurse preceptor. It is the role and responsibility of the faculty from the academic institution to educate and guide the student on the various aspects of conducting a scholarly project (Staffileno et al., 2019). The role of the preceptor is to assure that the scholarly topic aligns with the institution's strategic goals and healthcare needs. The chosen approach must be conducted safely, with risk *no greater than* that which is provided during usual patient care. The student is expected to develop their idea and approach, present a well-developed plan to the preceptor, and incorporate constructive input as needed.

Nonresearch Scholarly Projects

DNP programs evolved in response to a call from the National Academy of Sciences (NIH, 2005) for nursing to prepare expert practitioners by developing a "non-research clinical doctorate" (AACN Fact Sheet, 2023). As a result, most DNP programs advocate for scholarly projects that are nonresearch in nature. Engaging in nonresearch projects prepares students to regularly integrate scholarship into their clinical practice postgraduation.

PRECEPTING DNP SCHOLARLY PROJECTS WITH A PERSPECTIVE ON HEALTH POLICY

Natasha North, Cynthia A. Danford, and Petra Brysiewicz

Attention to health policy is often omitted when planning and implementing research or non-research scholarly projects. The thought of addressing policy can be overwhelming, as nurses may be unfamiliar with the process and might incorrectly only view policy as occurring on a grand scale (i.e., nationally or internationally). Consequently, whether one is undertaking a research or nonresearch endeavor, health policy has often been viewed as an afterthought. What is forgotten is that policy development or change is what guides and sustains healthcare change for individuals and families. Preceptors need to embrace this perspective and help learners to identify and advocate for policy development or change (North et al., in press).

Policy action is not limited to a global, national, or governmental level. Policy often starts locally on a small scale (i.e., department or unit-based, institutional, or organizational) and builds over time. Practically speaking, policy is *a set of ideas, plans, or guidelines* that have *officially been agreed upon* by a group of people or an organization (Cambridge University Press & Assessment, 2023). Consider the following steps when guiding learners to integrate policy into their scholarly work:

- Identify the idea or plan (*What* should be done? *What* needs change? *Why* is the change needed?).
- Map the process (*How* will the plan be implemented? *Who* needs to be involved?).
- Frame the approach when thinking about the proposed change. Be practical. Incorporate four aspects from the Health Policy Triangle (Walt & Gilson, 1994). Note the process is iterative:
  - **Context**: Why is the change needed? What system factors will influence whether your proposed change

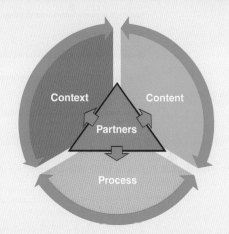

The Health Policy Triangle. Modified Health Policy Triangle © 2023 North, Brysiewicz, Danford, International Family Nursing Association. All rights reserved; Adapted from Walt, G. & Gilson, L. (1994). Reforming the health sector in developing countries: The central role of policy analysis. *Health Policy and Planning, 9*(4), 353–370.

is 1) agreed to and 2) implemented? Do the conditions and capacity for change exist?
- **Content**: What is the content of your proposed policy change?
- **Process**: How will the policy be brought forward and implemented?
- **Partners**: Which individuals and groups are affected by your policy change? Which individuals or groups will influence or decide whether your proposed policy change is 1) agreed to, and 2) implemented?

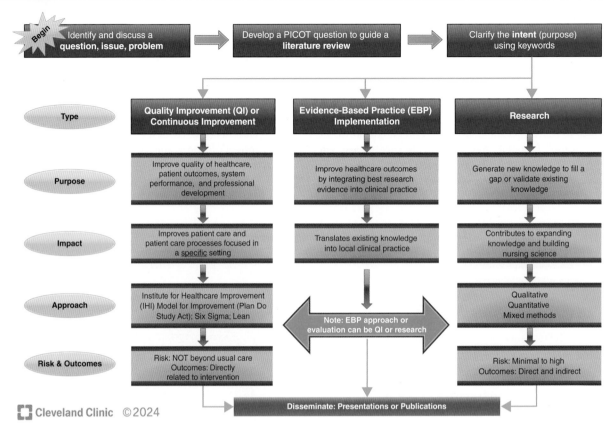

Figure 24.6 Pathway to Dissemination. Reprinted with permission, Cleveland Clinic Foundation ©2024. All Rights Reserved.

Common nonresearch projects include quality improvement (QI), needs assessment, program evaluation, policy analysis (Box: Precepting DNP Scholarly Projects With a Perspective on Health Policy), and evidence-based practice (EBP) implementation. These endeavors are to be distinguished from research, which is intended to generate new knowledge or validate existing knowledge (Ginex, 2017; Kawar et al., 2023) (Figure 24.6). To further differentiate, QI projects are localized to a specific setting, unit, or department, whereas research is intended to be generalizable. Nonresearch projects such as QI projects should have risk no greater than assumed when providing usual care, may not require approval by the Institutional Review Board (IRB) or may be considered exempt, and have outcomes directly related to the proposed intervention. Research studies usually have minimal to high risk, require IRB approval, and include direct and indirect outcomes.

Evidence-based practice implementation projects are used to integrate or apply best evidence into practice. Depending on approach, outcomes, and risk, EBP projects may be considered research or nonresearch. No matter what type of scholarly project, the student must begin the process with a question, problem, or topic of interest. Guiding the student to formalize a written problem statement relevant to a specific setting is a good place to begin. Once a problem statement is identified, a PICOT question can be generated (P = Population, I = Intervention or Issue, C = Comparison, O = Outcome, T = Time [optional]) (Fineout-Overholt & Johnson, 2023) (Appendix V). The PICOT question guides the literature review. Once a literature review has been completed and the evidence synthesized, the purpose can be verified and fine-tuned and the type of scholarly endeavor determined.

Approaches to Scholarly Projects

There are several approaches that students can use to implement nonresearch projects. The most common approach, Model for Improvement, developed by the Institute for Healthcare Improvement (IHI), is used to determine if a change is effective (AHRQ, 2020). Plan, Do, Study, Act (PDSA) or Plan, Do, Check, Act (PDCA) (Figure 24.7) is the cycle used to systematically track proposed change (IHI, n.d.; Langley, 2009). When developing a PDSA cycle, key questions driving the process include: What is to be accomplished? How will a change be determined to be an improvement? What change will result in an improvement? The PDSA is grounded in a "trial and learning" process using rapid change improvement (RCI), which implies testing interventions or repeating the PDSA cycle on a small scale (AHRQ, 2020).

Other approaches or models include Six Sigma, Lean, and Lean Six Sigma, which are commonly used in business environments but are being used with increasing frequency in healthcare management (AHRQ, 2020; Amaratunga & Dobranowski, 2016; Ninerola et al., 2020). Six Sigma is an approach often used to eliminate errors, improve processes, and decrease variability. Lean is a process used to streamline steps and minimize time, effort, and cost. Lean Six Sigma combines Six Sigma and Lean to more effectively improve process flow (Rathi et al., 2022).

Dissemination

Final nonresearch projects should be evaluated for appropriate dissemination. Some students choose to disseminate their work through institutional repositories or academic presentations. Other students choose to

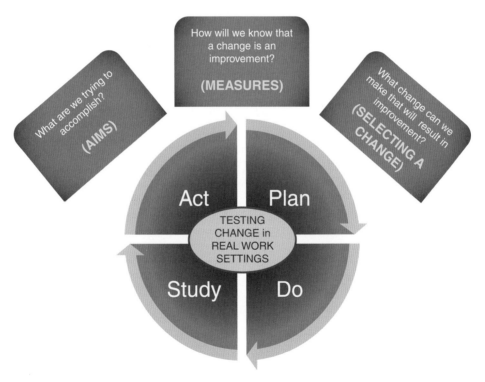

Figure 24.7 Model for Quality Improvement. This is a modified version of the Model for Improvement, developed by Associates in Process Improvement and adopted by the Institute for Healthcare Improvement (Langley et al. 2009). The model is commonly used by doctor of nursing practice (DNP) students as a framework to guide DNP project implementation. The model includes two parts: 1) Three questions asked in any order, and 2) A plan, do, study/check, act (PDSA/PDCA) cycle, which is used to test a change in a real work setting and helps to determine if the change constitutes an improvement. Gerald J. Langley, Ronald D. Moen, Kevin M. Nolan, Thomas W. Nolan, Clifford L. Norman, Lloyd P. Provost, April 2009, *The Improvement Guide: A Practical Approach to Enhancing Organizational Performance* (2nd Edition),Jossey-Bass.

Exemplar: Guiding DNP Projects

Kristen Marie Vargo

Planning doctor of nursing practice (DNP) scholarly projects can be challenging for DNP students. While planning my DNP project, I had to make multiple revisions of my PICOT question and proposal to ensure that my quality improvement (QI) project met the standards of the DNP program. My personal experience has informed my ability to precept and help students overcome challenges and barriers during their project development and implementation. Most students can identify a practice gap but struggle with formulating a QI project. Many projects are initially identified as "research" and require revision to meet the requirements of the DNP program. Additionally, many DNP students do not recognize the number of revisions necessary to plan and write their proposals. Students focus on the timeline of the program but do not realize that more time may be needed for the development of their proposals and completion of their projects.

After reflecting on my DNP project and precepting many DNP students, I have realized that more efforts are needed to evaluate the project and determine what outcome is being measured. Clarifying the outcome helps the learner to determine whether a project is classified as research or QI. For example, my project focused on the use of a music intervention in the preoperative setting. I originally planned to measure how music impacts patients' preoperative anxiety. With my focus on patient anxiety as an indirect outcome, the project was deemed as research. Through my many proposal revisions, I changed the outcome to focus on whether preoperative patients were interested in using the music intervention, the length of time they listened to the music, and the types of songs they preferred. With this revision, the project moved from being classified as research to QI.

As another example, I precepted a student who worked on a project involving taking stable ICU (Intensive Care Unit) patients off the unit to the hospital's rooftop pavilion, which allows access to a green space. Their original outcome was to assess changes in patient vital signs before and after leaving the ICU. After realizing that this was an indirect outcome with many possible confounding variables that needed to be controlled (research), we were able to alter her project. We identified a direct outcome, which included identifying the number of ICU patients that utilized the green space (QI).

As a preceptor, I have collaborated with students to help clarify their topic, outcomes, and methods of measurement during early stages of project planning. Sharing my own experiences has allowed me to more effectively precept students in the development of DNP projects that have impacted nursing practice.

Tips to Help Students Maintain Focus

1. Encourage students to select a topic they are passionate about, as considerable time will be spent on this topic during their graduate program.
2. Suggest maximizing resources as the student develops their project, including the research librarian, faculty advisor, members of the graduate project team, and site preceptors.
3. Remind students to set a realistic timeframe including multiple proposal revisions, approval of the project from the academic institution and clinical site, as well as potential IRB reviews.
4. Verify that desired outcomes are direct and measurable.
5. Provide encouragement and remind students that their project will have an impact on future nursing practices.

---

present a poster or oral presentation at a local, regional, or national conference. Journal publications are another option that require commitment to rigorous writing, editing, and rewriting. Preceptors may be invited to be an author on publications or presentations depending on the time and effort they have contributed.

Barriers to Quality Improvement

There are many barriers to implementing QI and EBP for both novice students and experienced nurses. Barriers identified include, but are not limited to, difficulty in differentiating research from nonresearch, inability to critique existing evidence, lack of skills or time, and decreased confidence in providing effective direction (Melnyk & Fineout-Overholt, 2023). One significant barrier for students in the implementation of EBP or QI is a lack of partnership with mentors or preceptors. Understanding the intent of nonresearch projects, differentiating between research and nonresearch work, and clarifying the process can strengthen the preceptor's capabilities and result in a positive experience for both the preceptor and the student learner (Exemplar: Guiding DNP Projects).

NOVICE NURSE EDUCATORS

Beth Heuer

Many nurses and advanced practice nurses enter academic practice and clinical nurse educator roles without formal preparation in teaching methodology, known as *pedagogy* (McQuilkin et al., 2020). Novice nurse educators benefit from mentoring relationships with experienced nursing faculty when transitioning to a faculty role in an academic or professional development setting. Mentoring helps to promote *bidirectional* awareness of educational roles and responsibilities, and increases retention of qualified nurse educators (Ephraim, 2020). Additionally, mentors can help new educators develop and solidify their new role identity (McQuilkin et al., 2020).

Mentoring relationships can be dyadic, with one experienced faculty member providing guidance to the novice nurse educator (NNE). According to Calaguas,

(2023) other mentoring relationships can include peer mentoring (with same-level colleagues), functional mentoring (for specific project-oriented assistance), and constellation mentoring (group mentoring with two or more faculty members) (Figure 24.8). Webber et al. (2020) described a "three-generational" model of mentoring in the academic setting that includes a new faculty member who is entering their first year of teaching, one who is at mid-career (faculty in their 2nd–4th year), and a senior faculty member who is tenured. For more information on mentoring, see Chapter 4.

Role acclimation for novice nurse educators is a multilayered experience. The orientation period includes learning the nuts-and-bolts of *how* to teach within the setting, as well as balancing the additional responsibilities of working in academia. Mentors can help set novice educators up for success by having regularly scheduled meetings to develop personal and professional goals,

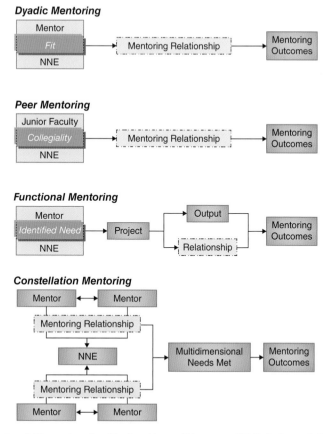

Figure 24.8 Models of Mentoring for Novice Nurse Educators (NNEs). From Calaguas, N. P. (2023). Mentoring novice nurse educators: Goals, principles, models, and key practices. *Journal of Professional Nursing, 44*, 8–11.

provide pedagogical support, and introduce them to the academic culture (Dahlke et al., 2021).

Setting Goals With the Novice Educator

Specific goals must be identified to help new faculty members develop educator competencies and to integrate these competencies into the role (National League for Nursing, 2022). Broad academic onboarding goals include balancing responsibility to teaching, research/scholarship, and service; setting short- and long-term career goals; disseminating one's work; understanding and navigating academic politics; avoiding career-limiting moves; and finding work-life balance (Clark and Sousa, 2019). Novice educators also benefit from specific advice by advanced practice mentors about balancing their educator role with ongoing clinical practice requirements. Targeted goals for new educators include development of skills to facilitate student learning and evaluation, and engagement in reflective self-evaluation. Faculty mentors provide guidance as novice educators learn to implement specific educational innovations, increase their scholarly activities, and establish their collegial network (Rogers et al., 2020).

Specific Orientation Needs: Teaching the Teacher

Novice educators require orientation to academic teaching expectations, including curricula, grading policies,

online learning management systems, library supports, simulation, and technology resources (Rogers et al., 2020). A nursing department-specific onboarding system can be used in combination with university- or system-wide orientation and personalized mentoring (Exemplar: Mentoring Novice Nursing Faculty). Multilayered orientation programs can help foster a sense of belonging and create a sense of collegiality and trust (Cotter & Clukey, 2019).

Learning the Educational Culture

New nursing faculty experience a significant culture shift as they move into regular academic teaching. Mentors should openly discuss cultural components within academia that include the need for individuals to formulate an academic career *strategy*; there is often a sense of *competition* for success and status amongst faculty. The goal is to ensure that novices do not "sink" but instead "swim" in the academic role (Cotter & Clukey, 2019). The educator-as-learner requires a network of support to thrive within the educational culture. Through enculturation, learners adapt to and accept the faculty values and norms. Enculturation can help enhance efficacy, competence, satisfaction, and retention. In academic settings, developing and maintaining a network of support creates an individual sense of belonging and a more cohesive faculty.

Exemplar: Mentoring Novice Nursing Faculty

Susan B. Dickey

During my many years of university experience, I have mentored countless new nursing faculty. Novice educators often lack understanding of the academic culture and landscape. New faculty can and should learn aspects of the new role from a variety of faculty members.

It is the mentor's responsibility to familiarize new faculty with institutional procedures, policies, and idiosyncrasies. An onboarding course that I developed included several topics: navigating university libraries; accessing instructional technology; obtaining faculty criminal background and child abuse clearances; introducing the University Faculty Senate; understanding faculty

governance and the professional union; and many more critical topics. This was a companion piece to human resource's institutional onboarding. The modules were made available continuously so that new faculty could come back at their convenience to review topics or refresh their knowledge.

Everyone is different, and novice nursing educators, similarly to students and orientees, will progress at their own pace. The American Nurses Association's (2015) *Code of Ethics for Nurses with Interpretive Statements* is another useful resource and framework to help guide new faculty orientation.

REFERENCES

Agency for Healthcare Research and Quality (AHRQ) (2020). Section 4: Ways to approach the quality improvement process. https://www.ahrq.gov/cahps/quality-improvement/improvement-guide/4-approach-qi-process/sect4part2.html

Amaratunga, T., & Dobranowski, J. (2016). Systematic review of the application of lean and six sigma quality improvement methodologies in radiology. *Journal of the American College of Radiology*, 13(9), 1088–1095. https://doi.org/10.1016/j.jacr.2016.02.033

American Association of Colleges of Nursing. (2021). *The essentials: Core competencies for professional nursing education.* American Association of Colleges of Nursing.

American Association of Colleges of Nursing (2023). Fact sheet: The doctorate of nursing practice (DNP). https://www.aacnnursing.org/news-data/fact-sheets/dnp-fact-sheet

Australian Institute of Health and Welfare. (2022). *Determinants of health for indigenous Australians.* Australian Institute of Health and Welfare. https://www.aihw.gov.au/reports/australias-health/social-determinants-and-indigenous-health

Bono-Neri, F., & Toney-Butler, T. J. (2023). Nursing students' knowledge of and exposure to human trafficking content in undergraduate curricula. *Nurse Education Today*, 129, 105920. https://doi.org/10.1016/j.nedt.2023.105920

Calaguas, N. P. (2023). Mentoring novice nurse educators: Goals, principles, models, and key practices. *Journal of Professional Nursing*, 44, 8–11. https://doi.org/10.1016/j.profnurs.2022.11.002

Cambridge University Press & Assessment. (2023). https://dictionary.cambridge.org/dictionary/english/

Cameron, R., & Mitchell, K. (2022). Shifting nursing students' attitudes towards Indigenous peoples by participation in a required Indigenous health course. *Quality Advancement in Nursing Education - Avancées En Formation Infirmière*, 8(3). https://doi.org/10.17483/2368-6669.1323

Centers for Disease Control and Prevention. (2018). Sex trafficking. CDC. https://www.cdc.gov/violenceprevention/sexualviolence/trafficking.html

Center for Health Care Strategies. (2021). *What is trauma-informed care?* Trauma-Informed Care Implementation Resource Center. https://www.traumainformedcare.chcs.org/what-is-trauma-informed-care/

Clark, A., & Sousa, B. (2019). *How to Be a Happy Academic.* Sage Publications.

Cotter, K. D., & Clukey, L. (2019). "Sink or swim": An ethnographic study of nurse educators in academic culture. *Nursing Education Perspectives*, 40(3), 139–143. https://doi.org/10.1097/01.nep.0000000000000434

Culturally safe and inclusive practice. (2021). https://nurses.ab.ca/media/sx3fb5z4/culturally-safe-and-inclusive-practice-practice-advice-2021.pdf

Dahlke, S., Raymond, C., Penconek, T., & Swaboda, N. (2021). An integrative review of mentoring novice faculty to teach. *Journal of Nursing Education*, 60(4), 203–208. https://doi.org/10.3928/01484834-20210322-04

Dawson, J., Laccos-Barrett, K., Hammond, C., & Rumbold, A. (2022). Reflexive practice as an approach to improve healthcare delivery for Indigenous Peoples: A systematic critical synthesis and exploration of the cultural safety education literature. *International Journal of Environmental Research and Public Health*, 19(11), 6691. https://doi.org/10.3390/ijerph19116691

Dudgeon, P., Derry, K. L., Mascall, C., & Ryder, A. (2022). Understanding Aboriginal models of selfhood: The National Empowerment Project's cultural, social, and emotional wellbeing program in Western Australia. *International Journal of Environmental Research and Public Health*, 19(7), 4078. https://doi.org/10.3390/ijerph19074078

Ephraim, N. (2020). Mentoring in nursing education: An essential element in the retention of new nurse faculty. *Journal of Professional Nursing*, 37(2). https://doi.org/10.1016/j.profnurs.2020.12.001

Fineout-Overholt, E., & Johnson, S. (2023). Asking compelling clinical questions In B. Mazurek Melnyk & E. Fineout-Overholt (Eds.), *Evidence-based practice in nursing & healthcare* (5th ed., pp. 45–47). Wolters-Kluwer.

Ford-Gilboe, M., Wathen, C. N., Varcoe, C., Herbert, C., Jackson, B. E., Lavoie, J. G., & Browne, A. J. (2018). How equity-oriented health care affects health: Key mechanisms and implications for primary health care practice and policy. *The Milbank Quarterly*, 96(4), 635–671.

Francis-Cracknell, A., Truong, M., & Adams, K. (2022). "Maybe what I do know is wrong…": Reframing educator roles and professional development for teaching Indigenous health. *Nursing Inquiry*, 30, e12531. https://doi.org/10.1111/nin.12531

Gee, G., Dudgeon, P., Schultz, C., Hart, A., & Kelly, K. (2014). Aboriginal and Torres Strait Islander social and emotional wellbeing In P. Dudgeon, H. Milroy, & R. Walker (Eds.), *Working together: Aboriginal and Torres Strait Islander mental health and wellbeing principles and practice* (pp. 55–68). ACT: Commonwealth of Australia.

Ginex, P. K. (2017). The difference between quality improvement, evidence-based practice, and research. *ONS Voice*, 32(8), 35. https://voice.ons.org/news-and-views/oncology-research-quality-improvement-evidence-based-practice

Government of Canada (2023). *Primary health care access among First Nations people living off reserve, Métis and Inuit, 2017 to 2020.* www150.Statcan.gc.ca. https://www150.statcan.gc.ca/n1/pub/41-20-0002/412000022023005-eng.htm

Hinch, B. K., Livesay, S., Stifter, J., & Brown, F., Jr (2020). Academic-practice partnerships: Building a sustainable model for doctor of nursing practice (DNP) projects. *Journal of Professional Nursing, 36*(6), 569–578. https://doi.org/10.1016/j.profnurs.2020.08.008

Hyett, S. L., Gabel, C., Marjerrison, S., & Schwartz, L. (2019). Deficit-based Indigenous health research and the stereotyping of Indigenous Peoples. *Canadian Journal of Bioethics, 2*(2), 102–109. https://doi.org/10.7202/1065690ar.

Institute for Healthcare Improvement (IHI). (n.d.). How to improve. https://www.ihi.org/resources/Pages/HowtoImprove/default.aspx

Kawar, L. N., Aquino-Maneja, E. M., Failla, K. R., Flores, S. L., & Squier, V. R. (2023). Research, evidence-based practice, and quality improvement simplified. *The Journal of Continuing Education in Nursing, 54*(1), 40–48. https://doi.org/10.3928/00220124-20221207-09

Langley, G. L., Moen, R., Nolan, K. M., Nolan, T. W., Norman, C. L., & Provost, L. P. (2009). *The improvement guide: A practical approach to enhancing organizational performance* (2nd edition). Jossey-Bass Publishers.

Lederer, L., & Wetzel, C. (2014). The health consequences of sex trafficking and their implications for identifying victims in healthcare facilities. *Annals of Health Law, 23*(1), 61–91.

Lee, H., Geynisman-Tan, J., Hofer, S., Anderson, E., Caravan, S., & Titchen, K. (2021). The impact of human trafficking training on healthcare professionals' knowledge and attitudes. *Journal of Medical Education and Curricular Development, 8.* https://doi.org/10.1177/23821205211016523

Longley, R. (2022). *What is chain of custody?* Definition *and examples.* https://www.thoughtco.com/chain-of-custody-4589132

Macy, R. J., Klein, L. B., Shuck, C. A., Rizo, C. F., Van Deinse, T. B., Wretman, C. J., & Luo, J. (2021). A scoping review of human trafficking screening and response. *Trauma, Violence, & Abuse.* 152483802110572. https://doi.org/10.1177/15248380211057273.

McAmis, N. E., Mirabella, A. C., McCarthy, E. M., Cama, C. A., Fogarasi, M. C., Thomas, L. A., Feinn, R. S., & Rivera-Godreau, I. (2022). Assessing healthcare provider knowledge of human trafficking. *PLOS ONE, 17*(3), e0264338. https://doi.org/10.1371/journal.pone.0264338

McQuilkin, M. A., Gatewood, E., Gramkowski, B., Hunter, J. M., Kuster, A., Melino, K., & Mihaly, L. K. (2020). Transitioning from clinician to nurse practitioner clinical faculty: A systematic review. *Journal of the American Association of Nurse Practitioners, 32*(10), 652–659. https://doi.org/10.1097/jxx.0000000000000295

Melnyk, B., & Fineout-Overholt, E. (2023). Making the case for evidence-based practice and cultivating a spirit of inquiry In B. Mazurek Melnyk & E. Fineout-Overholt (Eds.), *Evidence-based practice in nursing & healthcare* (5th ed., pp. 28). Wolters-Kluwer.

Mills, K., Creedy, D. K., & West, R. (2018). Experiences and outcomes of health professional students undertaking education on Indigenous health: A systematic integrative literature review. *Nurse Education Today, 69*, 149–158. https://doi.org/10.1016/j.nedt.2018.07.014

National Collaborating Centre for Indigenous Health, (2019). *Access to health services as a social determinant of First Nation, Inuit, and Metis health.* https://www.nccih.ca/495/Access_to_health_services_as_a_social_determinant_of_First_Nations,_Inuit_and_M%C3%A9tis_health.nccih?id=279

National Institute of Mental Health. (2020). NIMH» Coping with traumatic events. www.nimh.nih.gov. https://www.nimh.nih.gov/health/topics/coping-with-traumatic-events

National Institutes of Health (U.S.). Policy and Global Affairs. Committee for Monitoring the Nation's Changing Needs for Biomedical, Behavioral, and Clinical Personnel, Board on Higher Education and Welfare. (2005). *Advancing the nation's health needs: NIH research training programs.* National Academies Press.

National League for Nursing. (2022). *Core competencies for academic nurse educators.* NLN.org. https://www.nln.org/education/nursing-education-competencies/core-competencies-for-academic-nurse-educators

Nguyen, N. H., Subhan, F. B., Williams, K., & Chan, C. B. (2020). Barriers and mitigating strategies to healthcare access in Indigenous communities of Canada: A narrative review. *Healthcare, 8*(2), 112. https://doi.org/10.3390/healthcare8020112

Niñerola, A., Sánchez-Rebull, M. V., & Hernández-Lara, A. B. (2020). Quality improvement in healthcare: Six Sigma systematic review. *Health Policy, 124*(4), 438–445. https://doi.org/10.1016/j.healthpol.2020.01.002

North, N., Brysiewicz, P., Danford, C.A. (In press). International Family Nursing Association (IFNA) policy toolkit. International Family Nursing Association. https://internationalfamilynursing.org/

Pan American Health Organization (PAHO). (2019). *Strategic plan of the Pan American Health Organization 2020–2025.* https://www.paho.org/en/documents/paho-strategic-plan-2020-2025

Rathi, R., Vakharia, A., & Shadab, M. (2022). Lean six sigma in the healthcare sector: A systematic literature review. *Materials Today: Proceedings, 50*, 773–781. https://doi.org/10.1016/j.matpr.2021.05.534Get rights and content

Rogers, J., Ludwig-Beymer, P., & Baker, M. (2020). Nurse faculty orientation. *Nurse Educator, 45*(6), 1. https://doi.org/10.1097/nne.0000000000000802

Ruth, C., McLeod, L., Yamamoto, J. M., Sirski, M., Prior, H. J., & Sellers, E. (2023). Changes in prevalence and incidence at the population level of type 2 diabetes in First Nation and all other adults in Manitoba. *Canadian Journal of*

Diabetes, 47(5), 413–419. E2. https://doi.org/10.1016/j.jcjd.2023.03.005

Small-Rodriguez, D., & Akee, R. (2021). Identifying disparities in health outcomes and mortality for American Indian and Alaska Native populations using tribally disaggregated Vital Statistics and Health Survey data. *American Journal of Public Health, 111*(S2), S126–S132. https://doi.org/10.2105/ajph.2021.306427

Staffileno, B. A., Murphy, M. P., Hinch, B., & Carlson, E. (2019). Exploring the Doctor of Nursing Practice project facilitator/mentor role. *Nursing Outlook, 67*(4), 433–440. https://doi.org/10.1016/j.outlook.2019.01.005.

Subica, A. M., & Link, B. G. (2022). Cultural trauma as a fundamental cause of health disparities. *Social Science & Medicine, 292*, 114574. https://doi.org/10.1016/j.socscimed.2021.114574

The United States Department of Justice. (2023). What is human trafficking? Justice.gov. https://www.justice.gov/humantrafficking/what-is-human-trafficking

Turin, T. C., Saad, N., Jun, M., Tonelli, M., Ma, Z., Barnabe, C. C. M., Manns, B., & Hemmelgarn, B. (2016). Life-time risk of diabetes among First Nations and non–First Nations people. *CMAJ, 188*(16), 1147–1153. https://doi.org/10.1503/cmaj.150787

Walt, G., & Gilson, L. (1994). Reforming the health sector in developing countries: The central role of policy analysis. *Health Policy and Planning, 9*(4), 353–370. https://doi.org/10.1093/heapol/9.4.353

Watson, J., Smith, M. C., & Gullett, D. L. (2020). Jean Watson's theory of unitary caring science and theory of human caring: *In Nursing theories and nursing practice* (pp. 311–326). F.A. Davis Company.

Webber, E., Vaughn-Deneen, T., & Anthony, M. (2020). Three-generation academic mentoring teams. *Nurse Educator, 1*. https://doi.org/10.1097/nne.0000000000000777

World Health Organization (2023). *Historic resolution calls for action to improve the health of Indigenous Peoples.* https://www.who.int/news/item/29-05-2023-historic-resolution-calls-for-action-to-improve-the-health-of-indigenous-peoples#:~:text=Indigenous%20Peoples%20face%20significant%20health,levels%2C%20limited%20education%2C%20and%20political

25

Bringing Closure to the Precepting Experience

Beth Heuer and Cynthia A. Danford

CHAPTER OBJECTIVES

- Identify components of a professional identity mindset
- Describe learner readiness for transition into further precepted experiences or independent practice
- Review strategies to disengage from the learner
- Synthesize precepting concepts to create well-prepared and enthusiastic RN and APRN preceptors

Precepting novices involves commitment to building an effective nursing workforce grounded in evidence-based knowledge and skills. Flexibility is necessary in working with learners with varying abilities and experiences. While the preceptor is guiding the novice, they are also building their own expertise in educator, coach, and, sometimes, mentor roles. Each precepted experience has a beginning and a time to bring closure. The end of any precepting experience provides an opportunity to reflect on what was learned, how to move forward with new knowledge, and what changes to consider for future precepting experiences. Acknowledging successes brings a sense of purpose, motivation, and enthusiasm for future opportunities. Preceptors are encouraged to enjoy the process, embrace the perks of precepting, and appreciate the outcomes for themselves, learners, and the nursing profession.

A few themes emerge as preceptors move learners beyond the structured clinical education experience. These include fostering the development of professional identity, determining student readiness, and disengaging the learner.

THE PROFESSIONAL IDENTITY MINDSET

A preceptor mindset is one of growth in professional identity for both self and the learner. A growth mindset involves preceptors choosing to not only grow as teachers in the clinical setting, but also to continue developing updated, evidence-based, best practice skills as healthcare evolves and advances (Rager Huett & Wessel, 2022). Preceptors with a *growth* mindset believe that with persistence and nurturing, the learner can apply knowledge and build professional skills (Cooley & Larsen, 2018). Preceptors with a *fixed* mindset may be quick to judge and resistant to facilitating change. For example, the preceptor with a fixed mindset may tell the novice who makes an error that they do not have what it takes to be a good nurse. Alternatively, by sharing a growth mindset through discussion and role-modeling, the preceptor encourages the learner to focus on possibilities, and to see nursing as a career, not just as a series of tasks to be completed during a shift. The International Society for Professional Identity in Nursing (ISPIN) has identified domains that create an understanding of what it means "to think, act, and feel like a nurse" (What Is Professional Identity in Nursing?, n.d.) (Figure 25.1). Professional identity evolves and matures through clinical and leadership experiences, ongoing career development, and during role transitions (Joseph & Godfrey, 2023). Preceptors model professionalism-in-action and allow learners to envision themselves in the roles to which they aspire.

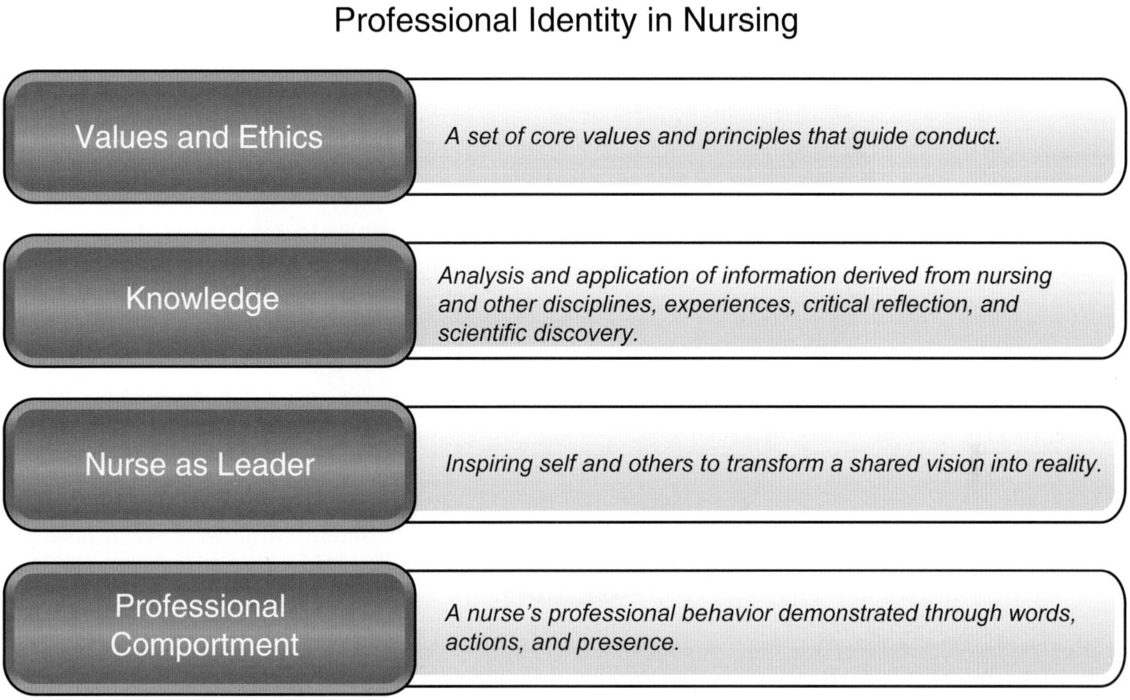

Professional Identity in Nursing

Values and Ethics	*A set of core values and principles that guide conduct.*
Knowledge	*Analysis and application of information derived from nursing and other disciplines, experiences, critical reflection, and scientific discovery.*
Nurse as Leader	*Inspiring self and others to transform a shared vision into reality.*
Professional Comportment	*A nurse's professional behavior demonstrated through words, actions, and presence.*

Fig. 25.1 Professional identify in nursing. (Adapted from Joseph, M. L. & Godfrey, N. (2023). A new mindset. *Nurse Leader. 21*(2), 183–187. © 2022 University of Kansas/ISPIN.)

LEARNER READINESS FOR INDEPENDENCE

Preceptors alone do not "ready" or prepare the learner for independent practice. The process of readiness conceptualized by Gruenberg et al. (2021) is an interactive blend of learner qualities, preceptor–learner relationships, and clinical experiences (Figure 25.2). Learner characteristics include initiative, responsibility, and self-awareness (Gruenberg et al., 2021). Some learners are able to actively apply these qualities during their clinical experience and excel quickly. Other learners may need multiple clinical experiences in a variety of settings to build readiness. One preceptor can only provide experiences in one setting and is not responsible for developing the learner into a fully safe and competent professional. Learners need to be able to acknowledge their own limits and take responsibility for their learning. They also need to develop skills to seek help and manage frustration. Preceptors can remind novices that learning occurs on a continuum and is attained through time and repetition. However, high-quality preceptor–learner relationships provide a foundation for professional growth through role-modeling and interdisciplinary interactions.

Learners need to be detail-oriented so that care is comprehensive, high quality, and safe. In the hospital setting, nursing professional development staff and unit leaders determine that nurse orientees have met specific competencies to complete their orientation. Faculty members assess that students have the knowledge, skills, and experiences needed to graduate and take the NCLEX or advanced practice registered nurse (APRN) certification examinations. Preceptor input is a critical component of determining learner readiness for a new professional role.

DISENGAGING FROM THE LEARNER

Precepting is about facilitating role transition at all levels. From novice learner to advanced learner within a specific setting, or from nurse or APRN orientee to acclimated, autonomous team member, preceptors provide valuable direction. The preceptor may take a "sink or swim" approach to increasing learner independence, yet they should always be ready to act as a "life raft" to keep both the learner and the patient safe. To facilitate transition, novices need to disengage from their

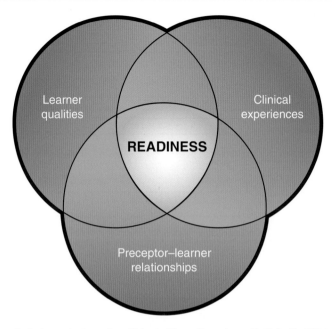

Fig. 25.2 Readiness for independent practice. (Adapted from Gruenberg, K., Hsia, S., O'Brien, B., & O'Sullivan, P. (2021). Exploring multiple perspectives on pharmacy students' readiness for advanced pharmacy practice experiences. *American Journal of Pharmaceutical Education*, *85*(5), 8358. https://doi.org/10.5688/ajpe8358)

previous role and advance into the new role. This change may include the matriculating student transitioning to new clinical experiences at a different site, the graduating student moving on for NCLEX examination or other certification, or the RN orientee transitioning into the role of a full team member within a new workplace setting. Successful precepted experiences will help students and new orientees successfully transition to new roles while reducing "reality shock" (Kramer, 1974). Learners may face heightened levels of fear, uncertainty, and curiosity as they face new challenges, and benefit from ongoing reassurance from colleagues and mentors who share their own stories of getting through new experiences.

ACCEPTING GRATITUDE

Precepting is time-consuming and often challenging. In the busyness that ensues with each clinical day, it can be difficult to stop and savor the benefits. There can be a genuine lift in taking a few moments while reading thank-you cards from previous students and remembering that efforts are appreciated. For nurses and APRNs who live in states that offer tax credits for preceptorship, this additional benefit can have great value.

Those who precept are encouraged to take advantage of all available perks offered by institutions and universities. The perks may include attending continuing education offerings, adding a faculty title onto one's resume or CV, or using clinical resources that are not otherwise available. By seeking out new learning opportunities as the precepting landscape changes, preceptors can remain up-to-date on clinical teaching skills. Changes in the education landscape may lead to financial benefits for preceptors in the future, although this will require ongoing advocacy efforts (Heuer et al., 2023). APRN preceptors should take advantage of the opportunity to utilize their precepting experience for credentialing renewal credit. Accepting recognition for work and effort is a well-deserved perk.

PIECING THE EXPERIENCE TOGETHER

Working as a preceptor shapes personal and professional growth for oneself and for the learner. The goal is to create a positive learning environment that has lasting benefits for all involved. Schools of nursing build partnerships with institutions and with individual nurses and APRNs who are dedicated to clinical teaching. Preceptors share their expertise and contribute to the growth of the profession while reaffirming their own knowledge and passion for their career. Learners receive on-site clinical training from experts in their field. Hospitals and clinical institutions subsequently benefit when hiring novice nurses who are acclimated to the job and the culture through their clinical education experiences.

Reflecting back on the visual image of a quilt, introduced in the first chapter, each preceptor contributes a "piece" to the learner's education, building rich "blocks" of knowledge and clinical experiences. When the education experience is complete, the learner will have attained a vibrant combination of didactic knowledge, assessment skills, clinical judgment ability, procedural acumen, and professionalism.

REFERENCES

Cooley, J. H., & Larson, S. (2018). Promoting a growth mindset in pharmacy educators and students. *Currents in Pharmacy Teaching and Learning*, *10*(6), 675–679. https://doi.org/10.1016/j.cptl.2018.03.021

Gruenberg, K., Hsia, S., O'Brien, B., & O'Sullivan, P. (2021). Exploring multiple perspectives on pharmacy students' readiness for advanced pharmacy practice experiences. *American Journal of Pharmaceutical Education*, *85*(5), 8358. https://doi.org/10.5688/ajpe8358

Heuer, B., Zeno, R., Woosley, C., Bartlett, H., Hueckel, R., & Sonney, J. (2023). NAPNAP position statement on incentivizing APRN preceptors. *Journal of Pediatric Health Care*, *37*(1), 85–89. https://doi.org/10.1016/j.pedhc.2022.09.001

Joseph, M. L., & Godfrey, N. (2023). A new mindset: From tasks to professional identity. *Nurse Leader*, *21*(2), 183–187. https://doi.org/10.1016/j.mnl.2022.12.007

Kramer, M. (1974). *Reality shock: Why nurses leave nursing*. Mosby.

Rager Huett, J. L., & Wessel, R. D. (2022). Exploring best practices in preceptorships: Preceptor selection. *Athletic Training Education Journal*, *17*(1), 106–116. https://doi.org/10.4085/1947-380X-21-004

What is professional identity in nursing? (n.d.). www.kumc.edu. https://www.kumc.edu/school-of-nursing/outreach/consulting/professional-identity/about/what-is-professional-identity-in-nursing.html

Mentoring Contract Example (Chapter 4)

CLINICAL MENTORING EXPECTATIONS AND CONTRACT

Mentoring is an essential component of career development, and is intended to be a rich, rewarding experience for both parties involved. The mentor role entails being committed to career development of the mentee and the mentee is expected to follow through based on the mutual agreement described. The mentoring contract is intended to be an agreement between mentee and mentor, which involves regularly scheduled meetings and may increase in number depending on need. We, as mentor and mentee, have mutually agreed upon the expectations within this mentoring contract.

EXPECTATIONS FOR MENTORS

- **Team meetings**: There should be a minimum of one meeting with the mentee per month.
- **Presentations**: The mentor will attend rounds, meetings, and seminars in which the mentee is presenting.
- **Evaluation**: The mentor will participate in evaluation of the mentoring relationship. The mentor agrees to provide honest, constructive feedback to the mentee.
- **Confidentiality**: The content of all exchanges between the mentor and the mentee are subject to the expectations of professional confidentiality.
- **Professional development plan (PDP)**: The mentor will review, approve, and monitor the progress of the mentee's PDP.

EXPECTATIONS FOR MENTEES

- **Team meetings**: There should be a minimum of one meeting with the mentor per month.
- **Presentations**: The mentee will present at leadership meetings or rounds with the mentor in attendance.
- **Evaluation**: The mentee will participate in evaluations of the mentoring relationship. The mentee agrees to be accepting of honest, constructive feedback from the mentor.
- **Confidentiality**: The content of all exchanges between the mentor and the mentee are subject to the expectations of professional confidentiality.
- **Professional development plan (PDP)**: The mentee will develop a PDP with mentor and review progress.

Exit Clause: If my mentor/mentee needs to terminate the contract for any reason, I agree to abide by their decision without question or blame.

We, acting as mentor and mentee, agree to enter into a mentoring relationship based on the expectations described above.

_____ (mentor's signature) Date____/____/____

_____ (mentee's signature) Date____/____/____

Checklist for Beginning the Precepting Experience

Example 1: Undergraduate Nursing Students

From the faculty

☐ Faculty contact information

☐ Expectations of precepting

☐ Course description and objectives; may include syllabus and course content

☐ Summary of student potential

☐ Level of student (e.g., first semester, first clinical experience, last semester before graduation)

☐ Previous coursework and skills acquired

☐ Projected time for a site visit as appropriate

☐ Plan for periodic progress evaluation

☐ Final clinical performance evaluation

☐ Pertinent articles to guide precepting

From the student

☐ Student contact information

☐ Schedule of hours

☐ Student learning profile (See Appendix M)

☐ Personalized objectives

Example 2: Advanced Practice Registered Nursing Students

Student Specific
- [ ] Student specialty track
- [ ] Anticipated graduation
- [ ] Start/End dates of clinical practicum
- [ ] Student contact information
- [ ] Required number of clinical hours

Academic Program Specific
- [ ] Academic faculty contact information
- [ ] Course syllabus
- [ ] Practicum objectives
- [ ] Diagnostic and procedural skill list
- [ ] Anticipated faculty clinic site visit date _____

Facility Specific
- [ ] Facility tour
- [ ] Staff introductions
- [ ] Parking
- [ ] Building access
- [ ] Appropriate professional dress
- [ ] Arrival/End times

Patient Care Resources
- [ ] Current clinical practice guideline/literature links
- [ ] Specialty-specific clinical tools/measures
- [ ] Specialty-specific pharmacology resources
- [ ] Site specific treatment protocols/algorithms
- [ ] Information technology/on-line resource links

Documentation Resources
- [ ] Documentations templates
- [ ] Electronic Health Record computer access
- [ ] Electronic Health Record computer training
- [ ] Evaluation & Management coding cheat sheets

(adapted from Dunn & Lofgren, Chapter 19)

Competency Sign-off Checklist for Nurse Orientees

Example: Checklist can include sections on central and peripheral IV lines, tubes and drains, ostomy care, phlebotomy skills, infection control, and other nursing care activities specific to the clinical location.

EQUIPMENT			
Topic	**Resource**	**Objective**	**Preceptor Signature/ Date**
Portable blood pressure monitor	Video module: Blood pressure	Demonstrate VS and pulse oximetry reading	
IV infusion pump	Video module: Infusion pump	Program pump to administer IV bolus	
		Program pump to administer continuous IV fluid	
	Procedure: Securing Luer lock connections	Secure Luer lock connection	
Syringe pump	Video module: Syringe pump	Program syringe pump	
Wall suction	Procedure: Use of wall suction	Assemble suction equipment	
Portable suction	Procedure: Use of portable suction	Demonstrate use of portable suction	
12-lead EKG	Video module: 12-lead EKG	Demonstrate 12-lead EKG	
I & O			
Topic	**Resource**	**Objective**	**Preceptor Signature/ Date**
Maintenance fluids	Nursing benchmark:Fluid calculation	Calculate maintenance fluid requirements	
		Calculate expected urinary output	
I & O	Procedure: Measurement of I & O	Accurately measures and documents I & O	

MEDICATION ADMINISTRATION			
Topic	Resource	Objective	Preceptor Signature/ Date
Oral medication	Procedure: Administration of oral medication	Administers oral medication	
Intravenous medication	Procedure: Administration of intravenous medication	Administers IV medication via piggyback	
		Administers IV medication via syringe pump	
Intravenous push medication	Procedure: Administration of IV push medication	Administers IV push medication	
Double-check high alert and controlled medications	Procedure: Performing a two-clinician check	Perform a 2-RN IV med check	
Enteral tube medication	Procedure: Administration of medication via enteral tube	Administers medication via enteral tube	

Developing a Philosophy of Clinical Education Statement for APRN Students (Chapter 3)

A philosophy of clinical education statement is a general affirmation that can be individualized to emphasize the preceptor's commitment to helping the advanced practice registered nurse (APRN) student encounter a variety of ages, a variety of differentials, and changing acuity according to the primary, acute, or specialty area.

Writing a philosophy statement and sharing it with APRN students is a way for preceptors to introduce themselves and to stress their commitment to the student and to their practice. These statements can be as simple as a sentence or two (see first example) or may be several paragraphs in length (see second example).

EXAMPLE #1

"As an APRN in pediatrics, I am committed to providing a supportive learning environment that will foster independence and help the NP student provide individualized, developmentally appropriate care to the children and families they encounter."

EXAMPLE #2

"My clinical education philosophy is rooted in my knowledge/expertise in evidence-based adult-gerontology care, respect for the learner, genuine enthusiasm, and a strong dedication to patient-focused and family-focused care. I love to teach and enjoy doing so outside of the formal classroom setting.

"Precepting APRNs offers me the opportunity to combine my dedication as a clinician with the opportunity to prepare students for their role as advanced practice providers. I bring a high level of respect for other adult learners to my preceptor role. Their time and experience are valuable, and I learn from my students and from the teaching process every day as I precept. Student questions often lead to review of new literature and existing clinical guidelines, so that both the student and I understand the rationale for the care that we provide. I love to help students connect the dots between classroom lectures/rote knowledge, evidence-based guidelines, and real-life patient care."

Site-Specific APRN Clinical Experience Checklist (Chapters 10 and 15)

PRIMARY CARE CLINIC

- [ ] Complete history and physical (H & P)

- [ ] Developmental evaluation or mental status exam

- [ ] Well patient exam

  - [ ] Infant

  - [ ] Toddler/preschooler

  - [ ] School-age child

  - [ ] Adolescent

  - [ ] Adult

  - [ ] Geriatric

  - [ ] Pregnant patient

  - [ ] Sports physical

  - [ ] Anticipatory guidance/patient education

  - [ ] Vaccination schedules

- [ ] Sick patient visits

  - [ ] Eyes, Ears, Nose, Throat (EENT): (upper respiratory infection [URI], sinusitis, otitis or pharyngitis)

  - [ ] Respiratory: (bronchitis, pneumonia)

  - [ ] Gastrointestinal (GI): (gastroenteritis, reflux)

  - [ ] Genitourinary (GU): (urinary tract infection [UTI])

  - [ ] Dermatology: (dermatitis, urticaria, fungal infections)

  - [ ] Other _____

EMERGENCY DEPARTMENT OR INTENSIVE CARE UNIT

☐ Orientation to department, staffing models and organizational structure

☐ Participate in daily teaching rounds

☐ Procedure overview: indications, equipment, processes, skills

☐ Code/arrest procedures

☐ Intubation

☐ Extubation

☐ Chest tube placement

☐ Arterial line placement

☐ Lumbar puncture

☐ Central line placement

☐ Other _____

☐ Review of critical labs

☐ Correction of fluid balance or acid/base balance

☐ Review of invasive ventilation and management parameters

☐ Review of noninvasive ventilation

   ☐ Bilevel positive airway pressure [BiPAP]

   ☐ Continuous positive airway pressure [CPAP]

☐ Sedation basics

☐ Suturing

☐ Critical management of fever, tachycardia, hypotension, hypoxia

☐ Critical management of status asthmaticus, status epilepticus, bronchiolitis, diabetic ketoacidosis (DKA), respiratory failure, sepsis

SPECIALTY CLINIC

☐ Procedure overview: indications, equipment, processes, skills

☐ Setting vagal nerve stimulator

☐ Other specialty procedures _____

☐ Assist in interpretation of forensic data in child abuse cases

☐ Calculation of chemotherapy or other specialty medication dosing

☐ Basic x-ray interpretation

☐ Interpretation of specialty testing

☐ Echocardiogram

☐ Pulmonary function testing

☐ Metabolic and genetic labs

☐ Basic MRI and CT scan interpretation

☐ Administration and interpretation of specialty developmental or behavioral assessments

☐ Orthopedic procedures

   ☐ Closed reduction

   ☐ Casting

APRN Student Welcome Poster for Clinical Site (Chapter 14)

TO OUR PATIENTS AND FAMILIES

We are pleased to participate in University of _____ School of Nursing clinical training program for Advanced Practice Nursing students

Please welcome the student(s) working with us in our clinic/department

Insert Photo

Student Name, Credentials

THANK YOU for your kind support of this program!

How to Be an Amazing APRN Student in Any Clinical Site (Chapter 15)

Preceptors and faculty: please feel free to share with your students.

☐ Student develops personal learning needs and clinical objectives

☐ Student practices how to effectively present patients to the preceptor (using SNAPPS, SBAR, OLD CARTS, or OPQRST mnemonics)

☐ Student is proactive and prepared

☐ Arrives early in order to review the daily clinic schedule, identifying specific learning opportunities

☐ Reviews patient history prior to the encounter and identifies relevant data pertinent to the visit

☐ Research articles or resources related to unusual diagnoses or different medications relevant to patient encounters

☐ Participates in goal setting in advance of patient visits (e.g., "What should we make sure to cover today?" "What immunizations are due today?")

☐ Student demonstrates positive attitude and respect toward colleagues, patients, and families

☐ Student writes down questions throughout the day so that they can be addressed together during a break or at the end of the day

☐ Student collaborates actively during visits to provide added value to the experience

☐ Calculates medication dosages and performs medication reconciliations

☐ Within the clinic setting, develops after visit summaries and reviews them with patients and families as allowed by the practice site

☐ Student effectively promotes shared decision-making

☐ Student is properly dressed and displays professional demeanor

☐ Student receives constructive feedback appropriately, asking open-ended questions in a non-defensive, nonjudgmental way

Adapted from: Winklerprins, V. (n.d.). *How to be awesome in an ambulatory clinic rotation.* https://www.stfm.org/media/2161/how-to-be-awesome-in-an-ambulatory-clinic_studenteducation_final.pdf

Examples of Reflective Journaling (Chapter 8)

When guiding learners in using reflective journaling, inform them that each step is only one paragraph. The entire journal entry is meant to take up only one page. Learners may expand on more ideas initially and then later pare them down. The learner practices writing succinctly and identifying only key elements in the encounter.

The following are steps in developing a reflective journal entry:

1. Frame the vignette or clinical scenario.

_____
_____
_____
_____
_____

2. Support the actions of the vignette using clinical judgment.

_____
_____
_____
_____
_____

3. Evaluate and identify a plan for future situations.

_____
_____
_____
_____
_____

EXAMPLE FROM A BEGINNING APRN STUDENT

In clinic, I saw a 7-year-old boy whose teacher had concerns that the child seemed to stare off into space during class. His mother described being worried about his classroom performance because of these new behaviors. I asked a few questions to help me determine if this child might have ADHD. His mother stated that these episodes have occurred for only 2 months. She described that her son seems to daydream for 10 or 15 seconds and then "snaps out of it." She did not feel confident that she could get his attention if she touched him. She stated that otherwise, the child does not seem overly distracted or forgetful. His physical exam seemed normal. When talking with my preceptor, I let her know that the office had not received any Conners or Vanderbilt rating forms to assess for ADHD. I sensed that this child might not have ADHD and that maybe a neurology evaluation (or EEG) might be needed. I shared these thoughts with my preceptor.

When we returned to the room, my preceptor clarified a few aspects of the history. My preceptor pulled out a pinwheel and had the child hyperventilate by taking deep breaths and blowing on the pinwheel. At the count of 23, he quit blowing on the pinwheel and just stared ahead for about 15 seconds. He then seemed to snap out of it and looked at my preceptor like he'd forgotten what he was doing. I realized I just witnessed my first absence seizure. My preceptor launched into a discussion with the parents about what she had just seen and how she would order an EEG and refer him for an appointment in pediatric neurology. She also sent home parent and teacher Vanderbilt rating forms and asked for a copy of his most recent grades and any comments from teachers to make sure that nothing else was missing in his clinical picture.

I felt really excited that I sensed that something else was going on with this child and remembered to ask more questions. I felt like I was formulating differential diagnoses in my head as his mom answered questions, and I was thinking about whether this child was just inattentive or if there was more to it. My preceptor helped me to understand what to do next, what to order, and how to best explain this to the family without worrying them excessively.

Example of Journaling Rubric (Chapter 8)

Student name: _____

Preceptor/instructor: _____

One way to structure journaling rubrics is to include the following domains: degree of reflection, application of theory, analysis for future improvement, development of values, and degree of completion.

	SCORING RUBRIC			
Domain	**0**	**1**	**2**	**Score**
Degree of reflection	No reflection; experiences are listed	Some reflection is evident	Deep reflection is evident	___/2
Application of theory	No theory components are correlated	Some integration from readings/lectures to experience	Strong integrations from readings/lectures to experience	___/2
Analysis for future improvement	No thought toward improvement	Some thought toward improvement, not well-developed	Well-thought plan for future improvement	___/2
Development of values	No value development indicated	Some value development mentioned but not well-developed	Full exploration of a change to one or more values	___/2
Degree of completion	Not completed	Not all questions answered, short response	Full journal entry meeting length requirement	___/2
Total score				___/10

Adapted from: Miller, L. B. (2017). Review of journaling as a teaching and learning strategy. *Teaching and Learning in Nursing, 12*(1), 39–42.

One-Minute Preceptor Exemplars (Chapter 8)

The One-Minute Preceptor (OMP) model was originally developed by Neher et al. (1992). This model is vastly popular because of how quickly and effectively the learner can present the case and the preceptor can provide feedback. There are two phases to eliciting clinical judgment skills using the OMP. In the inquiry phase, you want to inquire about what the student understands about the clinical case by asking open-ended questions. In the discussion phase, you can give targeted teaching points and provide positive and corrective feedback.

FIVE MICROSKILLS ASSOCIATED WITH THE ONE-MINUTE PRECEPTOR MODEL

1. Get commitment to diagnosis and treatment option, which encourages the student to process and problem solve.
   - What do you think is going on?
   - What do you do next?
2. Probe for supporting evidence
   - What are major findings that lead you to that conclusion?
   - Why would you choose that treatment?.
3. Teach general rules at level of students' understanding
   - When this happens, do this.
4. Give positive feedback
   - You did an excellent job of _____.
5. Correct mistakes; allow student opportunity to critique their performance first and provide constructive feedback
   - "Do you feel you addressed the patient's questions?
   - Next time this happens, try ___.

CASE EXAMPLES USING THE ONE-MINUTE PRECEPTOR MODEL

Case #1

The student has just evaluated a 3-year-old boy who came for a primary-care problem-focused visit due to parent concern for language delay and minimal interactive play at preschool. The physical exam was grossly normal, and the student described pertinent positives concisely. No developmental questionnaires were provided to the parent's child at today's visit.

Preceptor: "What do you think is going on? What do you want to do next?"

Student: "I think that this child has autism. He needs a more thorough evaluation."

Preceptor: "Can you tell me about what makes you think that he has autism? What points to autism over any other possible diagnosis?"

Student: "Well, he's not talking yet, and he doesn't seem to want to play with his classmates at school."

Preceptor: "Let's think about what to do next. Could he have just a developmental speech delay, and have trouble communicating with peers, leading to some social difficulty at school? Typically, we want to get verification of behaviors with rating forms like the M-CHAT, and we need to assess his hearing if he has a speech delay, right?"
Student: "I forgot about that! So, I want to get an M-CHAT and figure out getting audiology testing."
Preceptor: "Exactly! I like that you are thinking about possible developmental diagnoses. And nice presentation on the physical exam findings.
Student: "Thanks. I'm feeling better about my physical exams in kids."
Preceptor: "Do you feel that you addressed all of his parents' basic concerns with this plan? Next time you see a child with this combination of symptoms, it's easy to just think autism, but let's remember that we want to rule out other issues as well. And we can check the M-CHAT and find decide whether further testing is needed."
Student: "Great—that makes good sense."

Case #2

A 6-year-old male presents to his primary care provider for new onset staring spells. The primary care provider orders an EEG and refers to neurology. The EEG shows generalized 3 Hz spike and wave discharges. The nurse practitioner (NP) student in the neurology clinic completes a history that is unremarkable, aside from the staring spells, and a normal physical exam; they review the EEG results.
Preceptor: "What are you thinking for a potential diagnosis based on the presenting information?"
Student: "Based on the EEG and history, I think the patient has childhood absence epilepsy."
Preceptor: "So, what do you want to do next?"
Student: "I think we should order an MRI of the brain to make sure nothing is wrong."
Preceptor: "Why do you want to order an MRI of the brain?"
Student: "In case there is an abnormality causing the seizures."
Preceptor: "What specific type of abnormality would you anticipate being the cause of this type of seizure?"
Student: "I'm not really sure. It just seems like the right thing to do."
Preceptor: "When ordering neuroimaging, it is best to have an idea of what you are specifically looking for, or at least potential and feasible options. In a case of new onset seizures, imaging is indicated if there are focal findings in the history, physical exam, or on EEG. In those cases, you have an idea of specific regions and potential abnormalities that you are evaluating with imaging. Do you have questions about this?"
Student: "No, that makes sense. Since this patient has a generalized epilepsy, normal neurologic exam, and a nonfocal history, we don't need imaging. I think we should start the patient on ethosuximide to treat his seizures."
Preceptor: "Sounds like a great plan. Let's talk more about dosing for ethosuximide. You did a great job arriving at a diagnosis and creating a treatment plan. Next time, remember that imaging is best reserved for instances where you are looking for specific potential abnormalities based on the history, physical, and diagnostic evaluation."
Student: "Thanks."

Case #3

In your school-based health clinic, a child presents with sore throat, bilateral ear pain, and nasal congestion for 2 days. The student takes a full history and performs a focused exam. They mention that the pharynx is injected with +1 tonsillar hypertrophy, and nasal mucosa edematous. There is a little fluid behind the TMs, but no erythema or bulging. The preceptor asks the student their impression of what the diagnosis may be, and to also provide one or two other differential diagnoses.
Preceptor: "What do you think are the most likely differential diagnoses for this patient?"
Student: "An upper respiratory infection, strep throat, and allergies."

Preceptor: "Can you identify which symptoms and physical findings support each of the possible diagnoses that you listed?"

Student: (listing out the symptoms)

- "I thought of upper respiratory infection because this illness commonly presents with nasal congestion, sore throat, and ear pain."
- "It's less likely the patient has strep throat because this usually is not accompanied by nasal congestion, however, it is possible that the patient has both a URI and strep."
- "Allergies are also another consideration since the patient is complaining about a sore throat, which can be postnasal drip, along with nasal congestion, and ear pain."

Preceptor: "One thing that can be useful when you're presenting a case like this is to include whether the patient has any fever, malaise, or fatigue, which would help narrow down the differential list. For allergies, are you seeing rhinorrhea? Allergic shiners? And since you mentioned strep, let's talk about whether you saw any exudate on the pharynx or petechiae on the soft palate.

Student: Oh, I forgot to mention it. He is afebrile, which is why his mom sent him to school. He says that he is tired today because his nose was so stuffy last night that he couldn't sleep well. I didn't notice any exudate, but I don't think that I paid close attention.

Preceptor: You did a nice job of identifying the possible diagnosis for the case along with providing evidence to support each differential that you considered. Let's tie in the additional information about the lack of fever, and the nasal stuffiness that kept him awake last night. And you can double-check your exam findings.

Student: Great. I want to make sure that I'm being thorough...

Preceptor: Come back to me after you pull these few things together. We'll discuss it in more detail and come up with our plan of treatment. We'll keep working on helping you tie together your exam findings and your differential diagnoses.

Student: I appreciate it. I'll be back in a few minutes with the rest of the details.

Sample Letter From Preceptor to Faculty Regarding Nurse Practitioner Student Concerns (Chapter 17)

Date:

RE: (NP student name)

Dear (faculty name):

Thank you for the opportunity to precept for (Name of University) NP program. I am writing in reference to (NP student name), who has been assigned to work with me. I have been precepting (NP student name) for approximately (XX) weeks/days and have identified some concerns. Although I have provided directions [and (NP student name) has made some improvement], his/her performance remains problematic. Briefly, I am particularly concerned about: (provide 1–2 brief examples such as: time management, poor assessment skills, poor interviewing skills, unsafe practice related to foundational skills, lack of attention to developmental variations in children, lack of initiative to interact with child/family or preceptor, moving forward too quickly without collaborating)

I would like to set up a phone conversation (or an early site visit) to talk with you about (NP student name)'s progress and a plan to help him/her progress. I am available on (Mondays or Tuesdays from 8:30–9:00 am or 4:30–5:00 pm). I look forward to hearing from you.

Sincerely,

(Preceptor name)

Sample Learning Plan Addressing APRN Student Concerns

Learning contract needs should be discussed with the preceptor to determine if the plan is realistic for the preceptor and clinical site. This sample reflects a plan for remediation due to student concerns/deficiencies in multiple areas. Plans can be more or less detailed.

University of _____ School of Nursing Learning Contract

Course Number and Name: _____

Student Name: _____ Date: _____

In accordance with the course guidelines and as a result of a mid-semester performance evaluation of (student name), NP student, by (preceptor name) and (clinical faculty name), concerns have been identified regarding said student. Since (student name)'s performance has not progressed since the beginning of the semester, the following learning contract has been developed to facilitate clinical progression.

Learning Plan

The following learning plan, based on the (course number) Clinical Evaluation Form and Clinical Course Objectives, is recommended in order for (student name) to progress to a passing evaluation score of _____ by (date). It is strongly recommended that (student name) reread the clinical objectives, as they will be held accountable to them. In order to progress, (student name) must complete the objectives in each category below (taken from the evaluation form) and obtain an evaluation score of no less than _____ by (date). Failure to meet the expectations of this learning plan may result in failure of (course number) and prevent further progression in their NP program.

In order to obtain further evidence of competent or incompetent performance, (student name) will continue to work primarily with (preceptor name at respective clinic). The goal of this learning plan is to provide direction for (student name) so they can show progression in advanced practice nursing performance.

Objective Category 1: Data Collection

- Review chart before patient encounter.
  - ° Take several minutes to review chart before interviewing the patient.

- ° Identify pertinent history and plan.
- ° Present to preceptor before interviewing the patient.
- Report on pertinent history and assessment findings with preceptor.
- Demonstrate independence in data collection with minimal direction.
  - ° Take initiative in directing history and physical exam.

Objective Category 2: Assessment Process

- Identify variations in history and physical exam related to all systems during a comprehensive visit.
- Discuss exam findings and their potential meaning with preceptor.
  - ° Identify need to further assess or follow-up on concerns.
  - ° Bring pertinent information to the attention of the preceptor for discussion.
- Identify at least two differential diagnoses for episodic or ill visits.
  - ° Discuss rationale for at least two differential diagnoses based on assessment findings.
  - ° Discuss rationale for which differential diagnoses can be ruled out.
- Demonstrate a consistently organized assessment with minimal direction.

Objective Category 3: Management Plan

- Based on assessment data, propose a plan for further evaluation or treatment, and discuss with preceptor.
  - ° Take the initiative to:
    - – Present plan without prompting from the preceptor.
    - – Identify the need for an immediate action during office visit (e.g., peak flow, O2 saturations, nebulizer treatments, blood glucose monitoring, medication administration).
    - – Review treatments and plan to teach patient and family as appropriate, including prescriptions, follow-up, and referral.
  - ° Discuss rationale for proposed treatment, including relevant evidence.
  - ° Initiate discussion of development of a management plan with minimal direction. (Note: You are not expected to always have the correct response or the correct and perfect plan, but you are expected to be thinking through a plan and to be able to articulate your thinking.)

Objective Category 4: Communication

- Communicate primarily with preceptor and clinical faculty in a timely manner.
  - ° Discuss scheduling and hours with preceptor and clinical faculty a minimum of 2 weeks ahead of time.
  - ° Present patient to preceptor after history and assessment are complete. Organize your thoughts and include:
    - – Chief complaint using OLD CART or OPQRST
    - – Pertinent history and assessment
    - – Treatment plan
- Communicate with patient and family professionally.
  - ° Talk with the patient using eye contact and welcoming body language; get out from behind the computer.
  - ° Use of inclusive patient-centered and family-centered language.

- Documentation
  - ° Documentation should be thorough and completed independently, with minimal corrections from the preceptor.
  - ° Provide clinical faculty with SOAP documentation for subsequent patients until your charting is approved by clinical faculty and minimal additions are provided by preceptor.
  - ° Add depth to weekly reflections by incorporating evidence when addressing questions or presenting new information.

Objective Category 5: Professional Role

- Provide clinical faculty and preceptor with a schedule of available clinical practicum hours.
  - ° As part of your professional responsibility, you are on your honor to be timely and to fulfill the hours you have committed to and as agreed upon by the preceptor.
  - ° Failure to comply or falsification of hours could result in failure. Driving time to the site is not included in clinical time.
- Organize time to complete patient data collection in a timely manner.
  - ° A comprehensive patient visit should be completed in 20 to 25 minutes. Negotiate time with your preceptor for more complex issues.
  - ° Focused episodic/acute care visit should be completed in 10 to 15 minutes.
- Take initiative to review patient schedule at the beginning of the day. Work with preceptor to identify scheduled patient encounter that may help learner meet specific objectives.
  - ° Target one sports physical or comprehensive wellness exam per day.
  - ° Target two to three episodic or acute-care visits per day.
  - ° After proficiency is attained as identified by your preceptor and clinical faculty, increase to two comprehensive exams per day and three to four acute-care visits as appropriate.
- Take initiative to read and review in preparation for clinical and to follow-up on previous cases.
  - ° Present new knowledge or follow-up information to preceptor on subsequent clinic day.
  - ° Incorporate discussion of relevant evidence.

Signatures:

_____

NP Student/Date

_____

Clinical Faculty/Date

Student Learning Profile

Name:_____ Preferred name and/or pronouns: _____

E-mail: _____

Home Phone: _____ Cell Phone: _____

    Past and present clinical experiences (r/t work and student experiences) and length of time in each experience:

_____
_____
_____
_____

The following information will help faculty track your progress and insights as you develop in your nursing/advanced practice registered nurse (APRN) role. This information will be useful to faculty and preceptors as your learning experiences are planned in the classroom and clinical settings. It will also be helpful in focusing clinical evaluations. Please respond to the following:

1. Information my preceptor and clinical faculty should know about me (e.g., work, school, personal, health): _____

_____
_____
_____
_____

2. My areas of strength are: _____

3. My short-term goals/objectives (individualized and measurable) for this semester are: _____

_____
_____
_____
_____

4. My long-term goals are: _____

_____
_____
_____
_____

Examples of Nurse Practitioner Student Learning Needs and Clinical Objectives (Chapter 9)

Please note that when writing objectives, the objectives must be measurable and realistic, and based on the student level and course objectives.

ALL CLINICAL SETTINGS

- Obtain a complete comprehensive health history without prompting from clinical preceptor by the end of the 1st month of clinical experience.

- Complete an appropriate focused physical exam based on the patient's presenting symptoms and history by the 2nd week of the clinical experience.

- Report subjective and objective data to preceptor in an appropriate, organized, concise manner by the 5th clinical experience.

- Identify correct differential diagnosis more than 50% of the time by the end of the 2nd month of clinical experience.

- Identify correct diagnostic tests to confirm differential diagnosis with 50% or less assistance from the provider by 30 hours, or halfway through the clinical rotation.

- Assess and manage the care of the patient with chronic conditions with assistance from clinical preceptor by 50 hours of clinical experience.

- Provide patient/family health counseling as needed by 40 hours of clinical experience.

PRIMARY CARE

- Complete an annual well-patient exam and provide appropriate health education without assistance from clinical preceptor by end of clinical experience.

- Formulate a management plan for a "sick" patient visit based on correct differential diagnosis with 25% or less assistance by the clinical preceptor by 50 hours of clinical experience.

ACUTE CARE

- Integrate discussion of critical illness pathophysiology with patient lab values to develop a plan of action for (minimum of) one patient daily, beginning with 2nd week of clinical experience.

- Active participation in inpatient teaching rounds with 25% or less assistance by the clinical preceptor by 50 hours of clinical experience.

- Verbalize knowledge of indications, and preparation for and performance of critical-care skills (e.g., arterial line insertion, chest tube insertion, etc.) within 1 week of participating in each procedure with the preceptor.

- Demonstrate advanced provider communication skills by reviewing daily treatment plans with patient (as possible) and family at bedside or by phone by 16 hours of clinical experience.

SPECIALTY CARE

- Discuss findings from evidence-based practice and research based on one specialty-care patient by the 3rd week of clinical rotation.

- Verbalize knowledge of indications, and preparation for and performance of specialty care skills (e.g., skin biopsy, wound incision and drain (I & D), etc.) within 1 week of participating in each procedure with the preceptor.

NONPF/AANP Preceptor Expectation Checklist:
Faculty Expectations of Preceptors (Chapter 9)

(Directions: Check off and provide date when completed.)

Establishing Clinical Rotation   **Completed/Date**

☐ Review nurse practitioner (NP) program policies regarding student placement guidelines.

☐ Communicate start date and time with student.

☐ Review documents related to the clinical course (welcome letter, clinical hours requirement, syllabus, course objectives, etc.) and clarify, if needed.

☐ Review Family Educational Rights and Privacy Act (FERPA).

Orientation   **Completed/Date**

☐ Orient student to clinical site, clinical site policies, EHR, and clinical team prior to student's patient experiences.

☐ Discuss course objectives, course requirements, student learning goals, and clinical experience expectations with the student.

☐ Discuss with student his/her experience/background.

☐ Outline appropriate tasks, patient cases, and caseload for each clinical day.

☐ Establish plan for student progression from observing to conducting visits with minimal intervention.

Clinical Experience   **Completed/Date**

☐ Model clinical skills and professional/ethical behaviors for student learning.

☐ Be present to observe all student clinical activities.

☐ Include the student as a pertinent part of the healthcare team and encourage interprofessional collaboration between student and other team members.

☐ Encourage learning using direct questioning methods and allowing reflection on feedback.

☐ Verify student clinical hours.

Communication   Completed/Date

☐ Guide, counsel, and encourage active student learning through clinical experiences.

☐ Communicate to faculty pertinent feedback regarding student performance and learning progression related to course expectations and requirements.

☐ Be available for virtual or face-to-face site visits.

Evaluation   Completed/Date

☐ Complete appropriate evaluation forms at intervals outlined in course requirements.

☐ Discuss evaluation(s) with student, providing constructive feedback on strengths, weaknesses, and plans for improvement.

☐ Participate in faculty-initiated plans of remediation, if necessary.

Completion of Clinical Rotation   Completed/Date

☐ Submit all documents as outlined in the course.

From Pitts, C., Padden, D., Knestrick, J., et al. (2019). A checklist for faculty and preceptor to enhance the nurse practitioner student clinical experience. *Journal of the American Association of Nurse Practitioners, 31*(10), 591–597.

NONPF/AANP Preceptor Expectation Checklist: **Preceptor Expectations** of Faculty (Chapter 9)

(Directions: Check off and provide date when completed.)

Establishing Clinical Rotation	Completed/Date

☐ Communicate start date and time with preceptor/clinical site point of contact.

☐ Identify preceptor's preferred method of communication.

☐ Send documents related to the clinical course (welcome letter, preceptor handbook, clinical hours requirement, syllabus, course objectives, etc.) to preceptor/clinical site point of contact via mail or e-mail.

☐ Provide preceptor/clinical site point of contact with student's credentials and clinical clearance paperwork.

☐ Discuss course objectives, course requirements, student learning goals, and clinical experience expectations with the preceptor.

Orientation	Completed/Date

☐ Provide the contact number/information to the clinical faculty responsible for the student.

☐ Discuss the purpose, frequency, length, and number of site visits with the preceptor.

☐ Offer face-to-face or online orientation opportunities to address adult learning/teaching strategies and effective preceptor approaches.

Clinical Experience	Completed/Date

☐ Assume primary responsibility for the student throughout the clinical experience.

☐ Assess student's clinical skills, knowledge, and competencies throughout clinical experience and assess for appropriate progression as it relates to course and clinical objectives.

☐ Support students in connecting knowledge obtained in academic setting with their clinical experiences.

☐ Review and confirm student clinical hours.

Communication   Completed/Date

☐ Engage in open communication with preceptor regarding student performance and learning
    progression related to course expectations and requirements.

☐ Schedule virtual or face-to-face site visits.

Evaluation   Completed/Date

☐ Collect and review evaluation forms completed by the preceptor at intervals as outlined in
    course requirements.

☐ Collect and review preceptor evaluation forms completed by the student.

☐ Discuss evaluation(s) with student, providing constructive feedback on strengths,
    weaknesses, and a plan for improvement.

☐ Initiate plans of remediation based on evaluations, if necessary.

Completion of Clinical Rotation   Completed/Date

☐ Review final evaluation submitted by preceptor, as outlined in the course.

☐ Send preceptor or clinical site a thank-you letter or token of appreciation, per program
    or university policy, including but not limited to: continuing education credits, monetary
    compensation, adjunct faculty positions, or access to school library resources.

☐ Provide preceptor with documentation of preceptorship for national certification renewal or
    dossier.

☐ Provide preceptor with feedback about preceptorship performance based on student
    evaluation(s).

From Pitts, C., Padden, D., Knestrick, J., et al. (2019). A checklist for faculty and preceptor to enhance the nurse practitioner
student clinical experience. *Journal of the American Association of Nurse Practitioners, 31*(10), 591–597.

Preceptor Agreement Form Template: Example

PRECEPTOR AGREEMENT

Preceptor: Please fill out Parts A and B of the Preceptor Agreement form. Sign and return to faculty. Clinical affiliation agreements and preceptor agreements must be in place prior to the student being on-site for clinicals.

PART A

*Preceptor Name:*_____

*Preceptor Work Address:*_____
   (Street / City / State / Zip Code)

Telephone: _____ *E-mail:* _____

Clinical Specialty: _____

*Name of Facility or Employer:*_____

RN License #: _____ *APRN License #:* _____

Select All Degrees Held: Undergraduate: _____ *Graduate:* _____ *Doctoral:* _____ *Other:* _____

Certifications (please list): _____

Please attach the following documents: (Resume and/or CV, evidence of certifications)

Please initial here that you received a copy of the Preceptor Handbook: _____

PART B

I, _____, agree to act as a preceptor for
   (Print Preceptor Name)

_____, in _____, who will be
(Print Student Name)   *(Course Name and Number)*

completing a Clinical Rotation at _____.
(Location Where Clinical Affiliation Agreement Exists)

I agree to abide by all the rules and requirements set forth in the Preceptor Handbook.

Preceptor Signature / Date

_____

Student Signature / Date

_____

Faculty Signature / Date

_____

Other Approval (if applicable) / Date

_____

Preceptors' Orientation Competence Instrument (POCI)

Developed by Pohjamies et al. (2022), the Preceptors' Orientation Competence Instrument (POCI) is a self-evaluation checklist of competencies or actions (beyond clinical skills) required of preceptors. This tool allows the preceptor to reflect on their skills and abilities in order to provide a high-quality orientation for new registered nurses (RNs) or advanced practice RNs (APRNs) within the clinical setting.

The preceptor self-rates each area of competence on scale of 1 to 4, where "1" equals *completely disagree*, "2" equals *partially disagree*, "3" equals *partially agree*, and "4" equals *completely agree*. The tool helps the preceptor to review their individual strengths and to identify areas for further development.

Factor (describing a nursing orientation competence)	Competence	Rating (on scale of 1 to 4)
Preceptor characteristics	I am empathetic when precepting the new employee.	
	I am flexible when precepting the new employee.	
	I am encouraging when precepting the new employee.	
	I create a respectful preceptorship.	
	I am approachable for the new employee.	
	I am patient when orientating the new employee.	
	I create a reliable preceptorship.	
	I am fair when orientating the new employee.	
	I appreciate the new employee as a member of the work community.	
	I take into account the learning style of the new employee when precepting.	
	I take into account the individuality of the new employee when precepting.	
	I act as a role model to the new employee.	
Goal-oriented orientation	I make sure that the learning goals of the new employee are concrete.	
	I make sure that the learning goals of the new employee are suitable to work tasks.	
	I guide the new employee to set the learning goals for the orientation period.	
	I give feedback to the new employee's set learning goals.	
	Together with the new employee, I go through what is required to achieve the set learning goals.	
	I orient the new employee according to set learning goals.	
	I encourage the new employee to independently observe the set learning goals.	
	I evaluate the new employee according to set learning goals.	
	I participate in the evaluation discussion of the new employee.	
	I plan daily learning situations for the new employee according to the learning goals.	

Factor (describing a nursing orientation competence)	Competence	Rating (on scale of 1 to 4)
Guiding a reflective discussion	In the orientation discussion, I encourage the new employee to evaluate their own activities from varied perspectives.	
	I tell the new employee that during their self-evaluation, new thoughts, feelings, and performances that one is not aware of might surface.	
	In the orientation discussion, I guide the new employee to clinical judgment.	
	In the orientation discussion, I guide the new employee to address any negative emotions.	
	I encourage the new employee to recall the experience as it happened and to evaluate it.	
	I know how to use support questions to deepen the new employee's self-assessment.	
	I encourage the new employee to actively process their experiences throughout the orientation.	
	I encourage the new employee to actively process their experiences throughout the orientation.	
	I guide the new employee to question what is taken for granted.	
Knowledge of work unit's orientation practices	I am familiar with the commonly agreed orientation practices in my work unit.	
	I am familiar with the orientation process for a new employee in my own organization.	
	I act according to the joint orientation practices.	
	I am familiar with the responsibilities of a preceptor.	
	I am familiar with the responsibilities and duties of a person who is responsible for whole orientation process in the work unit (e.g., nursing instructor).	
Creating a supportive learning atmosphere	In the orientation discussion, I seek reciprocity with the new employee.	
	In the orientation discussion, I strive for creating a safe atmosphere with the new employee.	
	I encourage the new employee to share their experiences.	
	I am empathetic to the experiences of the new employee.	
	I realize that the experiences of the new employee are unique and relevant to their learning.	
	I believe that an orientation discussion about the new employee's experiences will promote the development of their competence.	
	I take into account the new employee's previous work experience when precepting.	

Factor (describing a nursing orientation competence)	Competence	Rating (on scale of 1 to 4)
Preceptor's motivation	Receiving constructive feedback on acting as a preceptor increases my motivation to orient new employees.	
	The encouragement from colleagues on acting as preceptor increases my enthusiasm to orient new employees.	
	I want to learn and develop as a preceptor.	
	Positive experiences of precepting increase my perceptions of my own abilities to act as a preceptor.	
	I am interested in orienting new employees.	
Giving developmental feedback	I give feedback to the new employee for future development.	
	I give constructive feedback so that the new employee can change their performance.	
	I give feedback to the new employee right after the performance.	
	I give a constructive overall assessment of the new employee's performance.	

Modified from Pohjamies, N., Mikkonen, K., Kääriäinen, M., & Haapa, T. (2022). Development and psychometric testing of the preceptors' orientation competence instrument (POCI). *Nurse Education in Practice, 64,* 103445.

Orientation Topics for School Nurses

Healthcare Conditions: Acute and Chronic

Asthma	• Asthma management plans
	• Use of nebulizers, inhalers, and spacers
Anaphylaxis	• Allergen identification
	• Allergen avoidance strategies
	• Epinephrine injections
	• School staff training
Diabetes	• Blood glucose checks/continuous blood glucose monitoring
	• Carbohydrate counting and meal planning
	• Glucagon administration
	• Insulin administration (vial, pen, pump)
	• Insulin pump monitoring
	• Newly diagnosed and noncompliant patient care
	• "Sick day" plans and treatment
Mental health	• Anger and aggressive behavior
	• Anxiety and depression
	• Bullying
	• Grief
	• Self-injurious behavior and suicidal ideation

Seizures	• Seizure plans
	• Emergency medication administration
	• Teacher and staff training

Social and Mental Health Needs

Risky behaviors	• Alcohol and/or drug use
	• Tobacco and vaping
	• Unprotected sexual intercourse

Social issues	• Student homelessness
	• Poverty
	• Food insecurity
	• Immigration issues

Student special needs	• Attention deficit hyperactivity disorder (ADHD)
	• Autism
	• Genetic disorders and associated disabilities

Common Skills

| Catheterization | • Male and female |
| | • Sterile and nonsterile technique |

| Tracheostomy management | • Tracheostomy care and suctioning |

| Tube feedings and management | • Gastrostomy tubes |
| | • Nasogastric tubes |

Adapted from Blackmon-Jones L. (2017). A strategy to promote successful transition to school nursing. *NASN School Nurse, 32*(1):50–55.

APRN Student Competency Evaluation Using the PRIME Model

Students are evaluated on clinical competencies in order to standardize their performance in clinical practice. The PRIME model provides a foundation for evaluation of competencies as outlined by AACN to bridge the gap between the classroom and clinical practice. The tool includes the following areas of proficiency: **Professional, Reporter, Interpreter, Manager,** and **Educator/Evaluator.**

PROFESSIONAL: DEMONSTRATES PROFESSIONAL BEHAVIOR PRE-C THROUGH C5	YES	NO	
Displays professional demeanor and attire.			**Novice**: Developing skills.
Displays personal insight and participates in self-directed learning.			**Advanced beginner**: Requires oversight from preceptor. **Competent**: Assuming greater responsibility. **Proficient**: Recognizing more complex situations.
Interacts appropriately with patient/ caregiver.			**Pre-C**: Preclinical courses (e.g., health assessment) **C1–C5**: Progressive clinical courses over 5 semesters
Demonstrates respect for patient values.			

	Novice	Adv. beginner	Competent	Proficient
REPORTER: ABLE TO GATHER AND PRESENT INFORMATION ABOUT THE PATIENT				
Student gathers patient information using strong interviewing skills.	Pre-C	C1	C2	C3–5
Student performs a focused physical exam relative to the history and recognizes abnormal findings.	Pre-C	C1	C2	C3–5
Student accurately conveys patient information through an organized oral presentation.	Pre-C	C1	C2	C3–5
Student accurately documents history and physical exam (H & P) findings.	Pre-C	C1	C2	C3–5

	Novice	Adv. beginner	Competent	Proficient
INTERPRETER: ABLE TO ANALYZE AND PRIORITIZE PATIENT PROBLEMS				
Student can formulate a problem list for assigned patients.	Pre-C	C1	C1–2	C3–5
Student develops differential diagnoses based on patient H & P.	Pre-C	C1	C1–2	C3–5
Student able to interpret basic ECGs and laboratory tests.	Pre-C	C1	C1–2	C3–5
Student can interpret advanced diagnostic tests (e.g., radiology, specialized testing).	Pre-C	C1	C2	C3–5
MANAGER: ABLE TO MANAGE HEALTHCARE NEEDS AND COORDINATE CARE WITH INTERDISCIPLINARY TEAM				
Student can develop diagnostic and therapeutic plans for patients.	Pre-C	C1	C1–2	C3–5
Student can verbalize benefits and risks of the patient plan.	Pre-C	C1	C1–2	C3–5
Student incorporates patient values and social determinants of health in care plan.	Pre-C		C4	C5
Student participates in interprofessional practice.	Pre-C	C1	C2	C3–5
EDUCATOR/EVALUATOR: DEMONSTRATES EDUCATOR AND EVALUATOR QUALITIES				
Student educates the patient and caregiver regarding the management plan and expected outcomes.		C1	C2	C3–5
Student uses appropriate communication and teaching methods.			C1	C2–5
Student shares learning with staff, patients, and caregivers.		C1	C2	C3–5

Jenkins-Weintaub, E., Goodwin, M., & Fingerhood, M. (2023). Competency-based evaluation: Collaboration and consistency from academia to practice. *Journal of the American Association of Nurse Practitioners, 35*(2), 142–149.

Human Trafficking Resources, Referrals, and Responses to Guide Patient Care (Chapter 24)

CONSIDERATIONS WHEN HUMAN TRAFFICKING IS SUSPECTED

- Call police or security department with any immediate concerns for safety
- Consult local law enforcement or human trafficking task force:
  ° If the patient is under the age of 17
  ° If an adult and they agree to talk with law enforcement
- Consult the on-call forensic nurse
- Consult a social worker
- Review hospital policy on suspected human trafficking
- Provide resources, including follow-up medical and mental healthcare and referral to outside organizations, such as rape crisis center, domestic violence center, and law enforcement

WEBSITES AND HOTLINES

National Human Trafficking Hotline
https://humantraffickinghotline.org/en; (888) 373-7888

U.S. Department of Justice
https://www.justice.gov/humantrafficking/resource

Shared Hope International
https://sharedhope.org/resources/

Human Trafficking Training
https://polarisproject.org/training/

National Domestic Violence Hotline
800-799-SAFE (7233)

Rape, Abuse, and Incest National Network (RAINN)/National Sexual Assault Hotline
800-656-4673

National Center for Missing and Exploited Children
800-THE-LOST (843-5678)

Johns Hopkins Nursing Evidence-Based Practice Question Development Tool

JOHNS HOPKINS NURSING EVIDENCE-BASED PRACTICE: QUESTION DEVELOPMENT TOOL

1. What is the problem and why is it important?

2. What is the current practice?

3. What is the focus of the problem?
☐ Clinical ☐ Educational ☐ Administrative

4. How was the problem identified? (Check all that apply)
☐ Safety/risk management concems ☐ Quality concerns (efficiency, effectiveness, timeliness, equity, patient-centeredness) ☐ Unsatisfactory patient, staff, or organizational outcomes ☐ Variations in practice within the setting ☐ Variations in practice compared with external organizations ☐ Evidence validation for current practice ☐ Financial concerns

5. What is the scope of the problem?
☐ Individual ☐ Population ☐ Institution/system

6. What are the PICO components?

P – (Patient, population, problem):

I – (Intervention):

C – (Comparison with other interventions, if applicable):

O – (Outcomes that include metrics for evaluating results):

7. Initial EBP question:

8. List possible search terms, databases to search, and search strategies:

9. What evidence must be gathered?   (Check all that apply)

☐ Literature search   ☐ Patient/family preferences

☐ Standards (regulatory, professional, community)   ☐ Clinical expertise

☐ Guidelines   ☐ Organizational data

☐ Expert opinion

JOHNS HOPKINS NURSING EVIDENCE-BASED PRACTICE: QUESTION DEVELOPMENT TOOL

Directions for Use of the Question Development Tool

Purpose: This form is used to develop an answerable question and to guide the team in the evidence search process. The question, search terms and strategy, and sources of evidence can be revised as the EBP team refines the EBP project focus.

What is the problem and why is it important? Indicate why the project was undertaken. What led the team to seek evidence? Make sure the problem statement defines the actual problem and does not include a solution statement.

What is the current practice? Define the current practice as it relates to the problem.

What is the focus of the problem? Is the problem a clinical concern (e.g., preventing blood stream infections); an educational concern (e.g., discharge teaching for patients); or an administrative concern (e.g., safety of 12-hour nursing shifts)?

How was the problem identified? Check the statements that describe how the problem was identified.

What is the scope of the problem? Does the problem look at an individual (e.g., clinician, patient, family member); a population (e.g., adult cardiac patients, recovery room nurses); or an institution/system (e.g., patient transportation, patient or staff satisfaction)?

What are the PICO components?

- **P** (patient, population, problem) e.g., age, sex, setting, ethnicity, condition, disease, type of patient, or population
- **I** (intervention) e.g., treatment, medications, education, diagnostic tests or best practice(s)
- **C** (comparison with other interventions or current practice) may not be applicable if your question is looking for best practice.
- **O** (outcome) stated in measurable terms, expected outcomes based on the intervention identified, e.g., decrease in fall rate, decrease in length of stay, increase in patient satisfaction.

Initial EBP Question. A starting question that can be refined and adjusted as the team searches through the literature.

List possible search terms. Using PICO components and the initial EBP question, list relevant terms to begin the evidence search. Terms can be added or adjusted as the evidence search continues. Document the search terms, strategy, and databases searched in sufficient detail for replication.

What evidence must be gathered? Check the types of evidence the team will gather based on the PICO and initial EBP question.

Note: Page numbers followed by *b*, *f*, or *t* denote boxes, figures, and tables, respectively.